AUDITORY
IMAGERY

Edited by

DANIEL REISBERG
Reed College

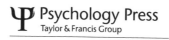

Psychology Press
Taylor & Francis Group

New York London

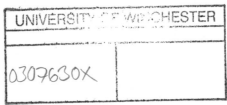
First Published by
Lawrence Erlbaum Associates, Inc., Publishers
365 Broadway
Hillsdale, New Jersey 07642

Transferred to Digital Printing 2009 by Psychology Press
270 Madison Avenue, New York NY 10016
27 Church Road, Hove, East Sussex BN3 2FA

Library of Congress Cataloging-in-Publication Data

Auditory Imagery / edited by Daniel Reisberg.
    p.   .cm.
Includes bibliographical references and index.
ISBN 0-8058-0556-7
1. Imagery (Psychology)   2. Auditory perception.   3. Sound—
Psychological aspects.   I. Reisberg, Daniel.
BF367.A83   1992
153.3'2—dc20   91-31965
                                                        CIP

Publisher's Note
The publisher has gone to great lengths to ensure the quality of this reprint
but points out that some imperfections in the original may be apparent.

Contents

Preface

The study of mental imagery has been a central concern of modern psychology, and, in the last two or three decades, we have learned an enormous amount about imagery. We have a rich corpus of data, gathered with an impressive repertoire of experimental techniques. There is a correspondingly impressive body of imagery theory. Central phenomena of imagery—mental rotation, mental scanning, the power of imagery mnemonics (to name just a few)—are standard fare in the psychology curriculum.

This wealth of information, however, has not been evenly spread. We know a vast amount about *visual* imagery (or, as some would have it, spatial imagery), but remarkably little about imagery in other modalities. While there are countless books and articles on visual imagery, the research literature contains a scant two or three dozen papers about imagery in any modality other than vision.

This volume constitutes a step toward remedying this information imbalance. The chapters here clearly do not inaugurate the study of auditory imagery. Instead, they celebrate the fact that research in auditory imagery has progressed to an extent that makes this volume possible. There are many reasons why we should welcome this research. At the very least, do the various claims made about visual imagery generalize to other modalities? For example, much has been written about the relation between imagery and perception; are these claims somehow unique to vision? Likewise, we know a great deal about image generation, but are different claims needed when we consider temporally defined auditory images, rather than spatially defined visual ones? To put all this more broadly, is it possible to have a theory of imagery-in-general, or does each modality of imagery have its own profile?

These are compelling reasons for broadening our research beyond visual imagery. Far more important, though, these other modalities demand study in their own right, and not merely as points of comparison to visual imagery. In particular, auditory imagery seems to occupy an intriguing position, at the intersection of several research domains. For example, psychologists have discussed the imagery that accompanies the composing and remembering of music. Psychologists interested in memory have noted the apparent relation between verbal rehearsal and auditory imagery. Psycholinguists have discussed the relation between speech perception and "inner speech." Psychologists have debated the role of inner speech in silent reading, and clinicians have discussed the nature of auditory hallucinations in schizophrenia and alcoholism. In addition, many scholars have discussed the role of the inner "monologue" that seems to accompany much of thought. For John Watson, this inner speech *was* thought. For Vygotsky, or Piaget, inner speech was a central mechanism through which instructions and plans became internalized as thought. Still other scholars have regarded inner speech as our best (or only) means of accessing the ongoing "stream of consciousness."

This richness of topics invites many questions. Is auditory imagery, in one guise or another, in fact involved in each of these domains? If so, then auditory imagery may turn out to have broad function indeed. Is the auditory imagery the *same* in each of these domains? We want to avoid proliferating species of auditory imagery, one per topic domain, but we also do not want to merge together phenomena that do not belong together.

Hence what role auditory imagery plays in these various domains seems an important empirical matter. Exploring imagery's function in each of these domains seems likely to illuminate these individual research areas. Examining imagery across domains seems certain to tell us a great deal about the form and function of auditory imagery. In the process, we will come to understand just what auditory imagery *is,* since this seems a matter to be settled by research, and not by stipulation.

I am happy to let the reader judge the worth of these many promises by considering the chapters in this volume—chapters deliberately selected to span from music imagery to imagery for speech, from the ordinary memory rehearsal of undergraduates to the delusional voices of schizophrenics. I have no doubt, given the contents of these chapters, that the reader will find this to be a rich and intriguing research avenue.

The chapters are organized roughly into three groups. Halpern, Crowder and Pitt, and Intons-Peterson address auditory imagery by building in important ways on what we know about visual imagery. A central concern in these chapters is the question of what information (pitch, rhythm, timbre) is depicted in an auditory image. The chapters by Campbell, Smith, Reisberg and Wilson, and MacKay raise questions about how exactly auditory imagery is related to hearing, and to covert speech. Finally, the chapters by Smith, Logie and Baddeley, Hubbard and Stoeckig, and Deutsch and Pierce all look at auditory imagery in a broader, more functional context, asking how this imagery is related to schizophrenic delusions, memory, and music. I say with pleasure, however, that this organizational sequence is somewhat arbitrary: The chapters cover diverse areas, but are all interconnected in many and intriguing ways. Discovering these interconnections has made editing this volume both instructive and also fun; I hope the reader shares these reactions.

Daniel Reisberg

Contributors

Alan Baddeley
MRC Applied Psychology Unit
15 Chaucer Road
Cambridge CB2 2EF England

Ruth Campbell
Department of Psychology
Goldsmiths' College
University of London
New Cross, London SE14 6NW England

Robert G. Crowder
Department of Psychology
Yale University
New Haven, CT 06520

Diana Deutsch
Department of Psychology
University of California, San Diego
La Jolla, CA 92093

Andrea Halpern
Department of Psychology
Bucknell University
Lewisburg, PA 17837

Timothy Hubbard
Department of Psychology
Eastern Oregon State College
La Grande, OR 97850

Margaret Jean Intons-Peterson
Department of Psychology
Indiana University
Bloomington, IN 47405

Robert Logie
Department of Psychology
King's College
Aberdeen AB9 2UB Scotland

Donald G. MacKay
Psychology Department
University of California, Los Angeles
Los Angeles, CA 90024

John R. Pierce
Center for Computer Research in Music &
    Acoustics
Department of Music
Stanford University
Stanford, CA 94305

Mark A. Pitt
Townshend Hall
1885 Neil Avenue Mall
Ohio State University
Columbus, OH 43210

Daniel Reisberg
Department of Psychology
Reed College
Portland, OR 97202

J.David Smith
Department of Psychology
New School for Social Research
New York, NY 10003

Keiko Stoeckig
Department of Psychology
Glassboro State College
Glassboro, NJ 08028

Meg Wilson
Psychology Department
University of California, Berkeley
Berkeley, CA 94720

1 Musical Aspects of Auditory Imagery

Andrea R. Halpern
Bucknell University

Convincing people that they experience auditory imagery for music is not diffi-cult. When I tell people that I study auditory imagery, be they psychologists, musicians, neither, or both, they often ask me how they can *stop* tunes from running through their head. Unfortunately, I have no expert answer for them. But anyone who has experienced such an annoyance will agree that auditory imagery, or "sounds in the head," is at least as vivid as the "pictures in the head" of visual imagery. This vividness is also illustrated by an item on an auditory imagery questionnaire that I employed in one of the studies described later on. It asked respondents to imagine the sound of fingernails scraping a chalkboard and to rate the image for vividness. You may not be surprised that many people reacted with shivers and remonstrations, as if I had actually done the obnoxious deed.

Despite this strong subjective experience, very little research has explored the nature of auditory imagery. From the subjective point of view, most people will agree that auditory imagery for music seems to extend in time, to have an identifiable tempo, and to have an identifiable pitch. The goal of my recent research has been to try to specify the characteristics of auditory imagery, partic-ularly for music. The success of such an enterprise would be a valuable addition to two extant literatures: that in music cognition and that in visual imagery research.

TESTING MUSICAL MEMORY

People interested in music cognition have naturally been concerned with the primary question: How is music represented in the mind? To answer this ques-

1

tion, the modal technique has been to present subjects a novel snippet of music, and then to ask some questions about it. Because asking for recall in music experiments invites problems in scoring (errors of representation versus production) and subject cooperation, typically the subject is asked to recognize or compare the recently presented extract with a new one. The independent variable is the extent to which the old and new selections are similar. For instance, if a listener fails to discriminate between a tune and one similar to it in contour, researchers conclude that the contour of both selections must have been abstracted and remembered (e.g., Dowling, 1978).

Two methodological principles are evident in this approach. One is that observing the learning of novel music is both instructive for the researcher and relevant to some of the subject's everyday musical tasks. Clearly, presenting experimenter-constructed music for learning confers all the usual advantages of experimental control. All subjects have uniform conditions for learning, and the characteristics of the stimuli can be precisely controlled. Also, learning and remembering stimulus melodies, despite their artificial construction, is in many ways similar to learning new music in real world situations. Simply understanding a later part of a new piece often requires memory of an earlier part, as in the theme and variation form (Pollard-Gott, 1983). And although no one probes memory for the new works as concert goers leave the hall, no doubt some memory traces are laid down during the performance, which probably could be assessed by implicit memory tasks.

Underlying this way of examining music cognition is the second principle, which is that memory in these situations is imperfect, and we gain insight by examining these imperfections. This is a standard approach to studying memory and one that has yielded much interesting information about the schematic nature of memory, that is, the order of priority in memory representations when only some information is retained. As an example of this type of research, I composed melodies that varied from one another only on one musical dimension, such as rhythm, contour, or modality (Halpern, 1984). After learning the melodies, subjects tried to identify them. The error pattern revealed that tunes of different contours were rarely confused with each other, whereas tunes identical except for modality (major vs. minor) were more frequently confused, especially among nonmusicians. Thus I concluded that contour was a salient dimension in the schematic memory representation but modality was less strongly encoded.

Thinking of music memory as schematic is probably accurate for many of the interactions that both trained and untrained people have with music. However, recently I have become interested in the nature of representation when memory for music is essentially perfect. Whereas it appears that the majority of work in music cognition has examined short-term memory, I would like to examine long-term memory. By this I mean that I am interested in the way well-learned music is represented. People are able to remember a large repertoire of music and retain it for many years (Bartlett & Snelus, 1980). What kinds of codes make this retention possible? Clearly, proposing verbal codes in the traditional sense is impractical when trying to understand memory for melody (as opposed to the lyrics in vocal music). Even if we assume that a small minority of musicians can encode tunes in terms of musical structure, motor commands, or musical notation, the successful retention of music by untrained people suggests the existence of other types of durable codes. The explication of those codes has been the goal of my current program of research.

The study of auditory imagery for music also dovetails with a second literature on visual imagery. Studies in visual imagery have often been concerned with the literal or analogue properties of visuo-spatial representations. So, for example, various authors have examined the size and shape of the mental visual field (Finke & Kosslyn, 1980), the subjective size of visual images (Kosslyn, 1978), the representation of depth (Pinker, 1980), and the order of construction of the images (Kosslyn, Cave, Provost, & von Gierke, 1988).

Some authors have proposed that visual imagery and visual perception share characteristics or even a common locus in the visual system (e.g., Finke, 1985). Farah (1988) has documented a number of physiological similarities between imaging and perceiving in both intact and brain damaged people. In addition to the intrinsic interest of this comparison, the extent to which we can compare visual imagery and perception facilitates studying the former because of the essentially private or introspective nature of imagery. On the other hand, at least part of the perceptual experience, the stimulus, is public and therefore measurable.

For these same reasons, the study of auditory imagery is not only interesting in itself, but invites fruitful comparisons with both auditory perception and visual imagery. The research reported here attempts to expand methods and findings from visual imagery research to auditory imagery, which is a comparatively unstudied phenomenon. Auditory and visual imagery are similar in that both are terms used for sometimes quite vivid quasi-perceptual experiences. However, intrinsic differences in the two modalities prevent a simple extension of methods from one to the other. The most obvious difference is that visual stimuli are extended in space, and we think that visual images represent that extension. Auditory stimuli are extended in time, and we may hypothesize that auditory images represent this corresponding extension.

This extension in time rather than space requires a different approach to experimentation. Auditory stimuli are ephemeral and dynamic, making mental manipulations more reliant on short-term memory and therefore more difficult than in the visual domain. For example, participants in an auditory experiment have to use short-term memory even to keep the recognition alternatives in focal attention, a trivial matter in most visual situations. Thus the questions an experimenter can put to subjects in an auditory imagery paradigm are more constrained than those in visual tasks. Particularly in auditory imagery for music, tasks might require a higher level of musical training for success than is desirable when the goal is to assess a general population.

The issue of training is another point of difference between the two modalities. One attractive aspect of studying auditory imagery for music is the opportunity to examine different levels of training in the subject population. For the most part, the research described here does not use subjects selected for their musical training. However, selecting people with various training levels can help answer whether auditory imagery abilities are universal, or if they are correlated with musical tuition.

The research described here derives from an interest in finding out to what extend the "tune inside the head" is a veridical experience. That is, does an auditory image of a tune exist in real time, with representations of tempo and pitch? Are these analogue representations used only in response to an experimenter's instructions, or are they spontaneously generated when mental comparisons of tunes are required? After describing work so far accomplished, I end by describing some studies in progress that extend the findings to the neuropsychological domain.

Temporal Extent

Just as the representation of spatial extension is of interest in studies of visual imagery, so is the extension and ordering in time important in auditory information processing. Consider the difficulty of trying to imagine "Jingle Bells" from the second phrase ("O'er the fields . . . ") *without* thinking of the first phrase of the song ("Dashing through. . .").

The approach taken in the first experiment of the series in Halpern (1988a) was modeled on the visual scanning study by Kosslyn, Ball, and Reiser (1978). In that study, subjects memorized a map of a fictional island that displayed features such as a beach, a hut, and a well. After subjects could accurately reproduce the map, Kosslyn and colleagues gave them a scanning task. As subjects heard the name of a map feature, they were to image the map and mentally focus on the feature. They then heard a second feature. If the feature was in fact included on the map, the task was to mentally scan to the second feature by imagining a little black speck moving from place to place. Subjects pressed a button when they "arrived" at the second place. If mental scanning is analogous to physical scanning, then time to push the button should increase with real distance on the map. This is in fact what happened, but only if subjects were specifically instructed to use imagery. If not, time to answer bore no relation to real distance between the features. I borrowed this technique in my initial series of experiments to see if temporal extent could be inferred in an auditory imagery task, as Kosslyn, Ball, and Reiser inferred spatial extent in theirs.

In most of these studies, undergraduates unselected for musical training or ability were employed, as the goal was to assess how ordinary people remember tunes. In the first study, lyrics to the beginning of three songs familiar to this population were used ("Do Re Mi," "The Star Spangled Banner," and "Hark the Herald Angels Sing"). These were chosen because each has the beginning or only syllable of a lyric falling unambiguously on odd-numbered beats. For instance, beats 1, 3, and 5 for "The Star-Spangled Banner" fall on the words "oh," "can," and "see," respectively. In addition, each song has unique words in its first phrase, so that a particular lyric refers to only one place in the song.

For each song, lyrics beginning on beats 1, 3, and 5 (variable that I refer to as "startpoint") were paired with lyrics 2, 4, 6, or 8 beats away ("stepsize") to comprise the "true" trials. In addition, a "false" trial was yoked to each "true" trial by replacing the second lyric in the pair by one resembling the true lyric.

Subjects were first asked about their familiarity with the songs and lyrics, so that we could be sure that participants were using long-term memory representations. Each trial consisted of presenting the name of one of the three songs, followed one second later by the first lyric of a pair and, after 750 msec, the second lyric. In the imagery condition, subjects were instructed to first "mentally focus" on the first lyric. Then they decided if the second lyric was a lyric in the song. If it wasn't, they were to press the False button on a response board as quickly and accurately as possible. If the second lyric was indeed in the song, subjects followed imagery instructions to "start" at the first lyric and "mentally play" the song until they "arrived" at the second lyric and pressed the True button. In the nonimagery condition, subjects were simply told to mentally focus on the first lyric, and when the second lyric appeared, to indicate whether it was or was not an actual song lyric by pressing the appropriate button.

Figure 1.1 shows the mean reaction time for each correct "true" trial. Note the main effect of group: The imagery group took longer to respond than the non-imagery group. This suggests that the imagery instructions caused that group to act differently from the non-imagery group, and is consistent with findings in the visual imagery literature that images take some time to form (Kosslyn, Cave, Provost, & von Gierke, 1988). As predicted, reaction time increased with stepsize. The increase had both linear and quadratic components, as it was positively accelerated with larger stepsizes. The fact that both groups showed the increase with stepsize implies that non-imagery subjects may also use analogue representations even when not so instructed.

One other difference between the two groups was that reaction time increased with startpoint, but only under imagery instructions. This implies that imagery subjects are slower to process parts of the song that occur farther from the beginning, as if they need to "run through" the initial part of the song before beginning the trial. Note that even the imagery instructions made no mention of starting the song from the beginning.

Thus, with or without imagery instructions, reaction time increased with increasing number of beats in the real stimulus song. This suggests that subjects

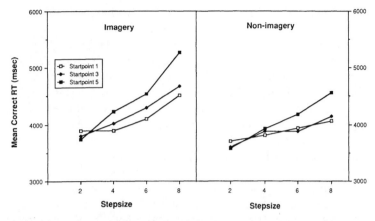

FIG. 1.1.   Mean reaction time as a function of startpoint, stepsize, and instruction group in the scanning experiment. Reprinted from Halpern (1988a).

were operating on a representation of the song in real time. The lack of a startpoint effect in the non-imagery group may mean that subjects do not always need to process the beginning of a song when mental work is required on a middle portion of it. However, I should also note that of the many versions and replications of this task conducted at about the same time, only in this instance did the startpoint effect fail to obtain. One is compelled then to consider this lack of an effect an exception.

In subsequent versions of the task, we showed that the results did not depend on auditory imagery ability, as assessed by the questionnaire mentioned earlier (the usual pattern with visual imagery), nor on the extent of reported imagery use during the experiment. And finally, subjects claimed to be unaware of the manipulations and hypothesis of the experiment, so that we are fairly confident that the data were not the result of mere subject cooperation.

However, the results in the scanning task do not imply a specifically musical representation. Subjects could have performed the task by looking up a list of the correct lyrics, or perhaps by using a list of visual representations of lyrics or notes. The next experiment probed specifically for a musical representation of the songs by using a mental pitch comparison task. The pitch comparison task *requires* subjects to process the first lyric in each trial, whereas previously, a subject could produce the correct answer without following instructions to "mentally focus" on the first lyric.

This type of task is modeled on another variety of visual imagery task, where imagery effects are elicited without necessarily giving imagery instructions. For instance, in the well-known mental rotation tasks first devised by Roger Shepard and colleagues, subjects are asked whether one object is the same as or different from another identical object that has been transformed by a rotation in the picture plane or depth (Shepard & Metzler, 1971). Subjects are not explicitly told about the transformations nor directed to use imagery. Nevertheless, the time taken to answer varies directly with the degree of rotation that separates the two objects in the real world. This finding has been interpreted as evidence for the analogue nature of visual imagery: imagining point A and then point C requires real-time processing of any intermediate points B.

Devising an auditory equivalent of mental rotation illustrates the difficulty, referred to in the Introduction, of traversing the two modalities. In the visual task, the two objects to be compared can be presented simultaneously on a screen, thus removing any memory load. Presenting two sounds simultaneously simply results in a confusing percept, or a third percept emerging from the two components, such as a major chord emerging from presentation of a C, E, and G sounded together. An additional problem results from the difficulty in labeling parts of an auditory representation. In the Kosslyn, Ball, and Reiser (1978) experiment, parts of the map were labeled with the feature name. For music, a convenient way to label is to use only songs (not instrumental music) and allow the lyrics to serve as labels for the notes. This unfortunately confines us to using sung music, which puts us at risk for actually testing text memory. But at least the pitch comparison task requires that the lyrics be used only indirectly as a means of locating the notes that are being compared.

Eight songs were selected that fulfilled the requirements of familiarity and beat placement noted in the previous experiment. For each of the 12 trial types (three startpoints and four stepsizes), the two component lyrics represented different pitches in the actual song. For instance, in "The Star-Spangled Banner" the note on the word "by" (beat 7) is higher in pitch than the note on the word "can" (beat 3).

Familiarization of the songs and lyrics, plus a demonstration of what "higher" and "lower" in pitch means, preceded the experiment. For each trial, subjects saw a song title, followed by the first lyric. The first lyric was always the closer of the two lyrics to the beginning of the song. After 500 msec, the second lyric appeared. To see whether imagery effects depended on instructions in this task, two groups were used. Subjects in the imagery group were told to "begin with the first lyric and play through the song in your mind until you reach the second lyric." Both groups were told to compare the pitch of lyric 2 with that of lyric 1, and press either the "higher" or "lower" button on a response board.

Although all subjects claimed to understand the task, this experiment differed dramatically from the previous one in its difficulty. Data from seven of 40 subjects were discarded because of error rates of 40% or over. The mean error rate of the remaining subjects was 24%, compared to 6% for the previous experiment. A *post hoc* division of the subjects by a median split of their years of training (*mdn* = 5.5 years) showed only that musicians were more accurate than nonmusicians (19% vs. 29% errors), but this factor did not interact with any others. As error rates in tasks like mental rotation are typically quite low, we see here an example of what I believe is the inherent higher level of difficulty in auditory imagery experiments. No differences in speed were found between musicians and nonmusicians.

Considering reaction time (RT), the type of instruction had absolutely no effect on the results, and so Fig. 1.2 shows data combined over groups in the left-hand panel. Reaction time increased as a function of both stepsize and startpoint, even more clearly than before. This effect is particularly compelling when one considers that only 76% of the data could be analyzed. The startpoint effect is quite clear for stepsizes 4, 6, and 8, but disappears at stepsize 2. This was also evident in Fig. 1.1 for the previous experiment. One explanation is that lyrics only two beats away from one another may be part of the same syntactic structure or musical motive. The two components may be so associated that the task may not require any time-consuming serial processing.

Turning now to the error pattern shown in the right-hand panel, once again instruction type made no difference in results, so the data are combined over groups. Error rate did change as a function of stepsize, but it only increased for Stepsizes 4 through 8. There was no effect of startpoint.

There was a Startpoint by Stepsize interaction, which appeared to show a decrease of errors at Stepsize 4. *Post-hoc* inspection of trials showed that the average pitch separation, in semitones, was largest for trials of stepsize 4. Perhaps this could explain the lower error rate if we assumed a symbolic distance effect. In auditory perception, tones close to one another in pitch are maximally interfering with one another (Dewar, Cuddy, & Mewhort, 1977). Thus a second-

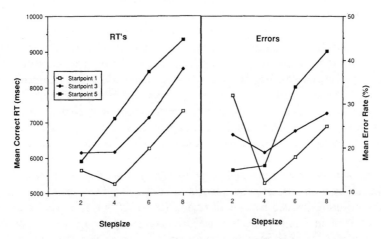

FIG. 1.2.   Mean reaction time and error rate as a function of startpoint and stepsize in the mental pitch comparison task. Collapsed across instruction groups. Reprinted from Halpern, (1988a).

ary analysis examined whether tones close together in pitch would be more difficult to compare mentally. In fact, error rates did decrease with increasing pitch separation, from 26% for pitch separations of 1 or 2 semitones, to 11% for pitch separations of 9 or 10 semitones. However, this was a weak relationship, as only the low 11% error rate was statistically different from the other rates by a Newman-Keul's test.

Because the pitch separation factor in the above experiment was added *post-hoc*, the next study in the series probed specifically for a symbolic distance effect in mental pitch comparison. In order to keep the stimulus set at a reasonable size and still fulfill the strict stimulus constraints necessary in all these studies, only stepsizes 4, 6, and 8 were used; and a new factor of pitch separation was added: 1 or 2 semitones, 3 or 4 semitones, 5 or 6 semitones, and 7 or 8 semitones. Startpoint was dropped as a formal factor (though startpoint was balanced over stepsize and pitch separation insofar as it was possible). Because imagery instructions did not interact with any factors in the previous experiment, only one instruction group was included, which did not receive imagery instructions.

Data from 2 of 20 subjects with error rates over 40% were discarded; the mean error rate of the remaining subjects was 22%. The usual stepsize effect obtained here in reaction times: They increased significantly from Stepsize 4 (4,787 msec) to Stepsize 6 (5,974 msec) to Stepsize 8 (6,486 msec). Means for the pitch separation categories appeared to be ordered in the predicted direction: They decreased monotonically from the smallest (5,910 msec) to the largest (5,400 msec) categories. However, this decrease was not statistically significant.

Mean error rates for the smallest to the largest pitch separation categories were 31%, 21%, 15% and 21%, respectively. These differed from one another, but a Newman-Keuls test revealed that only the 31% error rate for the closest pitch separation was statistically different from the other three.

We see then that the predicted effect of pitch separation was modestly supported, especially for error rates. One inevitable confound when using naturalistic materials is the inability to balance song over all the other factors. In the first experiment in the series, song was completely balanced over the other factors, but this confined us to using only three songs. In that study, there was a main effect of song and one interaction involving song, which fortunately did not prevent the emergence of the more interesting effects. Nevertheless, without balancing for song, weak effects like pitch separation may be obscured. A natural extension of this work would be to compose experimental materials where all the factors are neatly balanced. The challenge would be to show that participants can learn novel music and words as well as they know "Rudolph the Red-Nosed Reindeer," so that we can legitimately claim that we are still studying auditory imagery for well-known music.

One final unpublished study in the series examined whether the stepsize effect was merely an artifact of using serially-structured songs as stimuli. In this study, lyrics were either presented in the order of appearance in the song ("oh" followed by "dawn's" in "The Star Spangled Banner"), or in the reverse order. The mental pitch comparison task was run without imagery instructions. The hypothesis was that the reverse condition would prevent people from simply scanning the song in a serial fashion, leading to a slow and flat reaction time function with stepsize. This is in fact what happened. The reverse condition was slower than the forward condition, and reaction time did not vary as a function of stepsize with reverse presentation (the usual stepsize function obtained in the forward condition).

Comparing the two types of experiments described in this section, we see that changing the task so that a musical judgment is required considerably increased the difficulty level but did not substantially change the reaction time patterns from the scanning experiments. In this second task, reaction times increased with greater distance between the to-be-judged notes and also increased with the starting point of the first lyric, suggesting that intermediate notes were being processed, regardless of the instructions given to the subjects. Perhaps this more difficult task is almost impossible unless an imagery representation is employed. The apparent inevitability of this strategy is even more interesting considering that in actual pitch comparison tasks, intervening tones can have a large disruptive effect (Deutsch, 1970, 1972). Blackburn (cited in Dowling & Harwood, 1986) found the disruption even when the target tone was imagined. Efficient performance on a mental pitch comparison task ought to include bypassing the intervening tones in memory.

Also interesting is the weaker propensity to access an auditory image from its beginning regardless of what part of the representation is being probed. Again, efficient performance on the tasks ought to include being able to minimize short-term memory load by accessing the representation at the most appropriate place.

Taken altogether, the results of these experiments begin to support the claim that auditory imagery is not only a strong subjective experience (subjects never objected to carrying out auditory imagery tasks), but is also at least partly quantifiable. People indeed behave as if they were running songs through their heads. That is, the evidence seems to point towards a representation that codes extension in time, that unfolds in real time, that has strong links between adjacent elements, and that is unidirectionally ordered.

This should not be taken as a claim that serial processing is always obligatory. Thus I don't claim that we need to mentally play the first three movements of Beethoven's *Ninth Symphony* in order to think about the final "Ode to Joy" movement. It is very likely that hierarchical representations for music also exist that link motives to phrases to sections to movements. In the visual domain, researchers have proposed that these two types of representation coexist in our knowledge about maps. We have already seen Kosslyn's (Kosslyn, Ball, & Reiser, 1978) evidence that we can represent maps in analogue fashion. But others (Stevens & Coupe, 1978; Tversky, 1981) have shown that we encode maps symbolically as well. For instance, it is hard to convince people that Reno, Nevada, is *west* of Los Angeles, California, because we have encoded California as being west of Nevada on our simplified symbolic internal map of the United States. Clearly we have much propositional knowledge about tunes, and could answer many questions about "The Star-Spangled Banner" without activating an analogue image (composer, genre, nationality, emotion conveyed). But when answering questions about literal aspects of the music or words, imagery processing is apparently the strategy of choice.

Imagined Tempo

If a tune is extended in time, we may next ask whether the tempo, or the speed of that extension, is also represented in a consistent way. At least two types of anecdotal observations suggests that this is so. First, although people may believe that a synchronized musical performance requires the presence of a conductor, ensembles can function without a conductor at all. Ensembles such as rock bands, chamber choirs, string quartets, and church congregations may designate one member to begin and end pieces but otherwise operate without formal leadership. In order to synchronize their performances, members of musical groups must have some representation of the tempo of the piece in question. Second, people report anecdotally that their auditory images seem to have a specific tempo associated with them.

Clearly, representation of the tempo is hard to account for by using symbolic verbal codes. Perhaps tempo is represented literally in the auditory image. The question asked in the next studies was whether people represent a constant or preferred tempo of a tune when they claim to be imaging it. In one attempt to answer this question, Clynes and Walker (1982) had musicians tap their finger to imagined music that had been extensively studied in notated form (where tempo is specified by the composer), and found a very stable tapping rate compared to tapping without imagined music. Interestingly, they also found that most of the musicians imagined the tempo more slowly than when they actually played the music on the piano.

We may ask whether ordinary people have an experience of mental tempo when recalling familiar tunes that are known to subjects from many contexts and in many versions, and thus unlikely to have one tempo associated with them. In order to test the idea that tempo is consistently represented, we have to test several stronger hypotheses: that preferred tempo will be similar whether listening or imagining music, and that preferred tempos will be stable across time. Given that subjects show some stability in their selected tempos, we can see if constraints on the representation exist by asking people to mentally transform tempos until they reach upper and lower bounds.

The first study in the series (Halpern, 1988b) tested whether subjects preferred a particular tempo for familiar songs, both when the songs were actually heard and when they were merely imagined. The 19 stimulus songs were similar to those I used previously. Examples are "Do Re Mi," "Happy Birthday," and "Yesterday." Thus, the represented tempo should not be tied to a memory for any particular version, as might be the case with a current rock tune heard on one recording, or a symphony, where tempo is usually notated.

Even more than in the previous studies, it was important that the experimenter and the subject agreed on the placement of beats to the lyrics. Therefore in the familiarization phase subjects clapped along with the lyrics. Any clapping pattern different than the intended one was corrected by the experimenter. In the Perception task, participants interacted with a computer. They first heard the tune at a very slow tempo. The computer program allowed the listeners to change the tempo until the song sounded "correct" to them. In the Imagery task, subjects were given a list of song titles. They were instructed to imagine the tune in their head and to set a metronome to coincide with the beats in the imagined tune. All subjects performed both tasks in counterbalanced order.

The scattergram in Fig. 1.3 shows that people used a wide range of tempos: 70 to 140 beats per minute (bpm). The tempo settings for the 19 songs averaged across subjects differed from one another in both tasks, meaning that people were differentiating among the songs. Considering all the songs as a group, the means and variability of the imagined and perceived tempos did not differ.

Looking at individual songs in the two tasks, and as in evident from the Figure, perceived and imagined tempos were positively correlated ($r = .63$). Only 3 of the 19 songs had equal tempos in the two tasks (as measured by taking the ratio of imagined to perceived tempos and testing each against the hypothetical ratio of 1.00). For 7 of the songs, imagined tempos were faster than perceived; for 9, perceived tempos were faster than imagined, refuting Clynes and Walker's (1982) finding that imagined tempos are usually slower than per-

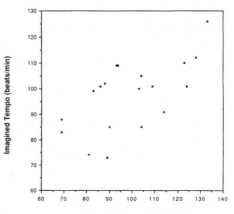

FIG. 1.3. Scatter diagram comparing mean perceived and imagined tempos for familiar songs. Reprinted from Halpern (1988b).

Perceived Tempo (beats/min)

ceived. However, the average absolute value of the difference between tempo setting in the two tasks was small, 20 bpm, relative to the range of tempos used in the tasks, 40 to 208 bpm. It is interesting to note that the average perceived and imagined tempos were about 100 bpm, or 600 msec per beat. This figure is commonly cited as being a "natural" or "preferred" rate for tapping, and the rate at which temporal discrimination is easiest (Fraisse, 1982).

The experiment demonstrates that the task of externalizing imagined pitch seemed logical to the subjects, and that imagining and perceiving tempo elicit quite similar results. The interesting question is whether people maintain a stable representation of tempo over time and repeated trials. If this strong hypothesis is supported, then we have evidence for the weaker position that the tempos are represented in the first place.

In the next study, previously unreported, participants imagined familiar songs, and then tapped a finger to match the beat of the imagined tempo. The tempos were tape-recorded and later matched to the nearest metronome setting to the produced beat. By having subjects tap, instead of setting a metronome as in the previous setting, we hoped to eliminate any possibility that verbal codes would be used to remember the tempo from one observation to the next.

Each song was presented four times for judgment: Half the songs (Same songs) were judged four times entirely within the first or second session; the other half were judged twice in one session and twice again two to five days later. The dependent measure was the average standard deviation of those judgments. Control judgments consisted of sets of four Different songs judged within or between sessions. This control set allowed us to determine whether people always tap at a uniform rate, perhaps due to constraints on the motor system. If people can only produce one or a few tempos, then naturally all their judgments will have low variability. Separate groups of musicians and nonmusicians participated. Because nonmusicians received slightly different instructions and more practice, results will be reported separately.

Instead of reporting results in units of beats per minute, each metronome setting was assigned a number from one to 40, to better capture the "closeness" of adjacent metronome settings in the analysis. As can be seen in Fig. 1.4, tempos for musicians were very stable both between and within sessions for Same songs, with standard deviations of about 1.7 metronome settings (about 6 bpm). Also evident was that the standard deviation for groups of Different songs was higher than that for Same songs. This shows that the subjects provided a variety of tempos when judging sets of different songs. But the standard deviation for Different songs remained unchanged within or between sessions. In other words, the range in tempo judgments among "Happy Birthday," "London Bridge," "White Christmas," and "Do Re Mi" was wider than that for four tries with "Happy Birthday," but the range remained stable within or over sessions.

The results for the nonmusicians apparently show less of an ability to keep a stable tempo. As seen in Fig. 1.4, Same songs within sessions were given the

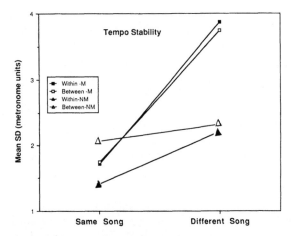

FIG. 1.4. Stability of imagined tempos for musicians and nonmusicians; for same and different songs, both within and between sessions.

same tempo most of the time, $SD = 1.4$ metronome settings. Nonmusicians were differentiating Same from Different songs within a given session, showing that they were sensitive to tempo stability under the easier condition. However, variability of settings for Same songs across the sessions was as high as the settings for Different songs.

A simple conclusion that nonmusicians can't maintain a stable tempo representation across sessions is hindered by the fact that variabilities were smaller in general for the nonmusicians compared to the musicians. Inspection of the data suggests that nonmusicians used a smaller range of tempos throughout the experiment. For example, the average difference between the slowest song ("White Christmas") and fastest song ("When the Saints Come Marching In") was 46 bpm for the musicians, but only 22 bpm for the nonmusicians. This difference in what we might call flexibility of mental tempo also shows up in the next experiment.

The stability of tempo across sessions is then evidence that at least musicians represent tempo with the auditory image. In the above two experiments, participants were asked to imagine the songs at a preferred or usual tempo. To what extent is this a rigid representation? Is the tempo subject to transformation under appropriate instructions? At one extreme, we may predict that the "speed" with which a song is imagined is subject to the same limits as auditory perception. Bolton (1894) found that the subjective feeling of rhythm broke down when internote intervals were shorter than 115 msec or longer than 1,580 msec. The fastest and slowest imaginable tempos may be of similar magnitude (or at the extreme metronome settings of 228 msec per beat to 1,500 msec per beat) and constant across song. At the other extreme, the representation of tempo may be so intrinsic to the song representation that subjects would have a difficult time imagining tempos too far removed from the preferred ones.

A third experiment attempted to answer these questions. Ten familiar songs served as stimuli, and participants were initially unselected for musical training. As in the first study in this series, the subjects first used the metronome to find the preferred tempo of the song. They then tried to imagine the song at faster and faster tempos until the task became too difficult, followed by imagining the song at slower and slower tempos (the order was reversed for half the subjects). For the fast/slow tasks, the subjects started with the metronome at the preferred tempo and moved the dial toward the fastest (208 bpm) or slowest (40 bpm) metronome setting, as appropriate. Each time the subjects changed the tempo on the metronome, they rated the difficulty of imagining the song at that tempo. The ratings were on a four point scale, where "1" signified "very easy" and "4" signified "very difficult". The subjects were told to record on their answer sheet the first metronome setting receiving a rating of "4".

For each of the three tasks, mean tempo settings differed significantly among the 10 songs. The mean fastest tempo of 164 bpm and slowest tempo of 65 bpm did not approach the metronome limits of 208 and 40 bpm. This implies that subjects were discriminating among the songs and not simply choosing the extremes on the metronome for their answers.

The mean preferred tempo was 109 bpm. This is significantly faster than the mean imagined tempo from Study 1 of 98 bpm. However, tempos in these two studies were strongly correlated, $r = .94$; that is, subjects set tempos faster but in a very similar ordering to the first study.

To answer the question of whether tempo representations are labile, we can note that the values recorded for the slowest and fastest tempos were dependent on the preferred tempo. Expressing this quantitatively, significant positive correlations were obtained among the different tasks here, as is obvious from Fig. 1.5. This implies that we are not dealing with an absolute limit on the speed with which a tune is imagined. For instance, the mean fastest imaginable tempo for "When the Saints Come Marching In" was 32 bpm faster than that for "White Christmas."

However, the extent of mental tempo transformation does seem to have limits dependent on both the song (as shown above) and the musical background of the subject. When asked, most subjects agreed that at least some of the songs had tempo "limits," beyond which it was difficult to imagine the songs. But the four subjects with the most extensive musical backgrounds also were able to imagine the songs at the most extreme tempos. The average difference between the fast and slow tempos was 153 bpm for the four musicians, versus 87 bpm for everyone else. What aspects of musical training may have allowed the greater flexibility shown by the musicians in the last two studies? It is doubtful that the musicians had had experience with this precise task in the course of their musical education. They may have had experience in other sorts of msucial transforma-

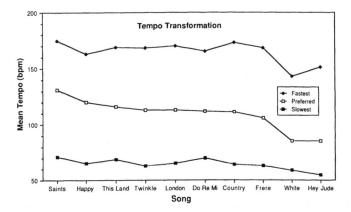

FIG. 1.5. Mean preferred, fastest, and slowest imaginable tempos for familiar songs.

tions, however, such as practicing a piece slowly before playing it up to speed. Also, good musicians need to be able to adjust tempos as a conductor searches for the appropriate speed of an entire piece or varies the tempo within a piece.

Conductors themselves probably find that being able to imagine the sounds of the orchestra from simply looking at the score to be a useful skill. Just as an interior decorator would value the ability to imagine the sofa in different colors in different locations before actually executing the plan, so would a conductor value being able to imagine adding or subtracting instruments to the ensemble or speeding up and slowing down the tempo. We may expect that conductors would show the most flexibility in auditory imagery tasks, and would make an interesting group to study.

In summary, these studies expand on the previous findings that temporal extent is represented in auditory imagery by specifying some of the characteristics of the temporal aspects of images. Ordinary people can externalize the "speed" of their internal images, and can differentiate among those tempos. To an appreciable extent, they, and even more so musicians, are able to replicate that tempo over long periods of time. These results strongly imply that tempo is encoded in the long-term memory representation of familiar tunes. The small advantage shown by musicians in maintaining that tempo may result from practice in being tempo setters for a group or for themselves. Nonmusicians less often produce their own music in a group, and singing in the shower does not require consistent adherence to any one tempo.

Imagined Pitch

Few people possess what is called absolute or "perfect" pitch, the ability to name a given played note or to produce a note when given its letter name ("A", "B flat"). Instead, almost all musicians and many untrained people possess a reasonably well developed sense of relative pitch. These people can recognize the correctness of a tune and perhaps produce good approximations of tunes they have heard. They can do this because Western music is based for the most part on the relationships of pitches to one another. For instance, when "White Christmas" is sung, the second note has to be one semitone, or 5.9% higher in frequency than the first note, regardless of where the tune is started. And in most musical contexts, the starting note of the piece is irrelevant. That is, "Happy Birthday" is, in all important ways, the same whether starting on a low note or a high note.

Yet in spontaneous singing, people do need to choose some starting pitch. Can we verify the subjective impression that the imaginal representations of these songs have something analogous to starting pitches? The next series of studies (Halpern, 1989) explores whether people maintain a representation of the starting pitch of familiar tunes. As was the case with imagined tempo, the strategy here was to adopt a stronger hypothesis: that people not only associate a pitch with imagined music, but that this pitch is fairly stable over trials and time. Keep in mind that these studies never use absolute pitch subjects, and the stimuli are traditional tunes like Christmas carols and children's songs, which are heard in many different keys.

In the first study, people hummed the starting pitch of familiar songs. We measured the variability of those judgments within sessions and between two sessions separated by 48 hours. Using the same logic as in the mental tempo studies, if pitch representation is stable, the variability of those judgments should be small and about the same whether the observations are gathered close together or far apart in time.

To select the subjects, a pre-test was used that screened out anyone who was truly singing-disabled; that is anyone who could not hold a pitch steady enough for us to measure. Otherwise, musical training was not considered, except that no subjects participated who admitted to possessing absolute pitch. Both males and females participated, and a comparison of their results will be of interest in several of the studies.

The procedure was as follows: Subjects were shown a list of well-known stimulus songs and asked to indicate familiarity. Then on each trial they were presented with lyrics from the first phrase of a song. They were then asked to run the first phrase of a song through their heads and think about the pitch of the first note. When they had comfortably obtained this pitch, they hummed it into a tape recorder, and the pitches were later transcribed into musical notation to the nearest semitone. Subjects could redo any trial where they felt that the produced pitch did not match the pitch they were imagining.

Several measures were taken to guard against the possibility that subjects were using their memory of one production to influence the production of another trial (either to produce the same pitch for the next observation of the same song, or to use relative pitch to produce a desired note for a different song). Each observation was separated from the next observation of the same song by at least three intervening trials. Between each trial, a different set of interfering notes was played on an electronic keyboard. To prevent vocalization of anything other than the starting pitch, subjects chewed gum (sugarless, with a choice of flavors). And finally, subjects were asked at the end of the study if they thought their responses on one trial were influenced by previous responses. No one so indicated.

Each song was presented four times for judgment: Half the songs were judged four times entirely within the first or second session; the other half were judged twice in one session and twice again 48 hrs. later. The dependent measure was the average standard deviation (variability) of those judgments. Control judgments consisted of sets of four Different songs judged across or between sessions. Like in the tempo studies, this control set allowed us to determine whether we were testing a bunch of "Johnny One-Notes," who would naturally show artifactual low variability.

As shown in Fig. 1.6, variability for judgments among the Same songs was low, whether between or within sessions. Variability among Different songs was much higher, showing that subjects were sensitive to different starting pitches where appropriate. This too did not depend on whether the judgments were between or within sessions. Also note that the absolute value of the variability was small for the Same songs, a little over one semitone.

As may be expected, males selected notes about an octave lower than did the females. The highest and lowest pitched songs were logical choices, in that the highest average pitch was for "Joy to the World," which descends a whole octave in its first phrase, and the lowest pitch was reserved for "Somewhere Over the Rainbow," whose first interval is an ascending octave.

If humming is an adequate externalization of mental pitch, then these results

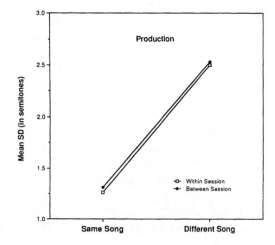

FIG. 1.6. Mean standard deviations of pitch productions for same or different songs, both between or within sessions. Reprinted from Halpern (1989).

point to a form of absolute pitch among ordinary people. But the use of the production technique has some disadvantages. Our surprisingly consistent results may have been partially due to the physical constraints imposed by using the vocal organs for a response. The gender and song differences described in the previous paragraph are consistent with this speculation. People may have produced only pitches that would have been acceptable if they were actually singing. On the other hand, perhaps stability was underestimated in subjects with poor singing ability.

To complement the production paradigm, a second study used a recognition task that eliminated the need for a vocal response. Subjects again thought of the first note in the tune, but this time they searched for it on an electronic keyboard. Since we wanted to make sure that participants couldn't see the note they picked and then simply remember (or misremember) the note name, the keyboard was placed upside down and hidden from view. In addition, all the other precautions to discourage explicit memory codes were repeated from the first study. The disadvantage of this paradigm is that playing all those notes while hunting for the correct one might cause memory interference, and so the variabilities might all be higher in this version. Two groups of subjects participated: an unselected group ("general subjects") and a group of musicians.

And indeed, the results in Fig. 1.7 shows that average standard deviations are about twice as high in this version. Although the two panels of the graph look identical, they in fact differ statistically. The results for musicians were the same as those in the previous experiment: Variabilities for Same songs were smaller than those for Different songs, whether between or within sessions. The general subjects also showed this main effect of Same vs. Different song, and vari-

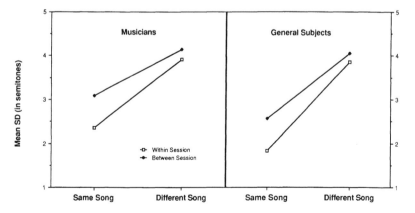

FIG. 1.7.   Mean standard deviations of pitch recognitions for same or different songs, both between or within sessions, for musicians and unselected subjects. Reprinted from Halpern (1989).

abilities were equal between and within sessions for Different songs. However, variabilities were significantly higher between than within sessions for Same songs.

One could argue that both production and recognition tasks are uninteresting from a cognitive point of view because subjects were just singing the songs to themselves, and using muscular or other physical cues to retrieve the starting notes of the pieces. Several secondary results argue against that claim. In the production task, recall that males and females produced different pitches for the songs. However, in the recognition task, gender had no effect on the pitches selected in either group. Also, the songs given the highest and lowest starting pitches were not obvious choices. "We Wish You a Merry Christmas" was given the highest note, but it *ascends* in the first few notes. "The First Noel" was given the lowest average pitch, and it *descends* in the first few notes.

Each of the two previous tasks might have favored people who are good at singing, or at note-finding, respectively. Even if mental representations of the pitches were adequate, a person with poor singing ability may have sung several extraneous pitches before settling on a satisfactory one in the first study. In the second study, a person with poor dexterity or one completely unfamiliar with keyboards may have played more pitches per trial before selecting the appropriate one, thereby again generating more interference. Accordingly, a third experiment used an initial rating task to remove any requirements for output skills in the main task.

First, subjects produced preferred notes for familiar songs, as in the first experiment of the series. Two to five days later, they were read the name of one of the four stimulus songs and told to imagine the first note of that song. A tone was then played, and they were to rate the tone's similarity to the starting pitch they were imagining. The presented tones included the subject's own preferred pitch plus pitches one to seven semitones higher and lower in a random order. Trials were not blocked by song so that successive trials created the usual desired memory interference. Additional interference notes were played between each trial. Each trial was repeated once, so each datum was the average of the two observations.

If subjects maintain a stable representation of starting pitch, they should rate their previously selected pitch as the most adequate note, and rate notes higher and lower as less adequate. Of secondary interest is the pattern of the remaining preference ratings. Krumhansl and Shephard (1979) found that two tones are judged to be more similar if the interval between them is considered musically small. For instance musical intervals of a fifth (7 semitones) and a fourth (5 semitones) are considered more highly related by music theoreticians and by subjects than physically closer intervals such as a major second (2 semitones). Returning to the current experiment, given that the previously selected preferred note would be rated most highly, would the ratings of other pitches correspond to the musical closeness of those pitches to the preferred one?

Musicians and nonmusicians participated, but musical training made no difference, and so Fig. 1.8 shows combined results.

The pattern of ratings resembles a series of peaks and valleys. Each peak was significantly different from the more distant of its adjacent neighbors, and the valleys were all different from their nearest peaks. Notice that the preferred note was rated highly, but so were tones 4 semitones (major third) lower, 3 semitones higher (minor third), and 7 semitones higher (perfect fifth), relative to the preferred note. This is interesting from a musical point of view because only the +7 peak is musically close to the preferred tone. So rather than solely reflecting musical closeness as defined by Western music theory, the pattern seems to reflect preference regions of pitch height. It appears that people are willing to pitch the entire piece up or down several semitones, but are less willing to accept a starting note only one or two semitones away. This suggests a quite good memory for the absolute pitch of the starting tone.

These results were essentially replicated in a follow-up study that omitted specific imagery instructions. All subjects claimed that they played the song to themselves before assigning a rating. Similar to the conclusions we reached after analyzing the mental pitch comparison task, imagery processing appears to be a highly preferred strategy when answering questions about the literal aspects of music.

The final study in this series returned to the question of limits on mental transformation of pitch, in the same way we explored the limits on tempo transformation earlier. If limits on such transformations exist, we should again see those limits being proportional to preferred pitches, rather than reflecting an absolute bound on imagined pitches. A recognition paradigm was employed here because one obviously wants to eliminate any constraints imposed by the vocal apparatus itself.

As a first phase, musically unselected subjects chose preferred notes for

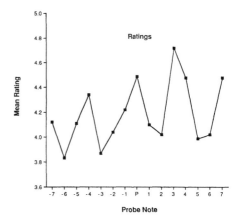

FIG. 1.8. Mean goodness rating on a 1 to 7 scale of subject's preferred note (P), and notes one to seven semitones above and below P. Reprinted from Halpern (1989).

familiar songs by hunting for the preferred note on a keyboard after imagining the song. To elicit the highest and lowest imaginable pitch, the experimenter played the previously selected preferred pitch, and then began playing successively higher (or lower) pitches in semitone increments. Half the subjects received each task first. As in previous paradigms, subjects rated the difficulty of imagining the song beginning on each presented pitch. And once again, interfering notes were played between each trial.

As was true in the earlier recognition paradigm, males and females selected the same pitches in all the tasks, confirming that subvocalization mechanisms are insufficient to explain the results.

Similar to the results of the tempo transformation study, highest and lowest imagined pitch depended on the preferred pitch (Fig. 1.9). Unfortunately, the pitch range over songs in this study was too narrow to show many differences between songs, but some information can be gained by looking at the songs pitched the highest ("Joy to the World") and the lowest ("Row Row Row"). The preferred, highest, and lowest settings for "Joy" were all higher than any other song. "Row" had the lowest preferred setting, and its lowest setting was two semitones below that for the next lowest songs. Thus we may tentatively conclude that no absolute upper or lower bound exists for the range of imagined pitches used here.

However, this study was the least informative of the series, and could be strengthened by selecting sets of songs with a wider range of preferred pitches. Alternatively, paradigms that don't depend on group averages would probably be able to maximize the chances of finding a wider range of preferred pitches.

To summarize this section, four experiments required people of varying musical backgrounds to externalize the pitch of an imagined tune. The tunes were all

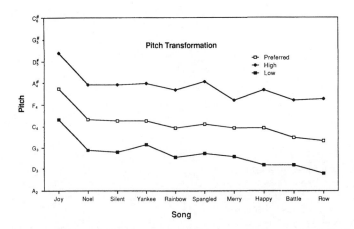

FIG. 1.9. Mean preferred, highest imaginable, and lowest imaginable pitch of familiar songs. Reprinted from Halpern (1989).

popular or traditional music, which had very probably been heard and performed at many pitch levels by the participants in their past. Considering that people without absolute pitch have difficulty remembering isolated tones, or tones in unfamiliar melodies, performance in these experiments was indicative of considerable memory for an arbitrary starting pitch of familiar tunes. This claim is also supported by data collected by Deutsch, Kuyper, and Fisher (1987). They found that untrained subjects reliably and consistently perceived a musical pitch illusion whose interpretation relied on some knowledge of absolute pitch.

Although the argument in this chapter is that ordinary people store absolute pitch to a greater extent than is commonly believed, this should not be taken to mean that everyone has a mild case of what is traditionally called absolute pitch. Clearly, verbal labels for notes were not used in these tasks, and consistency of pitch judgment was not up to the level shown by true absolute pitch possessors. When absolute pitch possessors make errors in pitch naming, they are frequently octave errors or errors of one semitone (e.g., Lockhead & Byrd, 1981). The third experiment showed that subjects were not inclined to equate notes separated by a semitone in preference ratings (although production attempts were sometimes only one semitone apart).

Neuropsychological Extensions

Within neuropsychology, some recent attention has been paid to the neuropsychology of music, or the search for understanding which brain structures may mediate musical tasks (for reviews, see Zatorre, 1984; Peretz & Morais, 1988). Although some would like to believe that musical skills "live" in the right hemisphere as a neat analogue to language in the left, the real situation is more complicated than that. The most common situation for finding musical deficits after right hemisphere (RH) damage, usually a right temporal lobectomy, has tended to be in musical discrimination tasks using unfamiliar material. As noted earlier, this is precisely the typical paradigm used in psychomusicology experiments. But one can argue that everyday musical experience more resembles the auditory imagery experiments I have been describing, where people recall and sometimes mentally manipulate a highly familiar tune. These experiments suggest that people have a very rich representation of everyday tunes.

It is this richness of representation that so far has not been examined in right hemisphere patients. Zatorre (1985) has shown that, like normals, RH patients can use the scale and contour of melodies to learn them, although they learn at a slower rate. But little work has explored what, if any, deficits occur in processing overlearned melodies. Will the type of high-level processing required in imagery tasks be affected by the impaired auditory discrimination that RH patients show? Or can we show a dissociation between perceptual and memorial skills in music?

Some work by Farah and associates (e.g., 1988) in the visual domain suggested that perceptual and memorial skills will be related. By analyzing evoked potentials in normal subjects, she has found that nearly identical brain areas are active in imagery and perception tasks. In brain-damaged patients, she reported that selective visual deficits are almost always accompanied by selective imagery deficits. For instance, patients who can recognize objects but not locate them in vision seem to show the same deficits when consulting a memory representation.

Zatorre and I are currently exploring these possible relationships in music. As a first step, we had thought to repeat the higher/lower pitch experiment described earlier, in both imaginal and perceptual versions. We anticipated two problems in extending this paradigm to the epilepsy surgery patients available to us. One was the very high error rate in that study, which would probably only increase with a less educated population suffering from the effects of epilepsy, medication, surgery, or all three. The second problem was that the task really requires processing of verbal (the lyric) and nonverbal (the imagined pitch) components. We thought this to be unwise if we wanted to compare left (LT) and right temporal lobe patients (RT), when we know that the former group has trouble with verbal information in general, and in retrieving the titles of familiar tunes specifically.

To reduce the error rate, we decided to present all trials blocked by song, instead of randomly. Pilot subjects from this population reported that thinking of "Puff the Magic Dragon," "Hark the Herald Angels Sing," and then "Happy Birthday" in rapid succession was difficult. Another decision was to present the perceptual version of whatever task we chose first, so it could serve as training for the imagery task. To solve the second problem, we attempted to devise versions of the task without any verbal components. However, pilot testing with completely nonverbal versions of the studies showed that even normal controls find it very difficult to make musical decisions without the benefit of some verbal cue to the song.

For our study now in progress, we reluctantly returned to a version of the higher/lower task that uses lyrics, but with minimal verbal memory demands. First, we screen subjects to make sure that they can make higher/lower judgments. Then they get a low memory load or "perceptual" version of the task where they will see the two critical lyrics highlighted in a line of text: "DASHING through the snow in a one-HORSE open sleigh. . . ." They simultaneously hear the tune being sung and decide if HORSE is higher or lower in pitch than DASHING. Finally, after presumably all subjects are very well trained on the lyrics, a true imagery task simply presents the two words DASHING and HORSE for judgment. Data gathered on the first small group of patients show that most people can at least perform these tasks at a reasonable level.

The theoretical problem with tasks having a heavy verbal component is that both RT and LT patients might show deficits, but for different reasons (impairment in verbal or musical skills, respectively). However, this is not a fatal flaw. Even if people are processing the lyrics as verbal units, the higher/lower judgment *requires* additional access to the musical image. So we can reason that even if both patient groups will be impaired relative to controls, RTs should still be worse than LTs on imaginal and perceptual versions if the right temporal lobe is "responsible" for the musical image as well as the musical percept. We will also be examining reaction time patterns to see if the groups vary qualitatively as well as quantitatively from one another.

Now, if, contrary to prediction, we find no impairment in the patients on the imagery task, but do find one on the perceptual task, we would then have evidence for a dissociation between imagery and perception, which would be in interesting contrast to the results from visual imagery. This would imply that auditory perception and imagery differ from one another more than is the case in the visual domain.

Conclusions

Referring back to the issues raised in the Introduction, the "tune inside the head" is in some ways an apt description of the representation of familiar tunes. These tunes seem to be stored with much exact or analogue information. People apparently need not rely only on such musical abstractions as contour or scale structure, as they do when processing unfamiliar tunes (Dowling, 1978). Real time passes while auditory images are activated, and the representations apparently include the fairly absolute information of tempo and pitch, in addition to the relative information of note and harmony relationships.

Few differences were found in most of the studies that compared imagery and nonimagery instruction groups. This suggests that imagery representations are the usual mode of processing familiar tunes. Of course this conclusion will be tempered by the task asked of the subjects. Thus if I asked a subject to decide whether the contour of a recently learned tune was the same as the tune I now present, he or she might very well be able to abstract and consult just the contours of the two excerpts. However, if I asked someone to draw the contour of a familiar children's tune (try it with, say, "Old Macdonald"), I propose that the rich imagery representation is consulted and the contour derived from that.

Some skills using auditory imagery are shared by musicians and nonmusicians alike. Both groups seem to process auditory images in real time and to perform judgment tasks equally quickly. Both groups showed evidence of auditory images containing pitch and tempo information. Musicians surpassed the nonmusicians in maintaining that information under more difficult memory conditions. Nonmusicians were susceptible to interference caused by the recognition foils in the pitch experiments, and were less able than musicians to maintain stable tempo judgments across sessions in the tempo consistency experiment. Interestingly, nonmusicians had more trouble overall with the tempo experiments than with the pitch experiments. One wonders if musical training in general improves understanding of tempo relationships more so than pitch relationships, an area for future research, perhaps.

Pragmatically, the analogies between visual and auditory imagery worked reasonably well in generating some of the research program outlined in this chapter. One intrinsic difficulty in comparing the modalities is the logical problem of presenting truly perceptual tasks in the auditory modality. Almost always, some memory component will enter into auditory comparisons. Simultaneous presentations of auditory stimuli are often not practical because of attentional and fusion effects. In the Introduction I noted that this was a methodological problem in that performance was likely to be worse on auditory versus visual versions of the imagery tasks. The theoretical problem, illustrated in the last section on neuropsychological extensions, is whether one can justifiably compare perceptual and imaginal tasks in the same way in vision and audition. I think the analogy cannot be strictly parallel, and the usual situation in audition will involve comparisons of high versus very low memory load tasks. Hopefully such comparisons will sometimes yield neuropsychological dissociations, so that componential analysis of auditory tasks can be made easier in future work.

ACKNOWLEDGMENTS

This research was supported by National Science Foundation Grant BNS-8607405. I wish to thank the many Bucknell students who worked as research assistants during the course of this project. Address correspondence to Andrea R. Halpern, Psychology Department, Bucknell University, Lewisburg, PA, 17837 or on electronic mail to AHALPERN@BUCKNELL.EDU.

REFERENCES

Bartlett, J. C., & Snelus, P. (1980). Lifespan memory for popular songs. *American Journal of Psychology, 93*, 551–560.

Bolton, T. L. (1894). Rhythm. *American Journal of Psychology, 6*, 145–238.

Clynes, M., & Walker, J. (1982). Neurobiologic functions of rhythm, time, and pulse in music. In M. Clynes (Ed.), *Music, mind, and brain: The neuropsychology of music* (pp. 171–216). New York: Plenum.

Deutsch, D. (1970). Tones and numbers: Specificity of interference in immediate memory. *Science, 168*, 1604–1605.

Deutsch, D. (1972). Mapping of interactions in pitch memory store. *Science, 175*, 1020–1022.

Deutsch, D., Kuyper, W. L., & Fisher, Y. (1987). The tritone paradox: Its presence and form of distribution in a general population. *Music Perception, 5*, 79–92.

Dewar, K. M., Cuddy, L. L., & Mewhort, D. J. K. (1977). Recognition memory for single tones with and without context. *Journal of Experimental Psychology: Human Learning and Memory, 3*, 60–67.

Dowling, W. J. (1978). Scale and contour: Two components of a theory of memory for melodies. *Psychological Review, 85*, 341–354.

Dowling, W. J., & Harwood, D. L. (1986). *Music cognition*. Orlando: Academic Press.

Farah, M. J. (1988). Is visual imagery really visual? Overlooked evidence from neuropsychology. *Psychological Review, 95*, 307–317.

Finke, R. A. (1985). Theories relating mental imagery to perception. *Psychological Bulletin, 98,* 236–259.

Finke, R. A., & Kosslyn, S. M. (1980). Mental imagery acuity in the peripheral visual field. *Journal of Experimental Psychology: Human Perception and Performance, 6,* 126–139.

Fraisse, P. (1982). Rhythm and tempo. In D. Deutsch (Ed.), *The psychology of music* (pp. 149–181). New York: Academic Press.

Halpern, A. R. (1984a). The organization of memory for familiar songs. *Journal of Experimental Psychology: Learning, Memory, and Cognition, 10,* 496–512.

Halpern, A. R. (1984b). Perception of structure in novel music. *Memory and Cognition, 12,* 163–170.

Halpern, A. R. (1988a). Mental scanning in auditory imagery for songs. *Journal of Experimental Psychology: Learning, Memory, and Cognition, 14,* 434–443.

Halpern, A. R. (1988b). Perceived and imagined tempos of familiar songs. *Music Perception, 6,* 193–202.

Halpern, A. R. (1989). Memory for the absolute pitch of familiar songs. *Memory and Cognition, 17,* 572–581.

Kosslyn, S. M. (1978). Measuring the visual angle of the mind's eye. *Cognitive Psychology, 10,* 356–389.

Kosslyn, S. M., Ball, T. M., & Reiser, B. J. (1978). Visual images preserve metric spatial information: Evidence from studies of image scanning. *Journal of Experimental Psychology: Human Perception and Performance, 4,* 47–60.

Kosslyn, S. M., Cave, C. B., Provost, D. A., & von Gierke, S. M. (1988). Sequential processes in image generation. *Cognitive Psychology, 20,* 319–343.

Krumhansl, C. L., & Shepard, R. N. (1979). Quantification of the hierarchy of tonal functions within a diatonic context. *Journal of Experimental Psychology: Human Perception and Performance, 5,* 579–594.

Lockhead, G. R., & Byrd, R. (1981). Practically perfect pitch. *Journal of the Acoustical Society of America, 70,* 387–389.

Peretz, I., & Morais, J. (1988). Determinants of laterality for music: Towards an information processing account. In K. Hugdahl (Ed.), *Handbook of dichotic listening: Theory, methods, and research* (pp. 323–358). New York: Wiley.

Pinker, S. (1980). Mental imagery in the third dimension. *Journal of Experimental Psychology: General, 6,* 58–66.

Pollard-Gott, L. (1983). Emergence of thematic concepts in repeated listening to music. *Cognitive Psychology, 15,* 66–94.

Shepard, R. N., & Metzler, J. (1971). Mental rotation of three-dimensional objects. *Science, 171,* 701–703.

Stevens, A. & Coupe, P. (1978). Distortions in judged spatial relations. *Cognitive Psychology, 63,* 390–397.

Tversky, B. (1981). Distortions in memory for maps. *Cognitive Psychology, 13,* 407–433.

Zatorre, R. J. (1984). Musical perception and cerebral function: A critical review. *Music Perception, 2,* 196–221.

Zatorre, R. J. (1985). Discrimination and recognition of tonal melodies after unilateral cerebral excisions. *Neuropsychologia, 23,* 31–41.

2 Research on Memory/Imagery for Musical Timbre

Robert G. Crowder
Mark A. Pitt*
Yale University

RESEARCH ON IMAGERY IN MUSIC:
PAST AND PRESENT

We have at hand eight recent books dealing with the psychology of music, all but one published in the 1980s (Clynes, 1982; Davies, 1978; Deutsch, 1982; Dowling & Harwood, 1986; Hargreaves, 1986; Howell, Cross & West, 1985; Serafine, 1988; Sloboda, 1985). To judge from their subject indexes, *none* makes reference to imagery in music, nor does Handel's recent monograph on speech and music entitled *Listening* (Handel, 1989). We don't want to insist too hard on this casual bibliographic scan. For one thing, the topic of imagery could have crept into these sources in disguised form, under another terminology. Further, the subject indices in these books may not be exhaustive, nor is our collection necessarily definitive.

But this absolutely thundering silence on imagery in music is in contrast with two factors. First, in *visual* cognition and perception, the issue of imagery has become increasingly central in the last two decades. Whole books on the topic have appeared, as has a journal, and in the larger domain of the cognitive sciences, imagery is recognized as a defining problem. One of us has commented elsewhere on the lag between visual and auditory scholarship (Crowder 1989a) and, because the present volume is intended to correct the imbalance, we shall not dwell further on it here.

Secondly, in contrast to the modern silence on musical imagery, it was not always thus: In the few earlier classics on music psychology, we found entries in the subject indexes of books by Seashore (1938/1967) and by Farnsworth (1958). Albeit decidedly pre-scientific, these treatments are thoughtful about musical

*Currently at Ohio State University.

29

imagery. Largely, they take the existence of imagery for granted and comment on its prevalence and use. In fact, both authors despaired of the lack of objective evidence for musical imagery and based their coverage instead on self-report studies and anecdotal descriptions. Seashore (1938/1967) devoted an entire chapter to imagery, speculating specifically on timbral color in images when he said of those possessing imagery, that "they can select out for hearing particular tone qualities in the manner than the organist manipulates his stops" (p. 167). To the extent that traditional organ stops affect the spectral balance between overtones accompanying a given pitch, this quotation anticipates issues and results of the research to be summarized later in this chapter.

Both Seashore (1938/1967) and Farnsworth (1958) distinguished various *different kinds of imagery* that are entailed by musical cognition, particularly between auditory (sensory) and kinesthetic (motor), as well as associated-visual imagery. This is another theme to which this chapter will return.

In the modern study of cognition, imagery is no longer the target of Behaviorist exorcism that it once was. The views of Hebb (1966, 1968) on imagery are not the latest word on the topic but seem to us to make good sense. Hebb's analysis may be seen as a form of *proceduralism* in memory; imagery is after all a form of memory. Imagery representation according to Hebb is the activation of the same central neural systems that played a role in the original event, but this time in the absence of the original sensory activity. His own favorite example of imagery was the experience of pain, itching, or cramping in a phantom limb, where the peripheral sensory activity cannot possibly even exist. Elsewhere (Crowder 1989b), the claim has been made that a useful model for memory in general is the persisting activity of the neural centers involved in the original experiences (Kolers & Roediger, 1984). Imagery, as a form of memory, would fall within that position.

Pitch, Loudness, and Timbre

This proceduralist attitude suggests that the experience of imagery is potentially as rich as the original event. For example, the non-temporal properties of a musical tone include its pitch, loudness, and timbre (Dowling & Harwood, 1985, p. 19). These properties, to be perceptible, must necessarily have neural consequences at some level. And those consequences could accordingly be activated in the absence of the original tonal input, as properties of imagery. (This is to say nothing about the potential dimensions of properties defined by two rather than a single musical tone.) As Hebb (1966, 1968) maintained, the difference between remembered events and images has to do with the completeness with which the peripheral and central activities of the original event are activated by the (spontaneous or deliberate) retrieval environment. Hebb (1968) believed that the differences in vividness of imagery (and memory) had to do with whether primary, sensory, or higher-order cell assemblies were activated.

But by another criterion these three potential dimensions of imagery for musical tones (pitch, loudness, timbre) are not equal. Frequency and amplitude are, within limits, under control of normal subjects. That is, for these dimensions a motor output matches much of the range of external stimulation that can occur. Crudely put, humming to oneself produces differences that could mimic either a pitch change or a loudness change in the true tone that was heard. (Of course, a physical source is not limited to the range of these that humans can produce, but this does not change the argument.) One would not know in principle whether obtained evidence for imagery were due to the *sensory* property of interest or to the *motor* system for controlling that property. Imagery for timbre does not share this ambiguity, as we shall argue below.

Two recent examples of musical imagery illustrate this ambiguity in assigning effects to sensory or to motor imagery. We allude to them before discussing imagery for timbre. But first, we should affirm that no ambiguity at all surrounds the central claim that these cases show *mental imagery* for musical stimuli. At stake is rather, in Hebbian terms, whether the content of the images owes more to the sensory system or to the motor system. Farah and Smith (1983) showed that maintaining an image of one pitch, rather than an alternative one, increased detection sensitivity of that first pitch as compared to the second, and vice versa. Both pitches were within humming range, however, and we don't know whether humming or some internal surrogate for it might have been operating in this experiment. Secondly, Halpern (1988) timed people's decision as to which of two lyrics from a well-known song ("Dashing . . . sleigh. . . ") started on the higher pitch. She found evidence for scanning of images in that the more distant the two lyrics were in the song the longer the decision time. The rates observed were consistent with a strategy of humming or singing to oneself (But see newer evidence in Halpern, chapter 1, this volume). Again, an auditory replay of the stimuli was possible, but so was a motor code.

Imagery for Timbre

Now, back to timbre: People can do little by way of vocally stimulating the sounds of a clarinet or an oboe. Besides differences in the reed, these instruments have different spectral elements in the overtone structures, because the former has a cylindrical bore and the latter a conical bore. In principle, to have a mental image of an instrumental timbre should indicate an auditory (sensory) representation rather than a motor one.

CURRENT RESEARCH ON MUSICAL IMAGERY

These considerations have motivated recent research on imagery for musical timbre (Crowder, 1989a, 1991). The original demonstration (Crowder, 1989a) comes in two parts, both entailing a same-different pitch judgment relating two successive tones. Part one of the demonstration shows that two successive instrumental tones are more readily judged as having the same pitch if they are also played on the same instrument than if played on different instruments. More specifically, the possible musical tones in this experiment formed a 3 × 3 arrangement with three diatonic pitches (F, G, and A) as one dimension, and three instruments (flute, guitar, and trumpet) as the other. The materials were digitized examples of actual instruments played under studio conditions.

On trials where the same pitch was played twice in a row, reaction times and accuracy to respond "same" were both superior when the two tones were produced on the same instrument than when produced on different instruments. This finding, by itself, is not without interest, showing that the memory trace that necessarily mediates the time between the two tones (half a second) carries information about timbre as well as pitch.

In the second part of the experiment, the first tone was always a sine wave set at one of the same three critical pitches. But during the interval between this sine save and the second tone, subjects were asked to form a mental image of a specified instrument playing that particular pitch. The instrument's name was presented on the CRT at the same time the sine wave sounded. Subjects pressed a button when they felt they had achieved the stipulated image, whereupon the second tone was presented, either the same or a different pitch, played on either the imagined instrument or on one of the others. Notice that the task does not guarantee the use of imagery: A pitch match between the sine wave and the second (instrumental) sound is all that perfect performance requires.

However, the image people were asked to produce affected performance reliably, and in the same way the first of two genuine instrumental tones did in the previous experiment. That is, when the first (imagined) tone and the second matched with respect to instrument, reaction times to the second tone were faster, and accuracy higher, than when they mismatched. Because our subjects were, like all of us, incapable of producing the timbres of a flute, guitar, or trumpet on their own, the case for true auditory, sensory, imagery rests on this demonstration.

The matching effect in both the two-tone comparison and the image-based comparison could possibly result from a "startle" response in mismatch conditions, delaying somehow the same-pitch responses. We acknowledge this interpretation here, although experiments described later rule out such a possibility.

In this discussion, we have steered clear of a formal definition of timbre (see Handel, 1989, chapter 6). But all sources are agreed that two classes of factor govern this property: (a) the *spectral* cues afforded by the presence and emphasis of certain harmonics differentially by various instruments, and (b) the *dynamic* cues afforded by different attack and decay characteristics of musical sounds. I have already alluded to the clarinet and oboe timbres as illustrations of the former. For the latter, we may imagine the same string instrument being either plucked or bowed, and the ensuing timbre differences. In the previous experiment, using naturalistic musical sounds, these qualities are confounded, as they are in the everyday world. But in the laboratory we can do better, in the sense of probing analytically for the operating principles on which the system depends. Accordingly, we have been arranging experiments to discover whether all aspects of timbre, especially (a) and (b), are equally conducive to mental imagery.

We first[1] wished to remain with naturalistic musical tones, but stressing this time the dynamic cues to timbre by using actual plucking and bowing sounds from a real violoncello. As before, we digitized a vocabulary of the same three pitches being plucked (abrupt attack) or bowed (gradual attack) by an experienced amateur. The actual pitches were calibrated as before. Each lasted a quarter second with a half second between the two. The results are shown in Table 2.1. With thirteen subjects, the 50 msec difference between the two conditions with same-pitch stimuli was statistically reliable, $t(12) = 2.00$. Moreover, this advantage for the same-timbre condition over the different-timbre condition was true of 10 of the 13 subjects, with three individuals reversed ($p = .0460$). In these data, other aspects of the results were entirely unremarkable except for the accuracy differences obtained when the true pitches were different: Of the ten non-tied subjects, eight showed more accurate performance when both pitch and timbre were different than when only timbre in the two tones was different, with two showing the opposite ($p = .055$). Across experiments this marginal difference for the "different" responses is not a consistent one, but the larger variance and poorer performance when pitch and timbre mismatch are not without theoretical plausibility or empirical precedent (Crowder, 1990).

The results for "same" responses are of the most interest here because they establish a precondition for the second member of the pair of experiments, in which a sine wave is used as the basis for a mental image of a verbally named instrument playing *that pitch*. Thirteen new subjects were used in this second experiment of the pair. In a training phase, they were first introduced to the 2 (articulations) $\times$ 3 (pitches) vocabulary of tones. Then they were given practice in forming the desired auditory image. After a sine wave was played, they were to press a button when they "had" the image of the specified timbre playing that pitch. Thus, the actual timbre playing that pitch was presented so as to provide feedback during the training period. This training phrase continued until subjects reported proficiency in image generation. The next phase of the training protocol was the same, except that a comparison tone was presented when the button was pressed, indicating that a satisfactory image had been generated. The test phase of the experiment proceeded in this same manner, except that the comparison tone was drawn from the 2 $\times$ 3 array of 'cello tones. The first block of trials counted as practice and was discarded.

---

[1]It is understood that the logical order of experiments does not always match the chronological order in which they were performed.

TABLE 2.1
Means and Standard Deviations from Two-Tone Comparisons of 'Cello Pluck and Bow
(n = 13)

	Same Pitch/ Same Timbre	Same Pitch/ Different Timbre	Different Pitch/Same Timbre	Different Pitch/Different Timbre
Reaction Time	647	697	827.3	794.9
(sd)	246.4	197.4	551.6	445.5
Percent Accuracy	93.2	90.3	72.4	84.6
(sd)	13.9	15.6	32.1	19.8

The results are shown in Table 2.2. The layout of information is identical to the previous table, except that quotes surround the timbre distinction to indicate that the timbres were only imagined, not actually presented. The first thing to notice is that reaction times were slower and accuracy lower in the second experiment as compared to the first. This is as we would expect for responding based on mental images as opposed to real stimuli. Secondly, the reaction times show little evident variability, except for an overall time advantage when the pitches were the same as opposed to different (not a statistically reliable effect, however). In this experiment, accuracy was the more sensitive dependent variable. An overall 2×2 ANOVA showed a reliable main effect of same/different pitch, $F(1, 12) = 6.55$, $p = .025$, reflecting generally more accurate performance when the two pitches were different than when they were the same. Note that this accuracy difference favors the condition with the slower times in the previously discussed reaction-time analysis, as we would expect from a speed-accuracy trade-off. On its own therefore, this outcome is uninterpretable.

TABLE 2.2
Means and Standard Deviations from Comparisons of Imagined 'Cello Pluck and Bow Tones with
Real Tones
(n = 13)

	Same Pitch/ "Same Timbre"	Same Pitch/ "Different Timbre"	Different Pitch/"Same Timbre"	Different Pitch/"Different Timbre"
Reaction Time	1230.9	1257.4	1338.6	1331.8
(sd)	608.1	595.1	743.3	654.7
Percent Accuracy	75.8	59.6	68.8	78.8
(sd)	8.9	20.6	18.9	16.6

Not so the reliable interaction between pitch and timbre identity, $F(1, 12) =$ 5.77, $p = .033$. Here, the accuracy pattern followed exactly the latency pattern, which was not reliable here but was in other studies in this series—better responding on "same pitch" trials when timbres also matched than otherwise. Tests of simple effects showed that the crucial difference, between 75.8 and 59.6 in Table 2, was highly reliable, $F(1, 12) = 9.24$, $p = .01$. (The other reliable simple effect, of pitch with different timbres, is not straightforward because the overt responses were different.) Thus, by far the main outcome of the experiment was that subjects seemed capable of generating images of musical tones with timbral properties of the bona fide tones they were asked to imagine.

The present demonstration is similar to that reported in Crowder (1989a) but extends it to timbral features inherent in one single instrument rather than among several. As such, it rules out interpretations of the effect that might be offered based on mediation of the visual appearance of the instruments used. A flute and a guitar look different, of course, and this factor might possibly have been involved in the original three-instruments effect. However, plucked and bowed sounds on a 'cello result from the same instrumental source. The results suggest that the matching effect can occur for dynamic timbre differences, because the spectral, resonant properties of the 'cello do not change as a function of how its strings are irritated.

Or do they? Close reflection reveals that dynamic and spectral cues to timbre are not so completely independent in the everyday world as they seem. For example, abrupt onset of musical tones produces what are called transients, which can add high frequency noise that is simply not present with ramped stimuli. In our 'cello tones, we performed acoustic analyses that confirmed major differences in plucked and bowed stimuli with regard to spectral properties.[2]

Accordingly, we turned to synthetic sounds, which permit the unambiguous separation of spectral and dynamic factors in timbre. Using the same three pitches, we made a "spectral pair" of instrumental sounds that differed only in the presence and absence of harmonics to effect the distinction, leaving overall intensity equal.[3] The tones used in the "dynamic pair" of synthetic tones had spectral components that were identical, but one was highly ramped at the onset and the other abrupt. We shall first describe the two parts of the "spectral" experiment and then the "dynamic" experiment.

We tested a large number of student volunteers on both the spectral and the dynamic parts of this project, in counterbalanced order, for reasons soon to be explained. We tested unselected subjects at the beginning, but soon found that many of them were not readily disregarding timbre in order to respond to pitch. After this became obvious, we still accepted all volunteers for the experiment but

---

[2]The prolonged bowing articulation altered the overtone structure to include many more, and much more intense high frequency components than the brief plucked articulation.

[3]Essentially, one emphasized harmonics above the fourth partial, and the other emphasized those below the fifth partial.

posted the study lists in the vicinity of Yale's music campus. We administered a musical-background questionnaire to everyone, which, it turned out, was a good tactic.

In counterbalanced order, some subjects completed the task with spectral timbres first and others the dynamic timbres first. The experiment was otherwise like the first one described here, with two tones successively presented, each from a 2 × 3 array of timbre and pitch. Subjects were given careful instructions and examples of what the same/different pitch discrimination was intended to mean. Timbre was always irrelevant to the task. Table 2.3 presents the overall results of the spectral portion of the experiment. The means are for the 50 subjects we tested. Clearly, we did not obtain the same pattern of reaction times we had earlier. In particular, times to the same-pitch/different-timbre trials were not slower than same-pitch/same-timbre trials; indeed they were a bit faster. However, the accuracy data show that the group as a whole was not appreciably better than chance (50% correct) in the condition with the same pitch and different timbres. This condition was nearly impossible for some subjects and easy for others. The distribution of accuracy scores for this condition is shown in Fig. 2.1, which emphasizes the bimodality obtained. No scores at all fell between 37% and 70% correct, which is exactly where the mean was (56%). Evidently, people differ sharply in the ease with which they can attend to pitch cues while disregarding timbre.

To elucidate these individual differences, we examined the results of the musical background questionnaire that had been collected for all subjects. This questionnaire targeted the following information: (a) how many years of formal instrumental or vocal training the student had had, (b) how recent this activity had been, and (c) how many academic courses, in subjects pertaining to music, had been taken. The overall correlation between musical experience (the sum of a, b, and c) versus performance in the same-pitch/different-timbre condition—the Fig. 2.1 index—was +.66. People with more musical experience were better

TABLE 2.3
Means and Standard Deviations from Spectral-Timbre Experiment
(N = 50)

	Same Pitch/Same Timbre	Same Pitch/Different Timbre	Different Pitch/Same Timbre	Different Pitch/Differnt Timbre
Reaction time	624.1	546.6	675.6	677.9
(sd)	142.6	429.9	186	182.8
Percent Accuracy	98.1	56.0	91.4	94.6
(sd)	5.3	46.0	19.5	15.5

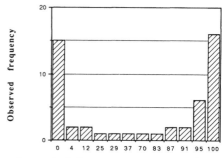

FIG. 2.1. Frequency distribution of scores in same-pitch/different timbre condition of spectral-synthetic experiment (n = 50).

able than their less experienced classmates to ignore timbre and process pitch on its own. Of course, we must not infer a causal relationship from this correlation: Young people who cannot abstract pitch from timbre might well discontinue their musical activities after a short time.

Restricting ourselves now to the 28 people in the higher-accuracy group for the same-pitch/different-timbre condition, we found that *every* individual had slower reaction times in this condition than in the same-pitch/same-timbre condition, exactly the same result that was found in the earlier study (Crowder, 1989a). The results are shown in Table 2.4. So even for subjects who could perform perfectly in separating pitch from timbre, a penalty in processing time was paid with a timbre mismatch. The probability of this outcome by chance alone is $1/2^28$, so we did not perform ANOVAS to back it up.

For the second part of this project—the part that depends on *imagery* for timbre—we contacted only subjects from the first phase who were among the 28 high-scoring subjects in Fig. 1. We were able to convince fifteen of these to return to the laboratory for a second session. The assigned task was more complicated than in the first session, although we knew that these subjects had no trouble understanding that the pitch comparison was the basis for the same–

TABLE 2.4
Means and Standard Deviations from 28 "Qualified" Subjects in Spectral-Timbre Experiment

	Same Pitch/ Same Timbre	Same Pitch/ Different Timbre	Different Pitch/Same Timbre	Different Pitch/Different Timbre
Reaction Time	576.2	732.8	630.7	682.7
(sd)	117.8	176.5	133.3	190.4
Percent Accuracy	99.3	95.7	94.5	92.8
(sd)	1.8	7.0	17.3	19.6

different judgments, because of their performance in the companion study just described. They were trained as in the imagery portion of the Crowder (1989a) experiment: They first listened to the six tones that could occur as the second comparison tone (3 pitches × 2 synthetic, spectrally defined timbres). During this demonstration phase, we suggested that the timbres could be called "organ" and "car horn," but subjects were free to substitute other terms if they wished. In the next phase of training, they heard sine waves at various pitches, accompanied by a written indication of one of the two "instruments" and had as long as they wanted to form a mental image of how that pitch would sound as played in the designated timbre. As before, feedback was provided in the form of the specified timbre playing the pitch of the sinewave. In the experimental session, the second tone of the pair was presented in either the imagined timbre or the other one.

The results are shown in Table 2.5, which is organized exactly like the other tables. The timbre difference is again enclosed in quotes because the match concerns an imagined tone quality and the presented probe tone. The reaction times in the four crucial conditions were all within less than 30 msec of each other. Nevertheless the simple effect of timbre in the same-pitch condition (a difference of 25.3 msec) was statistically reliable ($p < .05$). (No other effect was reliable in the omnibus ANOVA for these times.)

In the accuracy data of Table 5 we find even stronger evidence that matching an imagined timbre to the second of two tones produced an advantage. Every single subject of the fifteen had higher accuracy in the match condition than in the mismatch condition, even though the mean in the poorer condition (72.33% correct) was comfortably above chance. These individuals showed a corresponding effect of timbre on the different-pitch trials; all fifteen subjects were more accurate when both pitch and timbre were different than when the pitches were different and timbres the same. But this effect on judgments of different pitch was not evident in the earlier studies of natural timbres. Our primary conclusion is that even for subjects who are minimally able to perceive pitch and timbre independently, a residual dependence exists in the form of poorer performance

TABLE 2.5
Means and Standard Deviations from the Imagery Session of the Spectral-Timbre Experiment

	Same Pitch/ "Same Timbre"	Same Pitch/ "Different Timbre"	Different Pitch/"Same Timbre"	Different Pitch/"Different Timbre"
Reaction Time	666.3	691.6	662.7	676.3
(sd)	259.1	261.2	237.2	253.5
Percent Accuracy	86.2	72.33	86	98
(sd)	1.6	3.1	3	4.6

when timbre and pitch do not match than when they do. In Garner's (1974) sense, then, listener's must process pitch and timbre integrally, and not as separable dimensions (Crowder, 1990). This integrality in processing is assignable here to a mental image of the first comparison tone.

The dynamic half of the project on synthetic tones is easily described: Although we ourselves had thought the two timbres discriminable, our subjects gave no evidence of noticing the difference. In the initial session, with 50 subjects, neither reaction time nor accuracy was affected by timbre matching, and so we cannot deny the claim that this was a truly fictitious manipulation on our part. Without evidence that the dynamic timbral cue was potent in part one of the procedure, it made no sense to ask whether mental images were capable of mimicking this result.

In our most recent experiment, we produced two more conspicuously different timbres using only dynamic changes. These tones were either broadly ramped, with gradual onsets, or were more sudden in onset. We refer to them hereafter as "abrupt" and "gradual." Fourteen new subjects were tested in the first phase of this experiment, in which the two presented tones varied both in pitch and in timbre. Results are shown in Table 2.6. A little reflection makes obvious our reason for splitting the data according to whether the second tone was one of the abrupt ones or one of the gradual ones. Take an extreme case of a gradual-onset tone—one more exaggerated than those we used: As regards pitch, the stimulus would not, for such a tone, even begin until some appreciable time after the onset of the nominal tone. This is because in the first moments such an exaggerated ramped tone could actually be inaudible. This would obviously depend on stimulus parameters, but we can take the general point that people might be delayed in responding to gradual tones, relative to sudden tones, for psychologically uninteresting reasons.

Table 2.6 bears out this suspicion by revealing overall slower (and less accurate) responses when the gradual tone was the response signal than when the abrupt tone was. In an overall ANOVA the main effect of response was reliable for the accuracy data, in support of this evident trend in the results, $F(1, 13) = 8.27, p = .013$. For the latency data, this main effect did not achieve statistical reliability. As noted above, this result should not be at all surprising, any more than it would be to find that reading times for letters were less when a dark screen were abruptly illuminated as opposed to being gradually illuminated. This main effect does however vindicate that our manipulation of dynamic timbre cues was effective at least at some level, unlike the situation in the earlier experiment on dynamic cues to timbre.

Such vindication of our choice of stimuli is more telling in the rest of the data in Table 2.6. Again, as before, pitch differences interacted with timbre differences, $F(1, 13) = 12.0, p = .0042$, such that same-pitch trials led to worse performance when timbres differed than when they matched. This interaction was not reliable for the latency data. It was true for only 7 of the 14 subjects in

TABLE 2.6
Means and Standard Deviations for Dynamic Synthetic Timbres

		Same Pitch/Same Timbre	Same Pitch/ Different Timbre	Different Pitch/Same Timbre	Different Pitch/ DifferenTimbre
Abrupt second	Reaction time	857.6	1036.7	928.1	900
	(sd)	238.2	473.7	376.6	277.5
	Percent Accuracy	95.8	84.5	84.5	95.2
	(sd)	5.4	24.0	21.9	6.3
Gradual Second	Reaction Time	970.6	1146.1	1425.1	868.5
	(sd)	350.0	626.0	1593.3	265.4
	Percent Accuracy	94.0	73.3	77.4	91.0
	(sd)	6.8	29.7	24.6	10.6

the latency data, but 9 of 10 of the nontied subjects in the accuracy data, $p = .011$. Perhaps the most crucial result for the present is the simple effect of timbre differences when the two pitches were the same. For the latency data, this effect was just short of statistical reliability, $F(1, 13) = 4.3$, $p = .058$; whereas for the accuracy data it was solidly reliable, $F(1, 13) = 8.37$, $p = 013$.

The more elusive (in these experiments) effect of timbre differences in the different-pitch trials was not so close to reliability in the latency data, $F(1, 13) = 2.4$, $p = .150$, but it was highly reliable for the accuracy data, $F(1, 13) = 8.9$, $p = .01$. We confess to not understanding why in some experiments latency seems to be the more sensitive dependent variable and, in others, accuracy does. The main conclusion from the data of Table 2.6 remains that we have again satisfied the precondition for examining possible imagery effects in a companion experiment.

Fourteen fresh subjects were tested in the imagery version of the dynamic timbre experiment. They were led through the same training sequence as used in the other imagery experiments. First, the 2×3 (timbre $\times$ pitch) array of possible stimuli was presented with the explicit suggestion that some of the tones were "abrupt" and others "gradual." These subjects were given practice generating either of these two timbres in response to sine-wave cues matching the three pitches. Feedback was provided. The experimental session began immediately after the training phase.

The results are shown in Table 2.7. As in the previous experiment, we have partitioned the data according to whether the tone to be responded to was gradual or abrupt. The main thing to notice in Table 2.7 is that a consistent matching effect, favoring the same-pitch/"same"-timbre condition over the same pitch/

TABLE 2.7
Means and Standard Deviations for Imagery of Dynamic Timbres

		Same Pitch/"Same Timbre"	Same Pitch/ "Different Timbre"	Different Pitch/"Same Timbre"	Different Pitch/ "DifferenTimbre"
Abrupt second	Reaction time	1025.4	1130	1190	1205
	(sd)	412	439.5	455.4	426.7
	Percent Accuracy	76.1	74.6	68.2	69.1
	(sd)	26.3	27.8	28.2	32.6
Gradual Second	Reaction Time	1198.4	1024.8	1127.8	1162
	(sd)	425.4	320.2	334.0	422.9
	Percent Accuracy	74.4	77.1	66.8	69.6
	(sd)	27.3	24.1	31.3	29.3

"different"-timbre condition was *not* obtained here, as it had been for both latency and accuracy in the data of Table 2.6. It looks from the latency data as if such an effect had occurred for the abrupt target tones but it was reversed for the gradual tones. However, even the 104.6 msec effect in the abrupt data was not close to reliability on its own, $t(13) = 1.34$. In the gradual data, the effect was actually reversed by a larger amount.

An overall ANOVA on the latency data showed no reliable effect except for a statistically significant triple interaction of probe tone (abrupt/gradual), pitch (same/different) and timbre (same/different), $F(1, 13) = 8.16, p = .0135$. The means in Table 2.7 indicate that the opposite effect of a timbre "match" for abrupt and gradual test stimuli provides a convenient perspective on this interaction. We think a special circumstance makes it interpretable in this particular experiment. *The sine waves used as generation cues had abrupt onsets.* In other words, for the first time in these experiments, the cue to generation was itself not neutral with respect to the property being generated. (When we realized this feature of the experiment, we concluded that no alternative sine wave would qualify as neutral either, obviously not one with a gradual onset, for example.) For this reason, one should approach the data of Table 2.7 as performance resulting from a three-tone sequence, always an abrupt sine wave, then a putative imagined tone of either abrupt or gradual onset, and finally the probe tone, which was abrupt or gradual, respectively, for the top and bottom halves of Table 2.7. Thus, a three letter sequence such as A- "A" -A[4] specifies the circumstances

---

[4]The letter A stands for the abrupt stimuli and G for gradual.

applying to the cell with the reaction time of 1,025.4 msec, with the middle letter referring to the imagined tone.

In light of this observation, the interaction noted in reaction times makes good sense. Let us restrict ourselves to the same-pitch trials. (By inspection, neither variation in pitch nor timbre had an appreciable effect on the different pitch trials.) When the imagined tone was to be gradual, in contrast to the uniformly abrupt sine wave, times were relatively slow. This was true in the A- "G" -A cell in the upper part of the table (1,130 msec) and in the A- "G" -G cell of the lower part (1,198.4 msec). Faster reaction times resulted when the imagined tone was consistent with the abrupt sine wave, in conditions A- "A" -A (1,025.4 msec) and A- "A" -G (1,024.8 msec). We may say, then, that the additional work of generating an image discrepant with the abrupt sine wave impaired performance to the second tone.

However, this extra work was insufficient to arrive at a mental image sharing the timbral properties of the real tones in this experiment. If it had been, then a matching effect would be present between the imagined and second tones, perhaps superimposed on the result just described.

The analysis of variance based on accuracy scores in Table 2.7 showed no effects even marginally reliable, except for a main effect of pitch, with performance on same-pitch trials consistently more accurate than on different-pitch trials, $F(1, 13) = 6.09$, $p = 028$. The 8% accuracy advantage for same-pitch trials over different-pitch trials is of course confounded with the response in our task, and is immaterial to the purpose of the experiment.

The main finding in this last experiment is that dynamic cues to timbre, on their own, provide no evidence for the production and use of mental images. This negative result takes on considerable authority in light of two contrasts: First, the very same stimuli used here produced reliable matching effects in the previous experiment (Table 2.6). Therefore, dynamic timbre is useful in pitch decisions when the quality of the current tone is to be compared with the quality of one heard a half-second earlier. Second, the negative results here cannot be attributed to an insensitive experiment, because highly reliable outcomes were observed in both the latency and accuracy data of Table 2.7 for non-crucial effects (the sine-wave-match interaction in the former and the main effect of pitch in the latter). Accordingly, we may conclude that the capacity to imagine different timbre qualities appeals to spectral properties of tones but not their dynamic properties. By the same token, the present results rule out the interpretation of the imagery-matching effect in our early experiments based on a "startle" response to mismatching tones. Expecting a gradual tone and receiving a sudden one, or vice versa, should then have produced the inhibitory startle reaction.

Imagery for dynamic cues may exist in some form but may be qualitatively different from imagery for spectral cues, because a temporal component is integral to the former but not the latter. Dynamic cues to timbre evolve over time, whereas spectral cues stay comparatively more constant. The representation of dynamic cues may possess this temporal feature, resulting in an image that evolves over time rather than remain constant like an image composed of spectral cues. Our failure to demonstrate imagery for dynamic cues may be due to the temporal constraints of the paradigm that we employed. After imagining a specified timbre, subjects had to make a speeded response to the second tone, a requirement that may not have led to a full comparison of the dynamic cues of the imagined and presented timbres. In addition, the temporal properties of dynamic cues may make them more difficult to compare than their spectral counterparts, although this was not a problem when two tones differing only in dynamic properties were presented in close temporal proximity (Table 2.6). Employing an experimental paradigm that does not emphasize speeded responding could be helpful in addressing these issues.

This leaves us with a curious logical sequence. Early in the chapter we defended the use of timbre in mental imagery because instrumental timbres, unlike pitch and other properties of musical tones, cannot be simulated vocally and must therefore be based on sensory rather than motor images. Having then made a case for imagery for musical timbre, we set out to analyse whether the *spectral* or the *dynamic* cues to timbre are more susceptible to mental imagery in our task. We found that for subjects able to process pitch independently of timbre, the spectral features of tones were indeed represented in images. Now, we have just concluded that the dynamic cues, on their own, seem not to be represented in images. Yet, of the two, the dynamic cues are to some extent under the subjects' productive control and the spectral cues not! We can start to hum a tone suddenly or gradually, but we cannot readily change the spectral properties (except as the articulation of certain vowels does so in a limited way).

CONCLUSION

From these experiments we infer, first, that musical imagery can be brought into the laboratory successfully. We have furthermore begun to isolate the particular sensory qualities that form the basis for this imagery. From our studies here, we conclude that spectral, rather than dynamic, cues are the ones that underlie this memory process. This marks a clear difference between audition itself and auditory imagery, for both qualities are obviously salient in the former.

ACKNOWLEDGMENTS

The research described here was supported by NSF Grant GB 86-08344 to R. Crowder, who is at Department of Psychology, Box 11a Yale Station, New Haven, CT 06520. M. Pitt is currently at Department of Psychology, Townshend Hall, 1885 Neil Avenue Mall, The Ohio State University, Columbus, OH 43210.

REFERENCES

Clynes, M. (Ed.). (1982). *Music, mind, and brain*. New York: Plenum.

Crowder, R. G. (1989a). Imagery for musical timbre. *Journal of Experimental Psychology: Human Perception and Performance, 15,* 472–478.

Crowder, R. G. (1989b). Modularity and dissociations of memory systems. In H. L. Roediger, III, and F. I. M. Craik (Eds.), *Varieties of Memory and Consciousness: Essays in Honor of Endel Tulving.* Hillsdale, NJ: Lawrence Erlbaum Associates.

Crowder, R. G. (1991). Individual differences in the processing of auditory stimulus dimensions. In J. Pomerantz & G. R. Lockhead (Eds.), *The processing of structure.* American Psychological Association.

Davies, J. B. (1978). *The psychology of music.* Stanford, CA: Stanford University Press.

Deutsch, D. (Ed.). (1982). The *psychology of music.* New York: Academic Press.

Dowling, W. J., & Harwood, D. L. (1986). *Music Cognition.* New York: Academic Press.

Farah, M. J., & Smith, A. F. (1983). Perceptual interference and facilitation with auditory imagery. *Perception and Psychophysics, 33,* 475–478.

Farnsworth, P. R. (1958). *The social Psychology of music.* New York: Dryden.

Garner, W. R. (1974). *The processing of information and structure.* Potomac, Md: Erlbaum.

Halpern, A. R. (1988). Mental scanning in auditory imagery for songs. *Journal of Experimental Psychology: Learning, Memory and Cognition, 14,* 434–443.

Handel, S. (1989). *Listening: An introduction to the perception of auditory events.* Cambridge, MS: MIT Press.

Hargreaves, D. J. (1986). *The developmental psychology of music.* London: Cambridge University Press.

Hebb, D. O. (1966). *A textbook of psychology, Second Edition.* Philadelphia: W. B. Saunders.

Hebb, D. O. (1968). Concerning imagery. *Psychological Review, 75,* 466–477.

Howell, P., Cross, I., & West, R. (Eds.). (1985). *Musical structure and cognition.* London: Academic Press.

Kolers, P. A., & Roediger, H. L. III. (1984). Procedures of mind. *Journal of Verbal Learning and Verbal Behavior, 23,* 425–449.

Seashore, C. E. (1967). *Psychology of music.* New York: Dover. (Originally published by McGraw Hill, 1938)

Serafine, M. L. (1988). *Music as cognition: The development of thought in sound.* New York: Columbia University Press.

Sloboda, J. A. (1985). *The musical mind: The cognitive psychology of music.* Oxford: Clarendon Press.

3 Components of Auditory Imagery

Margaret Jean Intons-Peterson
Indiana University

Long considered a country cousin of visual imagery, auditory imagery is emerging as a phenomenon in its own right and as a process that can illuminate the general relations among imagery and other processes. Auditory imagery seems to incorporate some, but not invariably all, physical characteristics of sounds. Questions about the role of physical characteristics in imagery appear to be asked of auditory imagery; they have been pursued infrequently with visual imagery. Auditory imagery also may be used to compare its relation to auditory perception and cognition with those of visual imagery. These imaginal-perceptual-cognitive relationships are central issues in imagery.

The issue of the extent of parallelism between imagery and perception has dominated visual imagery research over the last few decades. Despite the dedicated and enthusiastic pursuit of answers, the results have been ambiguous. As becomes clear in a careful reading of some reviews (Finke & Shepard, 1986; Intons-Peterson & McDaniel, 1991), imaginal performance seems to be similar to perceptual performance when the tasks are highly unusual, when the tasks require the participants to engage in activities and responses that differ from their everyday lives. Imaginal and perceptual performance seem more likely to diverge when the tasks afford the opportunity to draw on real-world knowledge (e.g., Baird, Wagner, & Noma, 1982; Chambers & Reisberg, 1985; Evans & Pezdek, 1980; Giraudo & Peruch, 1988; Intons-Peterson & Roskos-Ewoldsen, 1989; Kerst & Howard, 1978; Maki, 1981; Moar & Bower, 1983; Moyer, Bradley, Sorensen, Whiting, & Mansfield, 1978; Nairne & Pusen, 1984; Reisberg & Chambers, 1991; Reisberg, Smith, Baxter, & Sonenshine, 1989; Stevens & Coupe, 1978; Tversky, 1981). One interpretation for these results is that imagery draws on processes that contribute to both perception and cognition (knowledge). This "dynamics systems" view is described more fully in Intons-Peterson (under review) for visual imagery.

Does auditory imagery show similar effects? Does auditory imagery reflect such perceptual attributes of auditory experience as loudness, pitch, and timbre? Does real world knowledge affect auditory imagery? The purpose of this chapter is to describe tentative answers to these questions by drawing on the admittedly scanty evidence now available in the auditory imagery literature. We begin with a definition of auditory imagery, then consider the components of auditory imagery and their interactions. Next is a comparison of the evidence from relatively "cognition-limited" and "cognition-rich" environments as a way of examining the relations among auditory imagery, perception, and cognition. We end with a brief sketch of a limited number of models that are applicable to auditory imagery and a discussion of the information needed to better understand auditory imagery.

What is auditory imagery? My preferred definition is that auditory imagery is the introspective persistence of an auditory experience, including one constructed from components drawn from long-term memory, in the absence of direct sensory instigation of that experience. This definition is intended to exclude auditory aftereffects, which result from a just-vanished auditory stimulus. The definition makes no claims about the physiological or biochemical underpinnings of imaginal representation, for such claims would be premature.

Before probing the components of auditory imagery, I digress to consider methodology. As suggested above, the particular materials used to study visual imagery may strongly affect, even determine, the outcome. The same may be true for auditory imagery. As with studies of visual imagery, research on auditory imagery has tested both familiar auditory events such as songs (Halpern, 1988, 1989), environmental sounds (Intons-Peterson, 1980; Segal & Fusella, 1970), musical instruments (Crowder, 1989a, 1989b), and voices (Geiselman & Bjork, 1980; Geiselman & Glenny, 1977; Johnson, Foley, & Leach, 1988; Nairne & Pusen, 1984) and unfamiliar auditory events such as pure tones (Farah & Smith, 1983), sine waves (Crowder, 1989a, 1989b), and unknown musical phrases (Weber & Brown, 1986).

Sometimes the time to generate auditory images has been assessed by simple image generation time (Intons-Peterson, 1980) or by reproductions of the relative pitch of imaginal tone sequences (Weber & Brown, 1986). Other paradigms have assessed detection of a signal coincident with imagery (Farah & Smith, 1983; Segal & Fusella, 1970) to ascertain the interfering or facilitating effects of auditory imagery on signal detection. In the same vein, other approaches have examined retention of words imagined or heard in one voice and tested in the same or another voice (Geiselman & Bjork, 1980; Geiselman & Glenny, 1977; Johnson et al., 1988). Finally, auditory imagery for unfamiliar (Weber & Brown, 1986) and for familiar (Halpern, 1988, 1989) musical selections has been assessed in various ways, which are described in detail in subsequent sections.

Like other types of imagery research, one must ask whether auditory imagery is invoked at all. In general, subjects report using auditory imagery, even when not so instructed (Halpern, 1988). Moreover, the possibility of demand factors or other contaminants was considered and rejected in most of the research cited in this chapter. These results strongly suggested that subjects generated and used auditory images.

Auditory imagery also is susceptible to demand characteristics associated with the task, the subjects, and the experimenters. That is, it is possible that some supposedly imaginal performance might be influenced to some extent by the demands of the task, by the subjects' guesses about the purposes of the research, and by inadvertent subtle cues given by hypothesis-knowledgeable experimenters (e.g., Anderson, 1978; Intons-Peterson, 1983; Intons-Peterson & White, 1981; Pylyshyn, 1981). Most of the research considered in this chapter has employed reasonable safeguards against such interpretations.

We now consider some components of auditory imagery, namely, loudness, pitch, and timbre. Information about the role of perception in auditory imagery stems in large part from experiments that manipulate physical cues known to affect auditory experience. The central contention is that if auditory imagery approximates audition, it will show the same dependence on perceptual attributes.

COMPONENTS OF AUDITORY IMAGERY

Two central determinants of auditory experience are loudness (intensity) and pitch (frequency). Hence, if auditory imagery relies on the same processes as audition these two components also will contribute to auditory imagery. Most of the research on auditory imagery has focused on pitch (frequency), which, by way of preview, clearly influences auditory imagery. More limited attention has been directed toward loudness and auditory imagery. We begin with the latter.

Loudness and Auditory Imagery

Do imaginal auditory representations encode loudness information? Research in my laboratory (Intons-Peterson, 1980) suggested that the answer is, "some of the time." In this work, subjects saw phrases describing environmental sounds. The sounds had been rated by an independent group of subjects on a scale of loudness that ranged from very soft (1) to very loud (7). When the main subjects read the phrases and when they generated the auditory images described by the phrases, their reading or image generation times were about the same for all of the phrases. Thus, the times to read or generate auditory images did *not* vary with the loudness ratings of the sounds. Perhaps auditory images do not encode loudness. This would be surprising for images of environmental sounds because these sounds often have varying onsets of loudness that depend on factors such as proximity and time. For example, the loudness of a train seems to increase as the train approaches and to fade as it recedes. Alternatively, auditory images might encode loudness but, for some reason, loud and soft images are generated with equal speed. Such a possibility does not explain why loudness cues are used only some of the time.

Two other tasks indicated that auditory images do encode loudness. In one task, the subjects saw pairs of the phrases. They were to match the loudness of the two phrases. For example, students were asked to imagine one sound described by the left-hand member of the pair, such as "wind chimes tinkling." Then they had to imagine and mentally adjust the right-hand member, say "popcorn popping," until it was equal to the loudness of their image of "wind chimes tinkling." Note that this task should induce the subjects to retrieve and include loudness information if at all possible, whereas the reading and image generation tasks made no such inviolate demands. Again, the phrases differed in their loudness ratings. For some pairs the ratings were very close. For others, the ratings were intermediate, far, or very far apart. In addition, the close, intermediate, and far distances were crossed with the actual ratings. Thus, some of the close pairs were rated as soft (quiet), others were rated as medium in loudness, and still others were rated as loud. I reasoned that if the imagined sounds included retrieved loudness information, the times required to match the loudness of the two members of a pair should increase with the distance between the loudness ratings of the sound phrases. The data did exactly that: The matching times increased by 163 msec from the "close" to the "very far" pairs, as shown in the lower panel of Fig. 3.1 (labeled "Exp. 2"). Thus, the results from matching task indicate that auditory images contain loudness information; those from the reading and generation tasks imply that this information is not always retrieved.

Further bolstering this conclusion were the results from the fourth task. In this case, the subjects were to generate images of the same pairs of phrases that had been used in the previous matching experiment, but their task was to identify the louder (or the softer) member of the pair. What would be expected here? For the matching experiment, we assumed that the differences in matching times occurred because the discriminability between two described sounds increases with the differential in their loudness ratings. This assumption accurately predicted that matching times would increase with increasing loudness-rating differentials. The assumption delivered a contrary prediction for comparative judgments of the louder (or softer) of two described sounds. In this case, the greater the loudness-rating differential, the easier the discrimination should be. Hence, I expected that the judgment times would decrease with increasing distances between the loudness ratings. Again, the results supported the predictions. As Fig. 3.2 shows, the judgments were slowest for the close distances. They became faster as the distance differential increased.

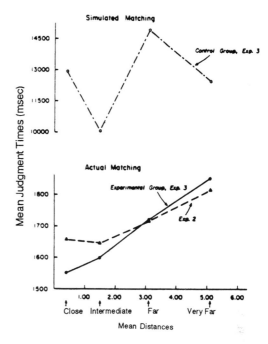

FIG. 3.1. Times to match auditory images and to simulate the matching or equalizing of the loudness of sounds, Experiment 3. From Intons-Peterson (1980). Copyright 1980 by the Psychonomic Society. Reprinted by permission.

These results seem quite compelling, but a possible confounding needs to be examined. Demand characteristics might have produced the results. That is, the tasks themselves may have encouraged the subjects to respond differentially. If this were the case, the results would not necessarily tell us anything about the representation of auditory imagery. To test this possibility, in another experiment new (control) subjects were asked to predict how long it would take them to match the loudness of two described sounds. Other (experimental) subjects also performed the matches, thus replicating the previous matching experiment. The results appear in Fig. 3.1. The Control group's prediction of the time to match is in the upper panel of the figure, and the Experimental group's actual performance is in the lower panel (labeled "Experimental Group, Exp. 3"). The simulated predictions were far from the actual performance, thereby challenging a demand characteristics explanation.

These results indicate that loudness information must be available in auditory imaginal representations, because it can be retrieved when the task demands it. This information is not obligatorily retrieved, however, for it does not invariably affect performance.

Indeed, the absence of loudness effects in the reading and generation times indicates that the likelihood of retrieving representations associated with louder sounds is not greater or faster than the likelihood of retrieving representations

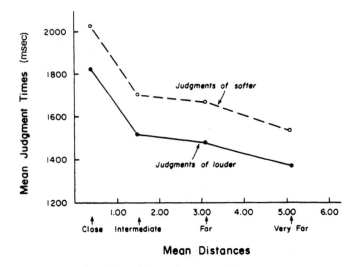

FIG. 3.2.   Times to identify the louder or softer member of an imagined pair of environmental sounds. From Intons-Peterson (1980). Copyright 1980 by the Psychonomic Society. Reprinted by permission.

associated with softer sounds. Once retrieved, the specific loudness cues may be used, as in the matching and comparative judgment tasks.

A serendipitous finding in this work was the common reports that participants reported "seeing" the images in addition to "hearing" them. In fact, for some stimuli, such as "popcorn popping," many participants said that they had to "see" the popcorn popping before they "heard" it! We will explore this cross-modality effect later.

Pitch and Auditory Imagery

In their recent review of the relation between imagery and perception, Finke and Shepard (1986, p. 37–48) concluded that pitch space is an important component of auditory imagery:

> [W]hat is most analogous in the auditory domain to the perception of visual objects in physical space is the perception of auditory objects in pitch space, rather than in literal physical space (see Attneave & Olson, 1971; Kubovy, 1981; Shepard, 1982). Pitch space primarily serves as what has been referred to by Kubovy as the 'indispensable attribute' of tones and by Attneave as the 'morphophoric' or form-bearing 'medium' within which such auditory objects as melodies and chords can be rigidly transformed while preserving their inherent structure. Moreover, there is increasing evidence that the space of auditory pitch is a complex medium containing circular as well as rectilinear components (see . . . Shepard, 1982). As a consequence,

many of the musically most significant transformations, including simple shifts up and down the scale and modulations between keys, correspond to rotations in that space. Indeed, all of the transformational phenomena of mental rotation and apparent movement . . . [of] visual imagery appear to carry over to the auditory domain when we investigate how listeners come to hear successively presented tones, melodies, or chords, as identical despite transpositions in pitch (Shepard, . . . 1982).

Obviously, Finke and Shepard (1986) assumed that pitch is a major component of auditory imagery. Investigations using a variety of imagined and real sounds support this assumption. These sounds include pure tones, relative and absolute pitch of notes in musical phrases, voices, and environmental sounds.

Pure Tones.   Farah and Smith (1983) used pure tones in a two-alternative forced-choice signal detection task. Although their primary focus was on possible facilitation and interference of auditory imagery on auditory perception, Farah and Smith's research also illuminates the role of pitch in auditory imagery. Their subjects imagined pure tones of one of two frequencies (715 or 1000 Hz) while listening for a target signal that was either one or the other of the same two frequencies. The dependent measure was the intensity (loudness) needed for the subject to be able to detect the signal. If pitch of an auditory image is an important component, performance should vary with pitch. But what form would the variation take? Farah and Smith argued that if auditory imagery and perception draw upon similar or even identical processes, the presence of the same pitch in an image might prime or facilitate detection of a target of the same pitch. This should be particularly likely if the image precedes the target. Further, the presence of an image of one pitch might interfere or impede detection of a target of the other pitch. In contrast, if pitch is not an essential and retrievable component of auditory images the pitch of the image should not affect detection of the targets.

The results showed the predicted interaction (see Fig. 3.3). Performance was better when the pitch of the image and the signal were the same (both were either 715 Hz or 1000 Hz) and poorer when the two pitches did not match. Moreover, performance was better when the auditory image preceded and thereby primed the auditory signal than when it was simultaneous with the signal. These results strongly implied the contribution of pitch to auditory images. Further reinforcing this conclusion, when the image preceded the signal, performance was slightly better when both pitches were relatively low (715 Hz) than when both pitches were relatively high (1000 Hz).

Farah and Smith's (1983) results suggest relative facilitation of matching pitches and relative interference of nonmatches, but these terms must be used loosely, because Farah and Smith did not include baseline conditions necessary to evaluate facilitation or interference. Nevertheless, the data tell us that pitch is an important component in representations of auditory images.

AUDITORY IMAGERY

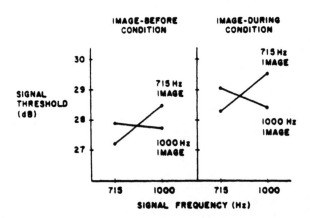

FIG. 3.3. Threshold (in decibels) for detaching signals. Left panel: Image precedes observation intervals. Right panel: Image coincides with observation intervals. From Farah and Smith (1983). Copyright 1983 by the Psychonomic Society. Reprinted by permission.

Farah and Smith manipulated single pure tones, but more complex stimuli deliver the same conclusion. For example, Hubbard and Stoeckig (1988) reported that imaginary tones are generated faster than chords and that images for tones and chords were recognized more often when compared with the same tone or pitch than when compared with different tones or pitches. These results held regardless of whether the different tones/pitches were harmonically or distantly related to the originals. Again, relative pitch of chords as well as individual tones seems to be an important feature of auditory imagery.

The absolute values of pitch did not appear to affect performance, however. Hubbard and Stockard tested the 12 notes of the chromatic scale and the 12 major chords based on the notes. Perhaps the envelope or dynamic series (space) corresponding to the image is critical, not its fundamental frequency.

I turn next to auditory imagery for songs (Halpern, 1989) and brief melodies (Weber & Brown, 1986).

Relative Pitch in Musical Phrases. Weber and Brown (1986) had college students learn 8-note musical phrases either with or without words. The students then imagined or sang aloud the phrases while they drew lines to indicate the height of each pitch relative to the preceding pitch. On half of the trials, the phrases were imagined or sung with words, and on the other half the phrases were imagined or sung as a series of hums or "*bas*," thereby completing a 2 (imagined or sung aloud) × 2 (words or hums used in imaginal or actual singing) design. If auditory imagery resembles auditory memory, performance should be similar when the songs are imagined and when they are sung or hummed.

The data supported this prediction, as the processing times to draw the lines indicating pitch heights were about the same when subjects imagined or sang the songs. It seems, then, that musical imagery for relative pitch is related to musical perception for the same stimuli.

Another issue was whether memory for songs depends more on the melodies, as Weber and Brown hypothesized, or on the words. If melodies are primary, performance should be better when melodies are imagined or hummed than when the words are sung imaginally or out loud. Interestingly, times were shorter when words were used than when they were not. This result, which did not interact with whether the stimuli were imagined or sung aloud, suggests that words (labels, familiarity) aid performance, perhaps because words made the individual tones more distinctive from one another than did humming or the use of ba. We later mention this finding in connection with the role of cognition in auditory imagery.

In a second experiment, Weber and Brown (1986) included a second response measure, using the designation "higher" or "lower" to indicate the relative position of the notes. They argued that the lines used in the first experiment might have suppressed visual imagery for the phrases. A spoken response should permit the subjects to draw on visual imagery if such imagery is a concomitant of auditory imagery or perception. In Experiment 2, students either drew lines or said "higher" or "lower" to indicate the relative pitches. The two experiments were highly similar in other respects. Processing times were longer for spoken than for drawn responses, but no differences for the other major conditions were significant. Thus, compared to a spoken response, the use of a written response does not handicap the subjects.

Finally, Weber and Brown (1986) stated that they found no evidence to indicate that kinesthetic or visual image coding aided performance. They concluded that "kinesthetic and visual image coding is unlikely and that the pitch generation of musical imagery shared resources with a more general auditory image" (p. 411). In brief, the authors interpreted their results as compelling evidence for a common representation underlying perceived and imagined musical memory. Relative pitch is a central component of this representation.

Absolute Pitch in Familiar Songs.   Absolute pitch also may be represented, at least for images of familiar songs typically played in the same key. For example, Halpern (1989) studied retention of absolute pitch for the first note of familiar songs, using college students without "perfect pitch." She used songs that typically were *not* played in the same key (see Halpern, chapter 1, this volume). An absolute value of the pitch was retained amazingly well, even by students without much formal musical training. Auditory images for familiar songs thus appear to contain information about absolute as well as relative pitch. This was true both when the participants were instructed to imagine the tunes and when they were not so instructed. As with Weber and Brown's (1986) research, apparently most people spontaneously imagine songs when asked to make judgments about the songs, even without explicit instructions to do so. Auditory imagery for music appears to be a robust and pervasive phenomenon.

Voices. In addition to pure tones and musical phrases, the pitch of voices varies. Hence, another way to manipulate the pitch of auditory images is to instruct people to imagine stimuli being spoken by a female or male speaker (Geiselman & Bjork, 1980; Geiselman & Glenny, 1977). Using this approach, Geiselman and Glenny had students listen to a tape recording of a female or male voice. They then saw word pairs and were told to imagine hearing words spoken by the female, the male, or their own voice. On a subsequent recognition test, which presented the words spoken by one or the other speaker, the subjects were more likely to recognize words spoken in the same voice during the test as the one they imagined during training than in a different voice. This same result was found in a second experiment when different male and female speakers were used for training and test, although performance was lower than for the first experiment. Once again, pitch of the imagined words aided retention when it matched or approximated the pitch of the tested words. Further, pitch mismatches produced lower performance. Clearly, a major result is the "same-voice-pitch" effect, which documents once more the significant role of pitch contours in auditory imagery. It is possible, however, that timbre, prosody, and related effects vary along with pitch.

The same-voice-pitch effect implies facilitation when the sex of the subject matches the sex of the test voice because, in general, the pitches of speakers of the same sex will be more similar than the pitches of speakers of the other sex. This implication is not supported by the data. In both experiments, performance was the same regardless of whether the sex of the subject matched or did not match the sex of the test voice. Geiselman and Glenny (1977) offered two explanations. The first was that a small number of attributes of an unfamiliar voice may be encoded in parallel with verbal attributes of the stimulus, perhaps all in propositional form. This alternative assumes that attributes of others' voices are encoded as part of a context that may be retrieved at the time of retention. Such an alternative assumes either that one's own voice is not so encoded or that the contexts involving one's own voice are less distinctive than those incorporating others' voices, two unsavory assumptions.

The second possibility is that the values of the attributes affect the meaning of the code. Thus, word pairs would assume slightly different connotations depending on the speaker. Reports of gender differences in language (e.g., Adams & Ware, 1989; Edelsky, 1976) suggest that the two sexes might differ in their interpretations. If so, we would expect to find the "same-voice-pitch" effect with the participant's own voice. Both explanations have difficulty with the absence of such an effect.

A third alternative comes from research by Johnson et al. (1988). Working within the Johnson-Raye (Johnson & Raye, 1981) reality-monitoring model, Johnson et al. predicted that subjects would have more difficulty identifying the origins of memories when the original subjects imagined or actually heard words spoken by another person than when the subjects imagined speaking the words in their own voice. This prediction stems from assumptions of the model that memories based on self-generated processes (e.g., imagery) differ from memories based on perception in their sensory and contextual information and in semantic detail. Words both imagined and heard in another person's voice will carry similar information, making it difficult to distinguish between them. In contrast, words imagined in the subject's own voice will have different cues from words imagined or spoken by another. In this case, the origins will be easily identified. Johnson et al.'s (1988) results supported these predictions.

Now let us consider the implications for the Geiselman-Glenny (1977) results. Suppose that when the targets are imagined in a particular voice, distinctive characteristics of that voice, including pitch, become part of the representation. Then presenting the same cues of voice at the time of retrieval will approach the training conditions and facilitate recall, in a manner proposed by Tulving and Thomson (1973) in their encoding specificity model. Presumably, the degree of match between the training and test situations will determine the extent of facilitation. Thus, when the same voice is used for both training and test, high cue overlap will facilitate retrieval. When the two voices mismatch (female-male or self-other) cue overlap is reduced and retrieval is lower, as Geiselman and Glenny found.

How does this view explain the superior recall of words imagined in one's own voice compared to recall of words imagined by one person during training and uttered by another person of the same sex during test? Both situations represent mismatches, so cue overlap and subsequent retrieval should be less than for matches. According to the Johnson et al. view, self-imagining gains an advantage because kinesthetic and other individualistic cues are added to those standardly elicited by imagining in another's voice. These extra cues are not sufficient to overcome the benefits of matches, but they outweigh those of mismatches produced by imagining in one voice during training and hearing the voice of another person of the same sex on the test.

In summary, the research on imagined voices supports the notion that pitch is a salient component of auditory imagery. But can it be used optionally, as was true for loudness? The research on imagined voices suggests an affirmative answer, but we sought a more definitive one by mimicking the experiments on the role of loudness in auditory imagery.

Environmental Sounds. We recently gathered data about the role of rated pitch of environmental sounds on the generation and use of images of those sounds. We used the same technique as that cited in Intons-Peterson (1980): Lists of environmental sounds were judged for their general pitch (on a scale of 1 = very low to 7 = very high). The times to generate images of these sounds were measured, in addition to the times to match sounds of different pitches and to identify the higher (or lower) pitched sound of a pair. The results are clear: Times to generate images of described sounds are not related to pitch. That is, it took longer to imagine a sound that is usually high-pitched (e.g., shrill whistle) than one that usually is low-pitched in nature (e.g., truck rumbling). However, as with loudness ratings, the further apart in rated pitch, the longer it took to match two imagined sounds in pitch and the shorter time it took to identify the higher or lower of the two described sounds. These results are similar to those for loudness ratings. These data suggest that a fundamental pitch, like loudness, does not necessarily affect auditory imaginal representation. Fundamental pitch seems to be no more obligatory than loudness for images of environmental sounds. An alternative explanation is that subjects rely on subvocalization when the task requires decisions about two images. Although this possibility is plausible in many cases (see discussions in many chapters in this volume), it seems unlikely to have had a pronounced effect on the described research because it is difficult to imitate many of the environmental sounds.

Timbre and Auditory Imagery

Crowder (1989a, 1989b) and his associates have been investigating the role of timbre as an attribute of auditory experience that is particularly close to its sensory correlates and relatively difficult to manipulate cognitively, at least within his paradigm (see chapter 2, this volume). He finds that when the pitches are identical, response times are faster and more accurate when the timbres match than when they differ. When the pitches differ, response times are nonsignificantly slower and less accurate with the same than with different timbres. Thus, differences in timbre impairs the detection of identical pitches. In the second experiment, a sine wave was substituted for the initial sound of each pair. The subjects were instructed to imagine a tone of the same pitch being played by one of the instruments. The second tone was played by an instrument with the same or different pitch in the supposed same or different timbre. Again, detection of identical pitches was impaired by timbre differences.

These results suggest that timbre may be a component of auditory images. Is timbre an essential component? It may be for some individuals, for Crowder found that a few of his subjects seemed to be unable to separate timbre from pitch. They responded as though the two aspects were integrally related. For most of his listeners, the dynamic cues of timbre did not seem to be invariably invoked as part of auditory images. Crowder and Pitt's chapter contains more information.

EVIDENCE FOR PARALLELISM
BETWEEN AUDITORY IMAGERY AND PERCEPTION

The relation between imagery and perception has long intrigued researchers in this area, as I noted at the beginning of this chapter. Many techniques have been used to try to resolve this question. One approach is to ask whether performance is approximately the same for imagery and perception. If the functions appear to be similar and if statistical analysis supports the null hypothesis, common conclusions are, in terms of increasing strength, that the two draw on the same processes, that they share similar processes, or that imagery uses perceptual mechanisms and processes. More precise quantitative comparisons have been made, but these comparisons used visual, not auditory, imagery (e.g., Intons-Peterson, under review; Kerst & Howard, 1978; Moyer, Bradley, Sorenson, Whiting, & Mansfield, 1978; Shepard & Chipman, 1970). Another technique is to use interference or facilitation paradigms to ascertain whether the effects are similar for auditory imagery and auditory perception. Further, theories may point to contrasting patterns of data.

As mentioned earlier, some exceptions notwithstanding, the results for visual imagery suggest that imagery and perception are most likely to be similar when the tasks are highly unusual. They tend to diverge as the tasks more closely approximate real-life activities (Intons-Peterson & McDaniel, 1991; Intons-Peterson & Roskos-Ewoldsen, 1989). Here we explore the evidence from studies of auditory imagery, focusing on the similarity to auditory perception. The first set of studies dealt with musical stimuli, the second set, with within-modality interference, and the third, with between-modality facilitation.

Musical Stimuli

Control groups are a problem for experiments on auditory imagery using musical stimuli, because subjects not instructed to use auditory imagery for these stimuli frequently do so spontaneously, at least when the auditory stimuli are songs or melodies (Halpern, 1988, 1989; Weber & Brown, 1986). Weber and Brown avoided this problem by having their perceptual groups sing or hum aloud melodies learned during the experimental session. As described previously, they found highly similar perceptual and imaginal performance, which led them to conclude that auditory imagery and perception draw on the same processes. This may be true, but there is a potential difficulty in using the above research as a critical test. Weber and Brown used only unfamiliar material. Research with visual imagery and perception (Intons-Peterson & Roskos-Ewoldson, 1989) suggests that this kind of situation would yield imaginal-perceptual parallelism; whereas familiar material might not. Halpern used familiar songs but had no satisfactory perceptual control. Hence, we recently investigated the role of familiarity of the material.

We tested memory for both familiar and unfamiliar song of various lengths, using Weber and Brown's (1986) technique of drawing lines to indicate relative pitches. Unfamiliar songs, counterbalanced through the singing aloud and imaginal singing conditions, contained five, eight, or twelve notes. The unfamiliar songs were taken from a collection of Hungarian folk tunes; the familiar songs were "Row, Row, Row Your Boat," "America," "Twinkle, Twinkle Little Star," "Star Spangled Banner," and "Auld Lang Syne." Half of the college students were assigned to singing the songs while drawing the lines, and half to imaginally singing the songs as they drew the lines. These groups were subdivided so that half began with unfamiliar songs and the other half with familiar songs.

If auditory imagery and perception rely on the same or similar processes, the times to draw the lines should be about the same for the imaginal and perceptual conditions, regardless of the familiarity of the songs. If, however, cognition significantly affects auditory imagery, any imaginal-perceptual performance differential should be accentuated for familiar songs compared to unfamiliar ones. That is what we found: The response times to correctly draw lines for relative pitch were reliably *shorter* when familiar songs were imagined than when they were sung, whereas the response times for unfamiliar songs (which presumably would be less likely to recruit ancillary cognitive cues) were almost identical for imagery and perception. Interestingly, this is a case in which cognition facilitated performance relative to perception. With visual imagery, the opposite usually is the case (Intons-Peterson & McDaniel, 1991).

Of course, the difference might be due to retardation by singing rather than to facilitation by imagining. Singing aloud requires more effort, including greater articulatory muscle involvement, than singing silently or imagining singing, and these greater demands might have slowed performance. To probe these possibilities, we told a new set of participants to imagine singing the familiar songs silently, to imagine singing the songs out loud, to sings the songs out loud from memory, or to sing the songs out loud with the lyrics in front of them. If articulatory movements, imaginal and actual, affect performance, then the second and third groups should be at a disadvantage compared to the first. The last group provided a standard for judging the completeness or accuracy of response in other conditions. All songs were familiar to all of the participants. Further, if musical perception of the songs (singing them aloud) approximates musical imagery for the same songs, the length of time required to "sing" various length songs should be comparable.

In fact, all of the groups singing the songs from memory took shorter times to complete the songs than the standardization group that used lyrics, and this main effect was significant. Most of the differences in singing times came from the relatively fast silent singing of the imaginal group not told about inclusion of articulatory movements. When the imagery group was told to include articulatory movements, the times were almost the same as those of the singing aloud from memory group and both of these approached the times of the standardization group. These results lead me to infer that the imagery instructions used by Halpern and by Weber and Brown probably encouraged inclusion of imaginary articulation. They also suggest to me that auditory imagery for musical phrases (and perhaps other forms of imagery, as well) may optionally encode kinesthetic and related cues (see also the chapters by Logie & Baddeley, Reisberg, Smith, & Wilson, this volume, and the article by Reisberg et al., 1989).

The results from musical stimuli thus suggest that auditory imagery closely parallels auditory perception when the material is unfamiliar. The parallels are substantially reduced when the material is familiar.

We turn next to studies that focused primarily on within-modality interference. The philosophy is that if imagery and perception share limited resources, engaging one will interfere with the other. Such interference would be interpreted as evidence of strong parallelism.

Within-Modality Interference

Segal and her colleagues (Segal & Fusella, 1969; Segal & Gordon, 1969) reasoned that imagery and perception share similar processes. It so, then imagining a visual scene different from a visual target should impede detection of the target compared to a control condition in which the target was detected without any imagery instructions. After obtaining positive results, Segal and Fusella (1970) extended the work to audition. Specifically, they compared detection of simple auditory and visual signals when the subjects simultaneously imagined visual scenes or environmental sounds.

This research was designed to explore two possible explanations for the previous findings. The first is that imagery interferes directly with perception of the signal, because the two processes have some sensory elements in common. The second possibility is that the image distracted the subjects. This notion implicates a central attention factor. Since there is no reason to believe that a visual image is more distracting than an auditory image, Segal and Fusella argued that visual and auditory images should block auditory and visual signals equally if the central attention factor is responsible. Note that if the two types of images produce differential blocking, the perception-imagery parallelism hypothesis would be supported over the central attention hypothesis.

Segal and Fusella (1970) began by testing the subjects' ability to detect the visual or the auditory signal against background noise in the absence of an imagery task. Thus, these results afford a standard against which possible facilitation or interference of the imagery condition can be evaluated. Then the subjects imagined images of common visual events or of common auditory events while they were engaged in either a visual or an auditory detection task. Different signals were used in two experiments. In the first experiment, the auditory signal was a harmonica chord (played on a tape loop), and the visual signal was a back-projected small blue arrow. In the second experiment, the auditory signal was a 250-cps pure tone, and the visual signal, a triangle composed of three parallel green lines of unequal length.

Imaging interfered with detection, in general, giving some support to the central attention hypothesis. More impressive, however, was the differential interference. Blocking was greater when the image and signal were in the same modality than when they were in different modalities. Thus, auditory signals were harder to detect when the subjects were simultaneously imagining an auditory event than when they were imagining a visual event (or when they were not imagining anything). The related result held for visual imagery and visual signals. Because the effects of differential blocking were much stronger than the generalized diminution from any imagery, Segal and Fusella concluded that their results supported the parallelism hypothesis.

This reasonable conclusion was further bolstered by Farah and Smith's (1983) finding of significant *facilitation* when the pitch of an auditory image matched that of a target auditory signal compared to mismatched image-signal pitches. In this case, the image and signal would be expected to recruit more similar sensory cues when the two matched than when they mismatched, so that the image would be an effective prime for the signal. As previously mentioned, their design offered evidence of relative, but not of absolute, facilitation and interference.

Crowder (1989a, 1989b) also found facilitation of the identification of identical pitches when the timbre of two sounds was perceptually identical and when it was imaginally identical. He noted a nonsignificant tendency toward interference in the same-different pitch discrimination task when the pitches had different timbres. This was true for actual or imagined sounds made by regular musical instruments (1989a) and for sounds whose spectral timbres were artificially manipulated, but only for subjects who were able to separate timbre from pitch. No such effect was found for individuals who were unable to ignore spectral timbre for participants in. another experiment that manipulated dynamic aspects of timbre. Crowder himself has doubts that the investigation of the role of dynamic aspects of timbre was sufficiently sensitive to warrant conclusions. He reports additional experiments in chapter 2.

In our experiment on the imaginal singing of familiar songs, the condition described earlier corresponded to the single-task situation in which the four groups sang the songs silently or aloud. In addition, a second task was imposed on the first to assess the potential interference of auditory images or of perceived songs on the imaginal or actual singing of other songs.

Again, we expected that occupying the auditory channel with two different messages would produce interference compared to a single task control. Moreover, the parallel imagery–perception hypothesis suggests that the extent of interference should be about the same for imagery and perception. These expectations were tested by having dual-task subjects imagine or listen to a concerto played either loudly or softly while imagining or singing different familiar songs. Thus, the dual-task subjects imagined singing or silently sang all of the songs (in an order balanced across the conditions) while listening to the concerto played softly, while listening to it played loudly, and while imagining it played softly and then loudly. The single task students either imagined singing or sang each of the five songs in a quiet setting. All of the orders were balanced across all of the groups and conditions. The subjects were acquainted with the intensity of the concerto played softly (mean = 58dB, range = 53dB - 64dB) or loudly (mean = 67dB, range = 61dB - 76dB) by listening to the two settings and imagining them before the experiment began.

As expected, the dual task of imagining the concerto played loudly or softly slowed the imagined or actual singing of the songs compared to the single task conditions of only imagining or singing the songs. To our surprise, however, actually hearing the concerto played loudly or softly speeded the times to imagine or sing the songs. These results were found for both primary tasks, imagining and singing the songs, an outcome that supports the hypothesis of auditory imaginal-perceptual parallelism.

Overall, then, with our within-modality tasks, we found significant interference from the process of imagining a second task but facilitation from actually hearing it.

How can these results be explained? The interference from a second task involving the same modality was predicted, of course, due to capacity limitations, but the facilitation from actually hearing the concerto was not predicted. Three possible explanations come quickly to mind. The first is that imagining the concerto requires more capacity than hearing the concerto or performing in silence. This explanation also implies that hearing the concerto requires *less* capacity than performing in quiet. This seems unlikely. The second possibility is that hearing the concerto produces a kind of priming. This alternative also is unlikely, because the concerto differed from any of the songs. Moreover, Rubin (1977, Experiment 4) found that subjects had difficulty writing the words of a familiar song while listening to the same song played at a tempo that exceeded the speed of writing because they could not keep up with the music. They also had trouble, and recalled fewer words, when a different song or no song was played. These considerations reinforce the expectation of interference, not facilitation.

A third possibility is that hearing the concerto does produce interference. The subjects handle the interference by abbreviating the primary task or by making it more elliptical. The result would be an apparent speeding of the primary task. Fortunately, we taped all productions of students singing aloud, thinking that they might adjust their tempi as a function of the interfering task. No such adjustment appeared. Instead, when the concerto was heard, the subjects dropped parts of the songs, particularly in the middle sections. In other words, the actual singing groups took shorter times to sing the songs because they abbreviated the songs, not because they speeded their singing. The imagined concerto groups might also have short-circuited their renditions, but their production times contradict such a contention.

The results discussed in this section suggest that auditory imagery and auditory perception are similar. This conclusion stems from research on musical memory and within-modality interference. Segal and Fusella (1970) also found some evidence for between-modality interference, for imagining either a visual or auditory event suppressed detection of visual and auditory signals compared to a control situation. Further, identifying the pitch relative to its predecessor suffers when the response is spoken compared to when it is written, an outcome Weber and Brown (1986) attributed to greater competition for processing capacity between auditory imagery for musical phrases and speaking (a verbal response mode) than for writing. I am not convinced by this argument, but it is clear that some forms of response to imaginal stimuli take more time than others. The data reviewed do not permit us to assume that auditory imagery actually shares the pathways and processes of auditory perception.

Imaginal-perceptual parallelism should not be restricted to interference, however. It seems plausible that facilitation would occur if an image or percept primed a subsequent event. We turn now to this possibility.

Between-Modality Facilitation

Between-modality imaginal facilitation may be obtained under special circumstances (Intons-Peterson, 1980). These special circumstances occur when an object elicits images in more than one modality. As mentioned previously, our subjects reported that when asked to generate an auditory image of a commonly experienced event they also generated a visual one. This was a pronounced effect, for visual images were spontaneously generated to 95% of the phrases. Sometimes the visual image preceded the auditory one, as with "popcorn popping," and the participants noted that they had to "see" the popcorn popping before they could "hear" it. The visual-image-before-auditory-image order was far more compelling than the reverse order: When given the task of generating *visual* images, another group indicated that they also produced auditory images 53% of the time. Thus, visual and auditory imagery clearly are related, perhaps even interdependent, with visual imagery having moderate primacy over auditory imagery.

The research discussed above used intentional tasks. The final work to consider in this section is Schacter and Graf's work (1989, Experiment 4) on the implicit memory task of stem completion. At issue is whether imagining a visual representation of the letters of two words in a pair prior to visual or auditory presentation of the word pair will facilitate word completion of the target word compared to baseline performance. It does. In fact, the difference in word completion between when the other word of the pair was or was not present was greater for the pairs presented auditorily than for the pairs presented visually. In this case, then, visually imagining pairs before their auditory presentation facilitated performance on an unexpected word completion task. Apparently, the similarity of the message is even more important than the modality of presentation.

Taken together, the explorations of the relations between auditory imagery and perception suggest that presentation of different imaginal and perceptual messages in the same modality produces interference. When an event elicits images in both visual and auditory imagery one image may prime the other, producing facilitation. These results implicate the auditory system in auditory imagery.

EVIDENCE FOR DIVERGENCES BETWEEN AUDITORY IMAGERY AND PERCEPTION: THE ROLE OF COGNITION

Although not fashionable, the question of the role of cognition (general world knowledge, expectations, etc.) in imagery needs to be raised. This question has been assiduously avoided by imagery researchers, perhaps because they wished to avoid the charges of using imparsimonious, fuzzy-minded "picture-in-the-head" models (or the auditory equivalent), leveled by Anderson (1978) and Pylyshyn (1981) against analog-type imagery models.

I consider this avoidance to be ill-founded, if for no other reason than that we rely on cognition, in the form of verbal instructions, every time we conduct an imagery experiment. It seems to me to be important to know how such instructions affect the subject's interpretation of the task. It also is important to determine how the participant's world knowledge influences their imaginal performance. These questions motivate this section of the chapter. In brief, I suspect that most images are "cognitively penetrable," to use Pylyshyn's term.

Whenever knowledge is retrieved to guide image construction, this knowledge may affect imagery by altering the meaning imputed to the task (Geiselman & Glenny, 1977). For example, stereotypic information about women and men may cause a word pair imagined in a female voice to be interpreted differently from the same pair imagined in a male voice. Further, the initial representation may differ because the subject perceives one voice to be that of a female and the other, of a male. These explanations imply that the representation of an auditory image will reflect the subject's cognitive interpretation of the image and what it signifies, in addition to perceptual aspects.

Although they called the issue "tonal primacy," Weber and Brown's (1986) work is relevant to this issue. These investigators compared the identification of relative pitch for songs with or without words. They defined *tonal primacy* as the "priority of tonal coding over verbal or word coding in musical phrases" (p. 411). In other words, they hypothesized that perceptual aspects (pitch coding) were more important than linguistic aspects (words for the songs). Pitch coding was somewhat faster for songs with words than for the same melodies without words. Thus, they found no support for tonal primacy.

This outcome may be interpreted differently: Cognition, as manifested here by the linguistic structure of the words, may play an important role in auditory imagery, at least in the identification of relative pitch.

Moreover, Halpern (1988) found that the time to determine whether a second word belonged in a familiar song after the first word had been given increased as a function of the separation of the two words in the song's lyrics. Each of the well-known songs had up to 13 distinctive beats. Each song had unique words in its phrase. After reading the name of the to-be-tested song on a monitor, subjects saw a word (lyric) from the song, followed 750 msec later by a second word. The college students pressed one button if the second word was in the song and another button if it was not. Imagery subjects were told to mentally play the songs in their heads until they arrived at the second word. A nonimagery control group was told to focus on the first word and, when the second word appeared, to indicate whether or not the word belonged in the song by pressing the appropriate button. Post-experimental inquiries and a subsequent experiment indicated that many of the supposed nonimagery control subjects actually used imagery; hence, the distinction between the groups will not be considered further.

In general, the farther apart the words in the real songs, the longer the subjects took to respond. This result was most pronounced when the initial word was not at the beginning of the song. Taken together, these data suggest not only that subjects use auditory imagery to respond to the task but also that they had to begin at the beginning of the song and "play it forward" to be able to respond—a cognitive memory function.

A second experiment separated the time to generate a representation of the first word (RT1) from comparing the first and second word (RT2). Even when RT1 was removed, the time to respond still increased with the distance between the two words and with the position of the first word. Apparently, even when the subjects had "arrived" at the first word, they still often had to return to the beginning. These results reinforce the dependence of imaginal performance on a cognitive-type scanning.

In a different approach, Nairne and Pusen (1984) explored the possibility that imagining digits in an experimenter's voice could produce the modality or suffix effects typically shown by actually hearing the items. It did not, implying that imagining the auditory production of items did not yield the same effect as actually hearing them.

Similarly, Segal and Fusella (1970) manipulated the familiarity of the visual and auditory images imposed on the signal detection task. Detection of the signals was impeded more by unfamiliar songs (e.g., seeing an elephant, hearing an oboe) than by familiar images (e.g., seeing a table, hearing a dog barking.) Presumably, images of unfamiliar objects are less distinct than images of familiar objects, and are more likely to be confused with the target stimuli. An alternative explanation is that it is harder to generate images of unfamiliar than of familiar objects, and the added difficulty of generating unfamiliar objects detracted from the attention allocated to target detection.

Regardless of the explanation, the outcome is clear: Cognitive factors may affect auditory imagery, just as they affect visual imagery (Intons-Peterson, under review; Intons-Peterson & McDaniel, 1991; Intons-Peterson & Roskos-Ewoldsen, 1989). Phrased differently, Neisser's (1972) observation that, "If memory and perception are the two key branches of cognitive psychology, the study of imagery stands precisely at their intersection" (p. 233) conveys the same message.

MODELS OF AUDITORY IMAGERY

This section could be as short as this sentence, for I have not been able to find a single model of auditory imagery, per se (save Hebb's 1966, 1968 early view, which was a general model of imagery). All other models of auditory imagery reviewed in the previous sections have been derived from models of visual imagery. To be more precise, the investigators have assumed that auditory imagery will be related to audition in the same way that visual imagery is to vision.

Consequently, I will review some of the major models of visual imagery, noting how they might apply to the auditory case, and then propose another model. It, too, is a general model of imagery.

Four current approaches have been labeled the Functional, Structural, Interactive (Finke, 1985; Intons-Peterson & McDaniel, 1991), and knowledge-weighted (Intons-Peterson & Roskos-Ewoldson, 1989) models. All four assume that imagery is related to perception, but the extent of the correspondence differs for the various models.

Functional Models

Models representing a functional view (e.g., Shepard, 1975) posit that imagery is functionally related to perception. Thus, images preserve general relations among perceptual components. They do not necessarily correspond in a one-to-one manner with each perceptual detail (or what might be called a "first-order isomorphism"). Instead, Shepard suggests that the relations are maintained in central events involved in both the perception and the image of an object (or what he has called a "second-order isomorphism"). Clearly, this model could accommodate auditory imagery. The notion would be that representations of auditory images bear a *general* relation to actual perception of the auditory event. The apparent dependence of auditory images on pitch is consistent with this model, of course, although the apparent optional coding of loudness and kinesthesis (at least for musical imagery) is troublesome.

Structural Models

Structural approaches adopt a stronger stand with respect to the relation between imagery and perception, holding that there is first-order isomorphism, to at least some extent. For example, Kosslyn's (1981) model hypothesizes some exact correspondences between the structural and surface features of perception and images. Memory for information to be imagined is retrieved from long-term memory into a spatial medium Kosslyn calls a "visual buffer." Presumably, the same type of structural relations could apply to the auditory case. If so, the model also would predict that the image affords access to surface properties such as timbre, as well as to structural features such as frequency and intensity. Once again, the seeming optionality of some attributes appears to be at odds with this model, although the data on pitch are consistent.

Interactive Models

The interactive approaches (Farah, 1985; Farah & Smith, 1983; Segal & Fusella, 1970; Weber & Brown, 1986) made even stronger claims about the parallelism between imagery and perception. The views postulated that the two processes are very similar, perhaps even using the same pathways. Further, as proposed by Hebb (1966, 1968), this imaginal-perceptual parallelism may arise primarily when coded at higher levels of the nervous system (see also Finke, 1985). The findings of comparable imaginal and perceptual performance bolster these views, as do the findings of greater within- than between-modality interference. More difficult to incorporate are the occasional divergences of imaginal and perceptual performance which seem to occur with familiar objects and the apparent optional features.

Knowledge-Weighted Model

The appearance of similarities with unfamiliar tasks and of discrepancies with familiar ones led Beverly Roskos-Ewoldsen and me (1989) to propose that images have a canonical form, a set of features essential to define the image. The activation of these features in long-term memory may simultaneously activate other, associated (ancillary) features. Obviously, the likelihood of activating ancillary features is greater for familiar than for unfamiliar objects. If activated, these ancillary features are effectively part of the image with respect to processing. These ancillary, as well as the canonical features, are available as part of the imaginal representation and may, but are not necessarily, accessed at the time of retrieval. Note that this model, which we called a "knowledge-weighted" model of imagery, can explain the loudness and kinesthesis results. It postulates that these attributes, like pitch, may be encoded, but that this information will be accessed during retrieval only if needed for the task. To date, our preliminary tests with auditory imagery are promising. More impressive, at this stage, is evidence that the model works well for various kinds of visual and haptic imagery, including imaginary carrying of weights, color and numerosity comparisons (Intons-Peterson & Roskos-Ewoldsen, 1989). This model shares some attributes with the Kosslyn-Shwartz (1977) model, although the knowledge-weighted view relies more heavily on the features initially retrieved from memory and less on subsequent memory searches than does the Kosslyn-Shwartz model.

General Systems Model

Finally, I mention briefly an even more general model (Intons-Peterson, under review). It proposes that the processes contributing to imagery may overlap with, or even be the same as, processes contributing to perception and to cognition. That is, imagery, perception, and cognition may not be defined distinctively, separately, and uniquely, but, rather, may recruit the similar processes to different extents, depending on the circumstances. Thus, certain imaginal tasks may require perceptual-like distinctions, whereas others demand more cognitive approaches. The processes induced imaginally will reflect these demands. This view resembles Neisser's (1972) approach.

This dynamic systems model was applied successfully to categorization based primarily on perceptual, on imaginal, and on cognitive (numeric) strategies. These strategies were fostered by having subjects learn to assign 2-line exemplars to one of two 4-line "parent" patterns (prototypes) shown in Fig. 3.4.

The two parent patterns were derived from the rectangle shown on the left in Fig. 3.4. Exemplars were constructed by sampling, randomly, two of the four lines from each parent pattern. Participants learned to classify the examplars as an instance of one of the two patterns, using one of three approaches. The imagery group first learned the number-line associations of the original rectangle. During the training, this group heard two numbers. Their task was to imagine the lines

FIG. 3.4. Rumelhart-Siple rectangle used to define the training and test items (left panel) and the two parent patterns (middle and right panels).

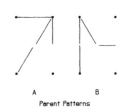

corresponding to the numbers and to then classify their image. The verbal strategy group heard the numbers only. The use of imagery or perception should have been minimized for the verbal strategy group because they never saw the original rectangle. The perception group had no training trials. Instead, to assess the ability of this group to perceive similarities between the test items and the two parent prototypes, pictures of the prototypes were present during all of the test trials. The pictures were not present during the test trials for the other groups.

The role of the three modes of learning, imagery, verbal strategy, and perception, was assessed by the test trials. When the test items contained only the lines or numbers used during training, all of the groups tended to assign the test items to the pattern with which they overlapped. When the test items introduced lines or numbers never shown during training or when they were reversals of the parent prototypes, the perceptual group responded on the basis of overall global similarity to the parent patterns, whereas the imagery and verbal strategy group continued to rely on overlapping features.

Do these results mean that imagery and the cognitive verbal strategy approach always stress specific rather than global features, and perception delivers the global? Clearly not; for when we changed the initial training to emphasize global aspects for the imaginal and verbal strategy groups and to emphasize specific features for the perceptual groups, we found reversed performance. These results display the versatility of imagery and its ability to mimic both perceptual and cognitive processes. They imply that the demands of the task may drive the kind of processing (imaginal, perceptual, cognitive) accorded. These results also illuminate the seeming paradox of similarities and differences between imagery and perception, for the characteristics of the task may determine the kind of processing, and ultimately, the outcomes.

CONCLUSIONS AND CHALLENGES

One striking observation is the diversity of tasks used to measure auditory imagery. The tasks range from detection or comparisons of pure tones to musical imagery for familiar songs. It would be easy to bemoan the absence of any kind of auditory imagery "scale" or standard of measurement, but to do so would be to ignore the richness of the paradigms tested. Although the diversity of tasks— and of results—is a challenge, it also offers the promise of a multifaceted understanding of auditory imagery. It would be particularly impressive if virtually all of the approaches conformed to some general model.

A major concern in all cases is whether subjects actually use auditory imagery. This seems to be more important with unusual auditory imagery tasks than with familiar musical phrases. Familiar musical phrases appear to spontaneously elicit auditory imagery. Most of the experiments reviewed in this chapter contained controls designed to circumvent problems of subject and experimenter-demand characteristics. Thus, the results probably reflect the operation of auditory imagery.

The evidence seems to proclaim that auditory images contain information about pitch. They also may contain information about loudness, timbre, and other ancillary features (e.g., kinesthesis) more often associated with familiar auditory objects than with unfamiliar ones. Loudness and other ancillary features affect auditory imagery when required by the task. The interference studies suggest that auditory images may invoke some of the same processes as perception. There also is evidence for a general interference effect from the imposition of a dual task. Further bolstering the parallelism between auditory imagery and perception is the occasional report of facilitation when the messages conveyed by the image and the percept coincide. Imagery reflects cognitive influences, as well, for Segal and Fusella (1970) found that the detection of signals was differentially sensitive to images of familiar versus unfamiliar objects. Similar results have been reported for visual images.

No model of auditory imagery exists. Instead, researchers have borrowed heavily from the visual imagery literature. Most of these models focus on the dependence of images on perception and are, therefore, not well equipped to handle evidence of the role of cognition on images. Two fairly recent models are designed to include imagery, perception, and cognition. Both of them are based on work with visual imagery, but can be applied to auditory imagery with ease.

Perhaps the biggest challenge is generating and testing models of both visual and auditory imagery. Such models presumably could be extended to other forms of imagery. We need principled research designed to ascertain the role of same- and cross modal effects in the two kinds of imagery, to examine specific predictions from models, and to identify the conditions under which auditory—and other—imageries are or are not dependent upon perception and cognition.

ACKNOWLEDGMENTS

I want to thank Robert Crowder, Andrea Halpern, Daniel Reisberg, Wendi Russell, and Robert J. Weber for reading and commenting on the chapter.

REFERENCES

Adams, K. L., & Ware, N. C. (1989). Sexism and the English language: The linguistic implications of being a woman. In J. Freeman (Ed.), *Women* (pp. 470–484). Mountain View, CA: Mayfield.

Anderson, J. R. (1978). Arguments concerning representation for mental imagery. *Psychological Review, 85,* 249–277.

Attneave, F., & Olson, R. K. (1971). Pitch as a medium: A new approach to psychophysical scaling. *American Journal of Psychology, 84,* 147–166.

Baird, J. C., Wagner, M., & Noma, E. (1982). Impossible cognitive spaces. *Geographic Analysis, 14*, 204–216.

Chambers, D., & Reisberg, D. (1985). Can mental images be ambiguous? *Journal of Experimental Psychology: Human Perception and Performance, 11*, 317–328.

Crowder, R. G. (1989a). Imagery for musical timbre. *Journal of Experimental Psychology: Human Perception and Performance, 15*, 472–478.

Crowder, R. G. (1989b, April). *Imagery for musical timbre.* Paper presented at the Conference on Perception of Structure, New Haven, Connecticut.

Edelsky, C. (1976). Subjective reactions to sex-linked language. *Journal of Social Psychology, 99*, 97–104.

Evans, G. W., & Pezdek, K. (1980). Cognitive mapping: Knowledge of real-world distance and location information. *Journal of Experimental Psychology: Human Learning and Memory, 6*, 13–24.

Farah, M. J. (1985). Psychophysical evidence for a shared representation medium for mental images and percepts. *Journal of Experimental Psychology: General, 114*, 91–103.

Farah, M. J., & Smith, A. F. (1983). Perceptual interference and facilitation with auditory imagery. *Perception & Psychophysics, 33*, 475–478.

Finke, R. A. (1985). Theories relating mental imagery to perception. *Psychological Review, 98*, 236–359.

Finke, R. A., & Shepard, R. N. (1986). Visual functions of mental imagery. In K. R. Boff, L. Kaufman, & J. P. Thomas (Eds.), *Handbook of perception and human performance*, Vol. 2 (Chapter 37, pp. 1–55). New York: Wiley-Interscience.

Geiselman, R. E., & Bjork, R. A. (1980). Primary versus secondary rehearsal in imagined voices: Differential effects on recognition. *Cognitive Psychology, 12*, 188–205.

Geiselman, R. E., & Glenny, J. (1977). Effects of imagining speakers' voices on the retention of words presented visually. *Memory & Cognition, 5*, 499–504.

Giraudo, M. D., & Peruch, P. (1988, September). *Distortions in the mental image of urban space.* Paper presented at the Second Workshop on Imagery and Cognition, Padova, Italy.

Halpern, A. R. (1988). Mental scanning in auditory imagery for songs. *Journal of Experimental Psychology: Learning, Memory, and Cognition, 14*, 434–443.

Halpern, A. R. (1989). Memory for the absolute pitch of familiar songs. *Memory & Cognition, 17*, 572–581.

Hebb, D. O. (1966). *A textbook of psychology*, (2nd ed.). Philadelphia: W. B. Saunders.

Hebb, D. O. (1968). Concerning imagery. *Psychological Review, 75*, 466–477.

Hubbard, T. L., & Stoeckig, K. (1988). Musical imagery: Generation of tones and chords. *Journal of Experimental Psychology: Learning, Memory, and Cognition, 14*, 656–667.

Intons-Peterson, M. J. (1980). The role of loudness in auditory imagery. *Memory & Cognition, 8*, 385–393.

Intons-Peterson, M. J., & McDaniel, M. A. (1991). Symmetries and asymmetries between imagery and perception. In C. Cornoldi & M. A. McDaniel (Eds.), *Imagery and Cognition* (pp. 47–76). New York: Springer-Verlag.

Intons-Peterson, M. J. Submitted. Imaginal classification.

Intons-Peterson, M. J., & McDaniel, M. A. (in press). Symmetries and asymmetries between imagery and perception. In C. Cornoldi & M. A. McDaniel (Eds.), *Imagery and Cognition.* New York: Springer-Verlag.

Intons-Peterson, M. J., & Roskos-Ewoldsen, B. B. (1989). Sensory-perceptual qualities of images. *Journal of Experimental Psychology: Learning, Memory, and Cognition, 15*, 188–199.

Intons-Peterson, M. J., & White, A. R. (1981). Experimenter naiveté and imaginal judgments. *Journal of Experimental Psychology: Human Perception and Performance, 7*, 833–843.

Johnson, M. K., Foley, M. A., & Leach, K. (1988). The consequences for memory of imagining in another person's voice. *Memory & Cognition, 16*, 337–342.

Johnson, M. K., & Raye, C. L. (1981). Reality monitoring. *Psychological Review, 88,* 67–85.

Kerst, S. M., & Howard, J. H. (1978). Memory psychophysics for visual area and length. *Memory & Cognition, 6,* 327–335.

Kosslyn, S. M. (1981). The medium and the message in mental imagery: A theory. *Psychological Review, 88,* 46–66.

Kosslyn, S. M., & Shwartz, S. P. (1977). A simulation of visual imagery. *Cognitive Science, 1,* 265–295.

Kubovy, M. (1981). Concurrent pitch-segregation and the theory of indispensable attributes. In M. Kubovy & J. R. Pomerantz (Eds.), *Perceptual organization,* (pp. 55–98). Hillsdale, NJ: Lawrence Erlbaum Associates.

Maki, R. H. (1981). Categorization and distance effects with spatial linear orders. *Journal of Experimental Psychology: Human Learning and Memory, 7,* 15–32.

Moar, I., & Bower, G. H. (1983). Inconsistency in spatial knowledge. *Memory & Cognition, 11,* 107–133.

Moyer, R. S., Bradley, D. R., Sorensen, M. H., Whiting, J. C., & Mansfield, D. P. (1978). Psychophysical functions for perceived and remembered size. *Science, 200,* 330–332.

Nairne, J. S., & Pusen, C. (1984). Serial recall of imagined voices. *Journal of Verbal Learning and Verbal Behavior, 23,* 331–342.

Neisser, U. (1972). Changing conceptions of imagery. In P. W. Sheehan (Ed.), *The function and nature of imagery* (pp. 233–251). New York: Academic Press.

Pylyshyn, Z. W. (1981). The imagery debate: Analogue media versus tacit knowledge. *Psychological Review, 88,* 16–45.

Reisberg, D., Chambers, D. (1991). Neither pictures nor propositions: What can we learn from a mental image? *Canadian Journal of Psychology.*

Reisberg, D., Smith, J. D., Baxter, D. A., & Sonenshine, M. (1989). "Enacted" auditory images are ambiguous; "Pure" auditory images are not. *Quarterly Journal of Experimental Psychology, 41A,* 619–641.

Rubin, D. C. (1977). Very long-term memory prose and verse. *Journal of Verbal Learning and Verbal Behavior, 16,* 611–621.

Schacter, D. L., & Graf, P. (1989). Modality specificity of implicit memory for new associations. *Journal of Experimental Psychology: Learning, Memory, and Cognition, 15,* 3–12.

Segal, S. J., & Fusella, V. (1970). Influence of imaged pictures and sounds on detection of visual and auditory signals. *Journal of Experimental Psychology, 83,* 458–464.

Segal, S. J., & Fusella, V. (1969). Effects of imaging and modes of stimulus onset on signal-to-noise ratio. *British Journal of Psychology, 60,* 458–464.

Segal, S. J., & Gordon, P. E. (1969). The Perky effect revisited: The influence of body position on judgments of imagery. *Perceptual and Motor Skills, 28,* 791–797.

Shepard, R. N. (1975). Form, formation, and transformation of internal representations. In R. Solso (Ed.), *Information processing and cognition: The Loyola Symposium,* (pp. 87–122). Hillsdale, NJ: Lawrence Erlbaum Associates.

Shepard, R. N. (1982). Geometric approximations to the structure of musical pitch. *Psychological Review, 89,* 305–333.

Shepard, R. N., & Chipman, S. (1970). Second-order isomorphism of internal representations: Shapes of states. *Cognitive psychology, 1,* 1–17.

Stevens, A., & Coupe, P. (1978). Distortions in judged spatial relations. *Cognitive Psychology, 10,* 422–437.

Tulving, E., & Thomson, D. M. (1973). Encoding specificity and retrieval processes in episodic memory. *Psychological Review, 80,* 352–373.

Tversky, B. (1981). Distortions in memory for maps. *Cognitive Psychology, 13,* 407–433.

Weber, R. J., & Brown, S. (1986). Musical imagery. *Music Perception, 3,* 411–426.

4 Speech in the Head? Rhyme Skill, Reading, and Immediate Memory in the Deaf

Ruth Campbell
Goldsmiths' College, University of London

Do people born deaf have inner speech? That is, can there be auditory (verbal) imagery without the experience of hearing speech? In answering this question we may cast light on the historically vexatious business of how language should be taught to those born with no useful hearing and also on the relative reliance of cognitive processes in normal hearing individuals on inner speech. It is this latter aspect that originally interested me and which is still the real focus of this chapter; the initiative for exploring this issue came not from experience with the deaf but with a normal university undergraduate (of whom more later). The importance to the deaf in this context is in shedding a different light on the nature of the development of inner speech.

One reason for my preoccupation with this subject is that a particular set of cognitive skills has been identified in hearing individuals that seem to be tightly linked both in development and in adult functioning and which are based on inner speech. The deaf do not, on the whole, master these skills, despite good intelligence and application. Since they cannot pick up acoustic information, the sense data for driving internal representations of speech are lacking and it would not be surprising if this led to a failure to develop inner speech. Not surprising, but, nevertheless, not proven. One aim of this chapter is to examine the extent to which congenital profound hearing loss (usually defined as a loss in the better ear of at least 85 dB) prevents the development of inner auditory-verbal processes, to examine to what extent it delays these processes, and to ask whether the deaf have a different sort of inner speech than hearing people have and whether alternatives to inner speech can be established. This does not aim to be a comprehensive review of the literature on deafness and cognitive processes; some current work is discussed (much of it using European sources), but a good deal is left uncited for the sake of brevity. In particular, this chapter, as I have already stated, is "phonocentrist"; it examines the deaf with reference to those processes used by hearing people. Therefore Sign as a communication system and a cognitive medium will be hardly discussed at all. The interested reader should consult Rodda and Grove (1987) for a dispassionate comparative account of research on the acquisition of cognitive skills as they relate to the language medium of the deaf. Detailed psycholinguistic studies of Sign (ASL) can be found in Klima and Bellugi (1979) or Siple (1978). Kyle and Woll (1988) describe recent studies in British Sign Language (BSL).

Lipreading and Inner Speech

Firstly, though, is it the case that speech cannot be "heard" without an acoustic input? Lipreading is, at best, a poor source of phonetic input; most phonemes are underspecified by vision alone, for their *place* of articulation cannot be discriminated if it is not at the front of the mouth, and *manner* of articulation is usually invisible. Nevertheless, lipreading can carry some phonetically relevant information clearly; several labiodental and labial speech sounds (b, th, v, m) are readily identified (or discriminated by sight from speech sounds of similar acoustic specification: viz /m/ and /n/); and the canonical vowels (/u:/, /i:/, /a:/) are as visibly distinctive as they are auditorily distinctive. Most people can identify pictures of some speech sounds without difficulty and, when context is constrained ("I am going to say a number between one and ten. . . three"), are 'good lipreaders.' When hearing is lost, it is not the case that phonetic discriminations are lost across the board. Silent lipreading specifically impairs certain discriminations while it may leave others intact. For someone born deaf, though, is lipreading more likely to confuse than clarify communication? Perhaps not: deaf people communicate face-to-face; sign languages use concurrent mouth movements; moreover, in the deaf as in hearing people, lipreading *is* speech reading. Lip-movements are interpreted as linguistic and communicative and not, for example, as breathing movements or as muscular tics.

However, perceiving is not the same thing as remembering; perhaps lipreading does not behave like hearing once the sensory input from the seen face has registered? Until recently it was widely believed that auditory speech leaves a useful "echo," an auditory image, that can provide a transient first stage in speech processing. By contrast, written words do not leave such a trace. Does lipreading leave a trace like a heard word or does it behave more like a printed word when recalled? There is no doubt that it leaves a trace (Campbell & Dodd, 1980) and that the trace looks the same in born-deaf as in hearing individuals (Dodd, Hobson, Brasher, & Campbell, 1983). The trace left by lipreading is specifically affected by heard, lipread (and possibly mouthed) speech, rather than by written material (see Campbell, 1987). Lipread material is processed as if it has been heard rather than read.

Thus, people—deaf and hearing—know that when mouths move speech is produced. While lipreading clearly cannot deliver all speech segmental information, it has pockets of usefulness; it helps in discriminating some speech sounds. For example, blind infants take longer to master the visible but hard to hear distinction between /m/ and /n/ in the development of their own speech (see Mills, 1987). Lipreading uses the same channels of processing as hearing for immediate memory. I do not claim that face-to-face language learning using lipreading alone (the Oral method) is a good way to induce the profoundly deaf child into language. The comparative evidence suggests it is not, and that for deaf people with absolutely no residual hearing, learning to lipread is difficult and frustrating (see Rodda & Grove, 1987) as well as "unnatural" (see Kyle & Woll, 1988).

The Three Rs: "Reading," "Rhyming," and "Remembering"

Most, it not all, language tasks typically show deaf school leavers aged 16 to 18 years at the level of 8- to 9-year-old hearing youngsters. In reading and spelling, in immediate recall and in metalinguistic tasks involving the segmentation and manipulation of parts of words, the deaf are usually poor. I highlight these skills here because, unlike syntactic, lexical and discourse-processing skills, which also tend to be poor in many deaf people, it is Reading, Rhyming (that is the ability to manipulate the speech segments of one's native language) and Remembering verbal lists that have been shown to be highly interrelated in normal hearers and where inner speech has been indicated as an intervening variable to capture the close correlations observed.

However, it is important to specify exactly what these three Rs mean in order to be sure of making sense of data and theories. *Reading* here will refer to the mastery of an alphabetic script. The acid test for skill in using such a script appropriately is in the reading and spelling of new and nonwords. This requires the correct identification and mapping of speech sounds to letters. It is such alphabetic reading skill that links with the ability to perform tasks reflecting phonological awareness such as phoneme counting ("Tap out the number of sounds in. . . . cat," Liberman, 1973), making spoonerisms ("Turn the first sound around in the following name. . . Pete Atkins", Perin, 1983) or phoneme deletion ("If I say fala, my friend says ala; if I say fooloo, what would my friend say?" Morais et al., 1979, 1986). It is this skill, the ability to manipulate sub-word-sized segments of ones native language, that I shall label *Rhyme* for the purposes of exposition in this chapter. In fact, the ability to detect rhyme itself is but a course indicator of such ability, for it only requires syllable matching rather than phoneme segmentation. It may not be quite as closely linked to developing literacy as phoneme segmentation (Goswami & Bryant, 1990). Non-alphabetic scripts, such as classical Chinese, which are word, not phoneme, based in their orthography, may be acquired without an increase in phonological awareness (Read et al., 1986).

Remembering is used here as alliterative shorthand for the ability to recall ordered lists of material verbally immediately after presentation. It is in such tasks that subjects typically recode and rehearse material into speech-based forms which are particularly useful for remembering lists of nameable items in the correct order (i.e., telephone numbers, new names). Memory in general, or in other ways, is not closely correlated with this skill (Morris, 1988). Nor is speech-based rehearsal the only means that people use to recall such lists. Depending on the type of material and the cognitive skills of the rememberer other codes may be used for rehearsal and can supplement inner speech. Thus a number of studies with deaf people who have Sign appear to show that sometimes they can use a sign-based system in remembering lists of 'words' (e.g., Bellugi, Klima and Siple, 1975). And it is well established that some lists can be helped by using a range of associative and imagistic strategies (e.g., Baddeley, 1990). The inner-speech aspect of remembering, though, has been under close scrutiny by psychologists. This is probably because it is the most usual strategy of normal, hearing adults and also the most effective for remembering nameable things *in order* for the purposes of immediate recall. This is worth testing for yourself: How do you "hold" a just heard telephone number? Almost certainly you will "say it to yourself"—at least until you can find a pen to write it down.

Now we take a look at some proposed components of this skill.

Immediate Verbal Memory: Subsystems

Baddeley and Hitch's (1974; and see Baddeley, 1986) model of verbal working memory has two components that can usefully serve the function of immediate repetition (whether written or spoken) of verbal material under the control of a central executive device; these are: (a) a phonological store of limited capacity that holds representations in phonemic form (whether these are derived from letters, heard speech or pictures); and (b) an articulatory loop, a slave system that maintains and refreshes material in the phonological store. These two processes can be distinguished by different experimental signatures. The phonological store corresponds with the inner ear. It is particularly disrupted when material sounds similar (phonemic confusability effects arise here). The articulatory loop corresponds with the inner voice; rehearsal is particularly susceptible to speaking while remembering; this shows most clearly in the abolition by concurrent speech of the word length effect. The word-length effect is the demonstration that span for lists of words that can be spoken quickly (i.e., short words) is greater than span for lists that take longer to say (i.e., long words; see Baddeley, Thomson & Buchanan, 1975). Concurrent speech is speaking an irrelevant speech sound aloud and continually while performing the memory task. Note that concurrent speech does not abolish *all* repetition ability: It just cuts span down in a specific way. In other words, the loop can be considered to have some storage properties.

A somewhat different conceptualization of immediate verbal memory (and one to which Baddeley and his collaborators recently appear to be moving; see Logie & Baddeley, this volume) has been advanced primarily by neuropsychologists who have observed dissociated abilities in patients with immediate verbal memory problems (Caramazza, Basili, Koller, & Berndt, 1981; Caramazza, Berndt, & Basili, 1983; Howard & Franklin, 1990; among others). They suggest that there are two functional phonologically-organized stores of limited capacity: The phonemic input buffer (PI, the inner ear) holds phonological representations of heard speech; The phonological output buffer (PO, inner voice) stores material that is about to be spoken. It is the mutual interaction (looping) between these two phonologically organized devices that constitutes rehearsal. Each buffer can be construed to be of limited storage capacity, estimated at approximately three syllables in adults. Studies with neurological patients suggest that both or either, or the links between them, can be affected by brain damage and lead to poor immediate memory span. In addition, it seems that it is the output buffer (PO) that is accessed by written material that is recoded for remembering. That is, this theorizing makes explicit a site for entry of written material to the system (see Franklin, 1989; Howard & Franklin, 1990; though explicit, it is contentious).

1) **Baddeley and Hitch's working memory metaphor**

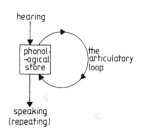

2) **A Two store model**

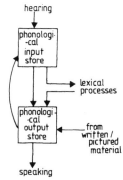

FIG. 4.1. Two ways to draw immediate verbal memory.

The difference between these views of what is involved in immediate memory are sketched out in Fig. 4.1.

It is possible that single loop models may not, as they stand, be sufficient to capture all the available evidence. We return to this at the end of this chapter, where evidence from the deaf is brought to bear on modelling phenomena in immediate verbal recall. It should be noted that both the Baddeley and Hitch (1974) and the two-buffer models indicate a role for "inner hearing" *and* a role for "inner speech" in effective short-term memory.

These, then, are my definitions of the three Rs for the purposes of this chapter. *Reading* refers to mastery of alphabetic orthography, in particular the ability to read and write new and non- words and evidence for alphabetically principled reading (regularity effects in reading, for example). *Rhyme* here refers to the ability to match and manipulate phonological segments in one's native language. *Remembering* is the word used in this chapter to refer to the immediate recall of verbal lists. All appear to reflect the ability to construct, manipulate and maintain a (segmented) phonological representation of speech. If the only source of seg- mented speech for the deaf is through lipreading, they surely will not perform immediate memory and alphabetic reading tasks with normal proficiency, for lipreading cannot deliver the segmental aspects of language in full. Thus, to the extent that reading is based on the use of alphabetic (sound-based) principles, the deaf will be bad readers and poor at verbal recall. That, at any rate, is the simple view of things. It rests, however, on two false assumptions. The first, as I have already pointed out, is that inner speech is the *only* means of recalling lists of nameable things. It is not. People use other available skills, including associative and imagistic ones, to support inner speech. As far as the deaf are concerned, one should know that a range of possible coding strategies (sign, finger-spelling) could be used (see Krakow & Hanson, 1985, to find out whether they are).

The second false assumption, with which I am directly concerned here, is that it is *only* through the acoustically based development of phonologically segmen- table representations (the development of Rhyme skill) that the magic triangle of the three Rs develops; that auditory input is paramount in driving the system by setting the ground for such representations and that Reading and Remembering will follow and then augment these audition-derived Rhyme skills.

To show that this is not the case, I present here two separate lines of evidence. One is to demonstrate the presence of phonological skills (and some boundary conditions on them) in the deaf in a range of reading, remembering and manip- ulation tasks. In connection with this I refer to two people who hear and speak perfectly well, but in whom there is no evidence that rhyming, remembering or reading alphabetically have developed effectively.

The other, with which I start, is to highlight the fact that, while the magic triangle indubitably exists, the prime cause—the driving force of hearing and speaking in setting up representations that allow rhyme-skills to operate—is by no means established.

The Magic Triangle: Interactive not Reactive

While rhyme and segmentation skills on aural speech were thought (Bryant & Bradley, 1983; Liberman, 1973) to predict progress in reading development, it has become clear that the relationship is more interactive and not necessarily causal. People who fail to acquire literacy because of inadequate schooling are poor at phonological segmentation tasks despite their excellent spoken language (Morais, Cary, Alegria, & Bertelson, 1979; Morais, Bertelson, Cary & Alegria, 1986; Morais, Alegria & Content, 1987). People who learn to read in a non-alphabetic language do not acquire the segmentation knack (Mann, 1986; Read et al., 1986). When illiterate adults are then taught to read, Rhyme skill (as defined here) follows. What about Remembering? Nonliterate adults with good spoken language could be poor at repeating nonwords. Morais and Mousty (in press) have observed that some adult illiterates are poor at repeating nonsense words. However, it is not yet established whether their problems will still be apparent when they are compared with appropriate matched controls, that is people of similar age and background who learned to read as adults. So it appears that learning to read, rather than being seen as the *product* of good segmented phonological representations, can also be viewed as *one way to improve them*. If we can get someone to read effectively in an alphabetic script, we stand a good chance of improving that person's Rhyme and Remembering abilities.

To the best of my knowledge, no systematic studies on teaching people to improve their repetition skills have yet been conducted that would parallel the studies on reading. The idea would be that by training illiterate adults in immediate repetition of ordered speech items (nonwords, phone numbers), Rhyme (phonemic segmentation ability) would improve. In children the skills develop together, with measures of span, of nonword repetition, and of reading showing a close relationship. However, it appears that the relationship is strongest in the early school years—at least in British schools (Gathercole, Emslie & Baddeley, 1990). It is possible that the mode of teaching may have an effect, too: whole-word teaching many not be so quick to "deliver" Rhyme and Remembering as more analytic, phonic methods.

Speaking and the Three Rs

If Remembering speech, and the ability to set up and manipulate phonological representations (Rhyming) are among the determinants of alphabetic Reading then, since Remembering depends on a loop involving speaking (articulation), we might infer that learning to speak fluently may be a critical (pre-) determinant of the magic triangle. After all, children normally become more fluent in their speech as they reach school age, and studies of auditory–verbal repetition in preschoolers and early school students show a very strong relationship between a child's rate of speech and immediate memory span (Hulme, Thomson, Muir, &

Lawrence, 1984; and see Hitch, 1990). The fluently speaking child is likely to be the one who plays sound-segmentation games and who would have a head-start in reading. Likely, but not necessarily. Bishop and her colleagues (Bishop 1985, 1988, Bishop & Robson 1989) have shown that congenitally dysarthric and anarthric youngsters in whom speech fails to develop because of cerebral palsy, nevertheless can be skilled at rhyme judgment on spoken, written and pictured words; can read and spell words and nonwords; and can remember lists of spoken and written material at a level commensurate with their measured intelligence and with every sign (word length and phonological similarity effects) that they are using inner speech to perform the task.

Failure of cortical control of the speech centres need not impair the development of the ability to use inner speech in reading and in rhyme judgment tasks, nor to develop auditory–verbal strategies (inner speech) for remembering.

Speaking and Listening but no three Rs?

A number of fluent speakers/hearers have been described who, nevertheless, seem not to make the triangular connection. They are not illiterate but, rather, their reading is "Chinese" in style. That is, they read words without any sign of sensitivity to sound-letter correspondence, so they show no regularity effects in reading and they are unable to read or write simple nonwords at a level commensurate with their general literacy. In the study of acquired reading disorder this is called phonological dyslexia, or if very severe, phonological alexia. The corresponding writing disorder is called phonological dysgraphia. As the "Chinese" sobriquet suggests, in the development of reading world-wide this is not an abnormal pattern. Indeed in non-alphabetic languages it is the *only* pattern. However, for youngsters exposed to alphabetic scripts who have good hearing and speech and who are at the senior secondary school level, it is unusual to find that YACHT would be correctly read or written to dictation, while ZUB may be stumbled over or not even attempted. Such students however can reach high levels of literacy: We encountered one five years ago (Butterworth, Campbell, & Howard, 1986; Campbell & Butterworth, 1985). Rebecca (a pseudonym) was then a 20-year-old undergraduate student whose only apparent problem was an inability to write to dictation a new name, or to read a new word/name aloud. She graduated with a good degree—in Psychology, as it happens. Rebecca spoke at an early age and her hearing was excellent. But her ability to handle inner speech was not good: she could not reliably match spoken rhymes, for instance, and she had a very small immediate memory span, which was better for written (4 digits) than for spoken material (3 digits). Her repetitions showed no sign of structuring by internal speech. For example, she repeated the spoken list "nought, one, oh, one" as "zero, one, zero, one," despite instructions to "repeat exactly what I say." Another graduate reader, Louise, described recently by Funnell and Davison (1989), shows a very similar pattern of phonological dyslexia accompanied by inferior-for-age performance on verbal memory and rhyme-type tasks. While Louise and Rebecca show some intriguing differences (Louise learned to rhyme and remember when she was taught a new, phonetic script explicitly; Rebecca learned a new phonetic script in order to master short-hand, but used literal, not phonological principles in its use), they are mentioned here because they show that the presence of good hearing and the development of normal speech do not always deliver the magic triangle—even when the orthography to be mastered is alphabetic and can give useful guidelines for constructing new words and for manipulating "speech sounds in the head."

Deafness and the Three Rs

We have seen that there is no *necessary* link between speech development and the three Rs, although there is certainly a statistical, predictable, and useful one. So now we can afford to be more relaxed about the relationship between the con-genital absence of hearing and the ways that Reading, Rhyming and Remember-ing may relate. In fact, the picture presented by the deaf, though varied, is clear. As with the congenitally speechless, it would be incorrect to say that the magic triangle cannot develop in the deaf. Nevertheless, some aspects of the three R's show idiosyncratic aspects.

I will look at each of the three R's in turn.

Remembering: Immediate Verbal Recall In The Deaf

Conrad (1979) showed that among profoundly deaf English schoolchildren some showed confusion in their recall of letter names that suggested reliance on the inner ear (the Phonological Store in Baddeley's model; the phonological input buffer, PI, in others). Like hearing youngsters, they showed smaller spans for lists of rhyming letter names (B,G,D,V) than nonrhyming ones (A,Z,L,F). This has been confirmed in deaf students who have sign available to them, as well as in strictly orally trained students. Indeed, there are now a number of studies showing that deaf college students can use speech information to remember lists of words and that this is often *more* effective for written list recall than using other coding strategies such as Sign or finger-spelling (Hanson & Lichtenstein, 1990; Krakow & Hanson, 1985; Lichtenstein, 1985; Waters & Doehring, 1990).

But by no means do all deaf students use the inner ear, and, moreover, while letters and printed words might be remembered using speech based codes, pic-tures and objects may not be. In a recent study we examined immediate recall of pictures (Campbell & Wright, 1990). We examined paired-associate memory in 8-year-olds. The task was this: Pairs of pictures were presented in a fixed order for subjects to remember. Then one of each pair was re-presented and the child was asked to find "the picture that went with this one." In one set of presentations (but not another) the pairs rhymed; an example was a picture of a fly paired with a picture of an eye. For rhyming, but not nonrhyming pairs, hearing children showed almost perfect matching: they used the (implicit) "rhyme-clue." But not a single deaf child was able to pick up on this *aide-memoire,* though their general ability on this task (for nonrhyming pairs) was equivalent to that of their hearing peers. Moreover, in another study in the same series, there was no indication that 17-year-old deaf youngsters remembered the correct presentation order of lists of pictured objects by naming them to themselves on presentation. Hearing subjects of similar age performed the task using inner speech, for where the objects had long names (umbrellas, binoculars, pyjamas) span was smaller than when the names were short (ant, pea, tent). No such word length effect (indicative of inner speech) occurred for the deaf, except when they were explicitly asked to recall the objects by naming them aloud rather than by sorting the pictures in order.

So it seems that the deaf provide ambivalent evidence concerning the necessity of hearing to activate a verbal immediate memory system. Some deaf people show evidence of the use of a phonological store (rely on an Inner Ear), and this is not a direct function of their primary language (Signing or Oral deaf can use the inner ear). In young deaf children, however, we found no evidence for the spontaneous use of such an input store when they were given pictures to recall (paired associate task). There is a similar situation for the inner voice (the articulatory loop or the phonological output buffer and its connections to phonological input). The evidence for the use of articulatory rehearsal (word-length effects) in the deaf is partial and ambivalent: deaf teenagers certainly use inner speech to recall words and to recall names of pictures if verbal recall is required, but not if recall is tested by ordered recognition.

It is likely that one aspect of this ambivalence reflects the slower development of such verbal memory systems in the deaf. On the other hand, I know of no evidence, either in signing or in speaking deaf groups, that deafness precludes the eventual development of inner speech and the inner ear.

Qualitative Differences in the Speech-Based Recall of Written Material in Deaf and Hearing groups?

Helen Wright and I recently performed a variant of the Conrad experiment with deaf teenagers. They were students at a school where Oral teaching was strictly followed; that is, the students were discouraged from using any means of face-to-face communication other than speaking (Campbell & Wright, 1989). If any students were likely to show speech coding, we thought they should be in this sample. The students were asked to remember and write down lists of written monosyllables like FA-BA-KA-TA, which appeared on a video screen long enough to read them (about one second, with two seconds between each list). The lists varied in length: some were three (FA BA TA), some four (DA THA

MA KA), and some five syllables long. We found that deaf and hearing teenagers were equally accurate. This is unusual. Memory span is generally worse in deaf than same-age hearing controls. Using Conrad's interpretation we could say that hearing youngsters were relatively impaired because they were using a speech code and, since the syllables all rhymed (they all ended in A), this caused confusion in the inner ear/inner voice maintenance system. The deaf, on this account, would have been doing the task without a speech code and so, although their repetition span is usually worse than that of hearers, in this case they achieved similar levels of performance.

Except that a closer look at the results revealed that this was not the right interpretation. We had designed our stimuli so that half of the lists had consonant letters in them that would be distinctive in terms of their lipreadability when spoken (e.g., THA is made with the tongue between the teeth in British English—the "TH" is very visible); while half the lists were of syllables where the consonants would be hard to distinguish as lipread items when spoken (e.g., "NA" could be "TA," "DA," "LA," or even "RA"). Hearing youngsters were not sensitive to this "lipreadability" dimension; deaf youngsters, however, were poorer at recalling "NA"-type lists than "THA"-type lists. The lipreadability of the *written* monosyllable was affecting their recall. So these deaf subjects seem to have been using a code in remembering written lists that is sensitive to a speech dimension that *they,* but not hearing students, are sensitive to. The lipreadability of the consonants disproportionately affected the deaf youngsters' recall, while rhyme (vowel similarity) did not seem to affect them unduly. This may not be too surprising; vowels have a powerful effect on hearing people because their acoustic amplitude and duration characteristics are greater than those of consonants; for the deaf without any residual hearing, this heard characteristic of speech may be less salient when it comes to internal recoding. That is, sensory characteristics of the speech input may leave their mark on the way that such input is coded for cognitive tasks. The implication is that speech codes vary with the acoustic and linguistic experience of the subject. Thus, some deaf people may develop inner speech but their code could be *qualitatively* different than that of hearing people; in particular lipreading-distinctive items may be relatively well coded and vowels less salient than in the corresponding speech codes that hearing people develop. This may be because they speak *or* because they perceive (lipread) certain speech sounds differently than hearing people; either produces the "lipreadability" effect.

Reading

If signs of phonological structure can sometimes be found in the immediate memory of deaf people, perhaps they can also be found in Reading. Are deaf children able to read and write nonwords? Do they show regularity effects in their reading? Or do they, rather, resemble the phonological dyslexic and read and write in a "Chinese" fashion? One problem in posing this question is to take into account the effects of alphabetic orthography at different stages of reading development. In hearing children, it is the younger readers who seem overreliant on letter-word mappings, for they tend to be faster at recognizing regularly spelled words and make regularization errors in reading and writing that tend not to be so marked in older, more skilled readers (i.e., see Waters & Doehring, 1990 for review). However, it is the older readers who are generally better at nonword analysis; that is, they can use the alphabetic principle in a skilled fashion but do not rely on it overmuch in skilled reading and writing. Another problem concerns the uses to which letter–sound mapping is put. Are phonological "readings" more likely when *overt* use has to be made, through speaking aloud or because of task demands to "use the sounds of the word" than when no such task demands exist (silent reading for meaning, word recognition in lexical decision)? Perhaps the deaf can use speech codes in reading when they have to, but not when they do not.

Unlike the phonological dyslexic, the deaf schoolchild can often spell (lipread) nonwords to dictation (Dodd, 1980) and can judge whether a homophone of a word (e.g., CHARE) matches a picture (Waters & Doehring, 1990). Rhyme and homophony in written words can be judged, though not with the accuracy of reading age-matched hearing controls (Campbell & Wright, 1988; Hanson & Fowler, 1987).

How sensitive are young deaf readers to the phonological structure of written words in speeded, silent recognition? Waters and Doehring (1990) examined the effects of spelling-sound regularity in visual lexical decision (e.g., Is the briefly displayed letter string a word or a nonword?). Unlike hearing children, who are faster at classifying regular than less regular words, the deaf of similar reading age showed no such effect. Another lexical decision task in Waters and Doehring's series of studies examined the role of inner speech more directly. The task was to decide whether *pairs* of letter strings were words or not. It has been shown (Meyer et al., 1974) that when the letter pairs rhyme (GOOD WOOD) the "yes" decision is made more quickly than when they do not (GOOD TREE). But to be sure that inner speech is responsible for the speeded response word pairs must be selected that look as if they rhyme but do not (PEAR FEAR), and one can also examine word pairs that rhyme but do not look as if they do (HEART PART). Waters & Doehring found that deaf, but not hearing, children were faster at pairs with similar visual endings, independent of rhyme. By contrast, Hanson and Fowler (1987) found that deaf college students showed the rhyme effect independently of visual similarity. It is reasonable to conclude that sensitivity to sound-regularity in reading may develop more gradually in deaf than in hearing readers and is therefore not evident in the deaf at the earlier reading stages. Waters and Doehring themselves report that it is in older (typically 13+), good deaf readers they find phonological structure may affect a range of reading tests.

More evidence that teen-age deaf readers can be sensitive to phonological structure comes from Leybaert's studies (Leybaert, 1987; Leybaert, Alegria, & Fonck, 1983; Leybaert, Alegria, & Morais, 1982) on the Stroop effect in reporting the color of printed color words. For normal hearing readers, the name of the printed word (e.g., BLUE) slows down the decision on the ink in which it is printed (e.g., black), when the two are not congruent. Moreover, BLOO—which is a homophone of the color word—also inhibits the "black" response to the ink color. Leybaert showed that deaf readers were as susceptible as hearing subjects to the effect of a homophone color carrier (like BLOO) in reporting the colour of the word. However, they did not show such an effect (here they were unlike hearing controls) when they performed a manual, rather than a vocal, response to the colored letter string.

So, to summarize, the deaf can construct phonological codes when they read and under certain circumstances they cannot avoid doing so. But, unlike hearing youngsters, such sensitivity seems more pronounced at later, not earlier, stages of reading acquisition. Thus it is possible that "inner speech" in the deaf may follow adequate learning of reading and writing rather than support it in the early stages. And I have already pointed out that the direction of the causal links between Rhyme and Reading development in hearing children is not clear. Alphabetic literacy, if effectively acquired, can give the deaf child a firmer picture of relevant phonological distinctions than unaided speech. When the deaf child has to speak what she reads aloud this may further "jog" a potential inner speech mechanism into action.

Similarly for Remembering, the educated deaf student can learn to make use of a speech code for recall quite efficiently, and this is, as we have seen, most marked for written and to-be-spoken lists rather than for picture lists for recognition. Once again, it could be that reading and writing have laid the path for this skill. Hanson et al. (1984) found a correlation between reading skill and susceptibility to phonemic similarity effects in recall in a group of deaf readers of reading age around 8 years. Waters and Doehring (1990) ran correlational analyses on their deaf subjects who had performed a battery of reading and remembering tasks. In the older, but not the younger deaf subjects (8–12 years), memory span and reading skill correlated. In hearing youngsters the correlations tend to be higher at younger ages. The important aspect of the different developmental relationships may relate to the deaf and the hearing child's speech vocabulary at school age. Deaf children often have a deficient vocabulary. (Waters & Doehring found that, on entering school, their deaf subjects were poor at picture naming— irrespective of their articulatory ability.) We could infer that for them reading is not primarily mapping names-in-the-head to letters-on-the-page but a new means of enlarging their vocabulary of names for things.

So deaf students do not, on the whole, resemble phonologically dyslexic students. The deaf may show regularity effects in reading, can read and write nonwords, can judge rhyme in written words. In other words they can often make use of the alphabetic principle quite adequately. They have short memory spans for their age but their spans can be shown—quite reliably (Hanson & Lichten-stein, 1990)—to be speech-structured and to be related to their reading skills—particularly in older deaf youngsters. What of the third R; Do the deaf show similar levels of phonological awareness ("Rhyme skill") to hearing children? The discussion presented here predicts that they may, but that it could develop through literacy rather than predict it or co-occur with the onset of reading. In one study, Waters, Morse, and Doehring (1984; cited in Waters & Doehring, 1990) compared deaf and hearing controls of reading age 6 years (the deaf children's chronological age was 10 years). The groups of children did not differ in their ability to perform a range of segmentation tasks, but segmentation skill ("Rhyme") correlated with reading ability only in the hearing children. Again, it should be noted that this task, so hard for the phonological dyslexic, was at least achievable by some deaf readers.

The magic triangle captures the usual close relationship between Reading, Remembering and Rhyming in normal hearing, speaking youngsters. But it can be entered with no speaking ability (Bishop's demonstration) and with no hearing ability, and useful bootstrapping of the other skills may then occur. A ped-agogical implication—assuming that a useful goal is to enable the deaf person to enter fully into a literate culture—is that it is therefore extremely important to teach the deaf child to read and to write and, if this training is alphabetic, that it may enhance the deaf child's skill in using inner speech. Of course, this discus-sion does not offer much that is useful in considering *how* to teach the deaf child to read and write, but three points may be made: Firstly, I would underline Waters and Doehring's (1990) comments on the poor vocabulary of deaf chil-dren. Where vocabulary can be increased, so reading skill may have a useful semantic/representational base on which written-word recognition could build. Secondly (and relatedly), there is no evidence that reading and writing are more difficult for the child who is brought up in Sign rather than speech; the potential disadvantages of having a different native language than the reading language appear to be outweighed by the rich conceptual/linguistic experience that the child with Sign as a native language could enjoy over the child with (im-poverished) spoken language (Rodda & Grove, 1987). Finally, it should be noted, in connection with Sign, that *finger-spelling*, where letters are signed to produce words, may, in theory, provide a "bridge" between signed and spoken/written language and a source of metalinguistic awareness, analogous to phonemic segmentation skill in hearing children. This is because finger-spelled words enter "silently" into the child's vocabulary; they are learned simply as new signs, not as a different type of item. Similarly, acronyms such as *USA* or *OK* naturally enter a hearing child's vocabulary. In both these cases there is potential for the child who is learning to read to be directed to the notion that there is a relationship between the finger-spelled letter (for the deaf) or the letter name (for the hearing) and a part of a previously known whole word. However, the evidence that finger spelling is *spontaneously* useful for the signing child in this way is negative, although it can be used under overt instruction (Hirsh-Pasek & Treiman, 1982; Krakow & Hanson, 1985; Treiman & Hirsh Pasek, 1983).

What is Happening in Rebecca?

But what of the phonological dyslexic; why doesn't Rebecca (and others like her) use inner speech, when all the outer apparatus is intact? Is her deficiency strategic (she chooses to read and remember this way) or structural (she must read and remember like this)? Probably both. If her problem is structural, then *which* structure involved in Reading, Remembering and Rhyming is a likely candidate? The looping model of Fig. 1 allows us some speculations. The first thing is to establish to what extent independent signatures for each of the proposed boxes and arrows can be supported. While this may sometimes be contentious, some minimal tasks can be suggested that could answer the question: Is this component functional? An intact input buffer (PI) would be indicated by unimpaired ability to discriminate spoken (and/or lipread) words; one test would be that of mispronunciation detection for known words. Rebecca was perfect at this. An intact output buffer (PO) is suggested because she can produce spoken words for pictures and for written words flawlessly. Furthermore she can repeat *single* words and *simple* spoken nonwords, indicating that PI–PO connexions are intact. The most likely cause of Rebecca's disorder and, by implication, the root problem for other phonological dyslexics with a developmental etiology, is a failure to develop an effective loop from PO to PI, which would serve to maintain and "refresh" the phonological record for purposes as many and varied as rhyme decision, repetition of lists and complex nonsense words, phoneme counting, etc. On this account, nonword reading failure reflects the critical role of PO to PI mappings in setting up an inner speech representation of what is read. Where phonological dyslexia coexists with good repetition, as in the adult acquired case described by Bisiacchi et al. (1989), the interpretation must be that the lesion has disrupted the mapping from vision (written words) to PO, while leaving the looping PO-PI function intact.

An Outer Loop in Inner Speech

However, the picture may be more complex than this. Just as, under the right conditions, a second arc may be seen around the rainbow, so, under careful inspection, a second phonetically-based system may be found to encircle the phonological system responsible for auditory verbal repetition, counting of sounds and assembly of speech sounds from letters. In auditory or lipread list recall, the last items are well remembered (recency) if no heard or lipread suffix follows them. A pre-phonological record, phonetically structured, would seem to be responsible for this (Campbell, 1987). That is, a phonetic input store (Pt.I) may be activated prior to phonemic categorization, through listening and/or

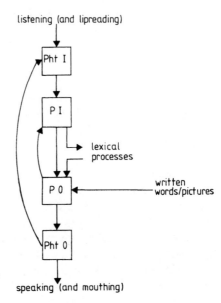

FIG. 4.2. The outer loop in inner speech.

lipreading. But a phonetically structured *output* device (Pt.O) is also involved in such recency phenomena. When the subject silently mouthes a written word this can produce a memory function with recency, just as if the list had been heard or lipread.[1]

One way to conceptualize this is in terms of linked phonetic buffers encircling the phonemic buffer stores, with auditory (also lipread, also mouthed) recency as a signature of this (outer) looped function. Fig. 4.2 sketches this possibility.

The following aspect of this system should be noted: It enables both a phonetic and a phonemic maintenance system to be activated for heard (and lipread, and mouthed) lists. All other things being equal, these may be additive and could help to give an advantage to auditory over silent visual span because written material (which is not spoken or mouthed) only uses the "inner circle." Just such a modality-specific advantage in favor of heard material is often observed in short-term memory experiments.

I would suggest that it is the outer loop that is primarily responsible for "modality specific" recency effects by providing an additional, short-lived,

---

[1]This position is an about-face from some of my earlier interpretations. I have resisted the idea, first proposed by Crowder (1983), that a phonetic loop (or something like it) is responsible for all recency-specific modality effects in speaking, lipreading and mouthing, because in some experiments (a) I find some purely orthographic stimuli that can sometimes generate these effects, and (b) there is not complete commonality of effect between different modes of presentation (e.g., a lipread suffix does not affect a heard list as much as a heard suffix does). I now think these problems are best dealt with as special cases that will moderate our views of the precise workings of the "outer loop."

coded trace. While the complete outer loop may be implicated in such recency, how might its functional components (Pt.I., Pt.O. and the Pt.I.–Pt.O. link) be tested? Normal phonetic categorization functions for synthetic speech would suggest whether phonetic perception is intact and phonetic tokens available for reflection. Speech pronunciation that shows no phonetic deviation from the language-specified norm would suggest that Pt.O. was all right. A measure of the Pt.I.–Pt.O. connexion would be the repetition of a simple phonologically illegal (but phonetically reasonable) utterance. Rebecca could do all of these. However she showed no auditory or lipread recency in her recall of spoken lists. Thus Rebecca appears not only to have a disrupted phonological rehearsal system, but also a disrupted *phonetic* loop (Pt.O.–Pt.I.).

The deaf, though, do not seem to behave like this. Although for them phonetic distinctions cannot be heard, and although the phonetic quality of their speech is poor, they nevertheless show recency for lipread recall (Dodd et al., 1983). The implication is that everything seems to be in place in the deaf for the outer loop in inner speech to be effective and to get to work on lipread phonetic inputs. However, it should be noted that the picture may be complicated by strategic differences between deaf and hearing people in the way they approach written and spoken recall tasks. The deaf often show visual (written) recall superiority in remembering word, letter or digit lists: they *may* use inner speech but do not *have* to. Rebecca is like this too. Her written span is greater than her span for spoken lists. She does not use inner speech—neither the outer nor the inner loop from the output to input store is functional: when she recalls words, whether written, lipread, mouthed, or spoken, there is reliance on maintenance systems in another (visual) domain. Outer speech and hearing do not guarantee the automatic development of inner speech, nor does congenital loss of hearing preclude it.

CONCLUSIONS

This chapter poses the following question: How does inner speech (including the inner voice) relate to the development of alphabetic reading, to the ability to perform speech segmentation tasks and to the development of immediate verbal memory? I have endeavored to answer this question using evidence from the deaf and from some data on normal and exceptional development of the three Rs.

It is easy to assume that the ability to play segmental speech games and to construct effective phonological representations lays the groundwork for mastery both of alphabetic reading and immediate verbal memory span. There are close relations in development between the three skills, but they are not necessarily linked causally in this way. Nor need reading—in the broader sense, which encompasses a mastery of whatever orthography one is taught—*necessarily* be linked to the other two Rs. Rebecca can read very well in the general sense - but can not use Rhyme (perform segmentation tasks) or Remember (use verbal rehearsal). Given that Rebecca has "broken free," one might predict that deaf people would tend to follow her "Chinese" reading route. While there may be such deaf individuals, the deaf people I have tested do not show this pattern. Rather, they show some ability in both Rhyme and Remembering and can Read using the alphabetic principle. Indeed, in the deaf the relationship between the three Rs may *tighten* as they become more literate (correlations between tasks tend to be higher at older ages in the deaf: see Waters & Doehring, 1990). This suggests to me that it is the development of literacy that encourages their development of "inner speech," and that could continue to support the development of their working memory span and ability to do some segmentation tasks, despite poor speech and absent hearing. The deaf, however, do not simply present a drawn-out, slowed-down version of linked processes that are usually observed much earlier in hearing people; the deaf are qualitatively different, too. They tend not to use a speech-based memory code when confronted with pictures or objects or when the task does not demand naming or other verbal responses (Campbell & Wright, 1990; 1988). Even when they seem to be using a speech code, it may bear the marks of having been seen rather than heard (Campbell & Wright, 1989).

"Inner speech," then, is a curiously abstract beast. It can be observed in those born without speech (Bishop's anarthrics) and in born-deaf people too. It does not, therefore, depend in any necessary or sufficient sense on "outer" speech or hearing. It can play a subtle role in a number of cognitive processes that are somewhat different in deaf and hearing people and which bear evidence of its sensory origins. It can be partitioned into subcomponents that can be independently tested. Does it clothe thought or engender it? That is a quite different question, for which very different answers will need to be sought. But I am convinced, as I hope you are, that it is a real beast, rather than a creature of fable.

REFERENCES

Baddeley, A D. (1986). *Working memory.* Oxford: Clarendon Press.

Baddeley, A. D. (1990). *Human memory.* Hove, U. K.: Lawrence Erlbaum Associates.

Baddeley, A. D., Thomson, N., & Buchanan, M. (1975). Word length and the structure of short term memory. *Journal of Verbal Learning and Verbal Behavior, 14,* 575–589.

Baddeley, A. D. & Hitch, G. (1974). Working Memory. In G. H. Bower (Ed.), *The psychology of learning and motivation. Advances in theory and research, Vol. 8,* New York: Academic Press.

Bellugi, U., Klima, E. S., & Siple, P. (1975). Remembering in signs. *Cognition, 3,* 93–125.

Bishop, D. V. M. (1985). Spelling ability in congenital dysarthria: Evidence against articulatory coding in translating between graphemes and phonemes. *Cognitive Neuropsychology, 2,* 229–251.

Bishop, D. V. M. (1988). Language Development in children with abnormal structure or function of the speech apparatus. In D. Bishop & K. Mogford (Eds.), *Language development in exceptional circumstances,* Edinburgh: Churchill - Livingstone.

Bishop, D. V. M., & Robson, J. (1989). Unimpaired short-term memory and rhyme judgment in congenitally speechless individuals: Implications for the notion of "Articulatory Coding." *Quarterly Journal of Experimental Psychology, 41A,* 123–141.

Bisiacchi, P. S., Cipolotti, L., & Denes, G. (1989). Impairment in processing meaningless verbal material in several modalities: The relationship between short-term memory and phonological skills. *Quarterly Journal of Experimental Psychology, 41A,* 293–320.

Bryant, P., & Bradley, L. (1983). Categorising sounds and learning to read: A casual connection. *Nature, 301,* 419–421.

Butterworth, B. L., Campbell, R., & Howard, D. (1986). The uses of short-term memory: A case study. *Quarterly Journal of Experimental Psychology, 38A,* 705–737.

Campbell, R. (1987). Lipreading and immediate memory processes. In B. Dodd & R. Campbell (Eds.), *Hearing by eye: the psychology of lipreading* (pp. 243–256). London: Lawrence Erlbaum Associates.

Campbell, R. (1990). Lipreading, neuropsychology and immediate memory. In G. Vallar & T. Shallice (Eds.), *Neuropsychological impairments of short-term memory* (pp. 268–286). Cambridge, U.K.: Cambridge University Press.

Campbell, R., & Butterworth, B. (1985). Phonological dyslexia and dysgraphia in a highly literate subject; A developmental case with associated deficits of phonemic processing and awareness. *Quarterly Journal of Experimental Psychology, 37A,* 435–475.

Campbell, R., & Dodd, B. (1980). Hearing by eye. *Quarterly Journal of Experimental Psychology, 32A,* 85–89.

Campbell, R., & Wright, H. (1988). Deafness, spelling & rhyme. *Quarterly Journal of Experimental Psychology, 40A,* 771–788.

Campbell, R., & Wright, H. (1989). Immediate memory in the orally trained deaf: Effects of "lipreadability" in the recall of written syllables. *British Journal of Psychology, 80,* 299–312.

Campbell, R., & Wright, H. (1990). Deafness and immediate memory for pictures; Dissociations between "inner voice" and "inner ear"? *Journal of Experimental Child Psychology, 50,* 259–286.

Caramazza, A., Basili, A. G., Koller, J. J., & Berndt, R. S. (1981). An investigation of repetition and language processing in a case of conduction aphasia. *Brain & Language 14,* 235–275.

Caramazza, A., Berndt, R. S., & Basili, A. G. (1983). The selective impairment of phonological processing: A case study. *Brain and Language, 18,* 128–174.

Conrad, R. (1979). *The deaf school child.* London: Harper and Row.

Crowder, R. G. (1983). The purity of auditory memory. *Philosophical Transactions of the Royal Society of London, B, 302,* 251–265.

Dodd, B. (1980). The spelling abilities of profoundly deaf children. In U. Frith (Ed.), *Cognitive processes in spelling.* London: Academic Press.

Dodd, B., Hobson, P., Brasher, J., & Campbell, R. (1983). Short term memory in deaf children. *British Journal of Developmental Psychology, 1,* 354–364.

Franklin, S. (1989). *A three phase model of auditory short-term memory: Evidence from three aphasic patients.* Paper presented to the Experimental Psychological Society, Cambridge, England.

Funnell, E., & Davison, M. (1989). Lexical capture: A developmental disorder of reading and spelling. *Quarterly Journal of Experimental Pyshcology, 41A,* 471–489.

Gathercole, S., Emslie, H., & Baddeley, A. D. (1990, January). *Differential Contributions of Phonological Memory to reading development between ages 5 and 7.* Paper presented at the 1990 meeting of the Experimental Psychology Society, London, UK.

Goswami, U., & Bryant, P. (1990). *Phonological skills and learning to read.* London: Lawrence Erlbaum Associates.

Hanson, V. L., & Fowler, C. (1987). Phonological coding in word reading: Evidence from hearing and deaf readers. *Memory & Cognition, 15,* 199–207.

Hanson, V. L., & Lichtenstein, E. (1990). Short term memory coding by deaf signers: Primary language coding reconsidered. *Cognitive Psychology, 22,* 211–224.

Hanson, V. L., Liberman, I. Y., & Shankweiler, D. (1984). Linguistic coding by deaf children in relation to beginning reading success. *Journal of Experimental Child Psychology, 37,* 378–393.

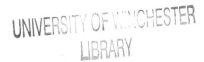

Hirsh-Pasek, K., & Treiman, R. (1982). Recoding in silent reading: Can the deaf child translate print into a more manageable form? *Volta Review, 84,* 71–82.

Hitch, G. (1990). Developmental fractionation of working memory. In G. Vallar & T. Shallice (Eds.), *Neuropsychological impairments of short-term memory* (pp. 220–246). Cambridge, U.K.: Cambridge University Press.

Howard, D., & Franklin, S. (1990). Memory without rehearsal. In G. Vallar & T. Shallice (Eds.), *Neuropsychological impairments of short-term memory* (pp. 287–318). Cambridge, U.K.: Cambridge University Press.

Hulme, C., Thomson, N., Muir, C., & Lawrence, A. (1984). Speech rate and the development of short-term memory span. *Journal of Experimental Child Psychology, 38,* 241–253.

Klima, E. S., & Bellugi, U. (1979). *The signs of language.* Cambridge, USA: Harvard University Press.

Krakow, R. A., & Hanson, V. L. (1985). Deaf signers and serial recall in the visual modality: Memory for signs, finger spelling and print. *Memory & Cognition, 13,* 265–272.

Kyle, J. G., & Woll, B. (1988). *Sign language: The study of deaf people and their language.* Cambridge, U.K.: Cambridge University Press.

Leybaert, J. (1987). *Le traitment du mot ecrit chez l'enfant sourd.* Doctor of Philosophy thesis, Université Libre de Bruxelles. transl: The treatment of the written word in the deaf child.

Leybaert, J., Alegria, J., & Fonck, E. (1983). Automaticity in word recognition and word naming in the deaf. *Cahiers de Psychologie Cognitive, 3,* 255–272.

Leybaert, J., Alegria, J., & Morais, J. (1982). On automatic reading processes in the deaf. *Cahiers de Psychologie Cognitive, 2,* 185–192.

Liberman, Y., I. 1973). Segmentation of the spoken word and reading acquisition. *Bulletin of the Orton Society, 23,* 65–77.

Lichtenstein, E. (1985). The relationship between reading processes and English skills of deaf college students. In D. S. Martin (Ed.), *Cognition, education & deafness.* New York: Gallaudet College Press.

Mann, V. (1986). Phonological awareness: The role of reading experience. *Cognition, 24,* 65–92.

Meyer, D. F., Schvaneveldt, R., & Ruddy, M. (1974). Functions of graphemic and phonemic codes in visual word recognition. *Memory & Cognition, 2,* 209–321.

Mills, A. (1987). The development of phonology in blind children. In B. Dodd & R. Campbell (Eds.), *Hearing by eye: The psychology of lipreading* (pp. 145–162). London: Lawrence Erlbaum Associates.

Morais, J., & Mousty, P. (in press). The causes of phonemic awareness. In J. Alegria, D. Holender, J. Morais, & M. Radeau (Eds.), *Analytic approaches to human cognition: Essays in honour of Paul Bertelson.*

Morais, J., Alegria, J., & Content, A. (1987). The relationships between segmental analysis and alphabetic literacy: An interactive view. *Cahiers de Psychologie Cognitive, 7,* 415–438.

Morais, J., Bertelson, P., Cary, L., & Alegria, J. (1986). Literacy training and speech segmentation. *Cognition, 24,* 45–64.

Morais, J., Cary, L., Alegria, J., & Bertelson, P. (1979). Does awareness of speech as a series of phones arise spontaneously? *Cognition, 7,* 323–331.

Morris, P. (1988). Memory Research: Past mistakes and future prospects. In G. Claxton (Ed.), *Growth points in cognition* (pp. 91–110). London: Routledge.

Perin, D. (1983). Phonemic segmentation in spelling. *British Journal of Psychology, 74,* 129–144.

Read, C., Zhang, Y., Nie, H., & Ding, B. (1986). The ability to manipulate speech sound depends on knowing alphabetic reading. *Cognition, 24,* 21–34.

Rodda, M., & Grove, C. (1987). *Language, cognition, and deafness.* Hillsdale, NJ: Lawrence Erlbaum Associates.

Siple, P. (Ed.) (1978). *Understanding Language Through Sign Research.* New York: Academic Press.

Treiman, R., & Hirsh-Pasek, K. (1983). Silent reading: Insights from congenitally deaf readers. *Cognitive Psychology, 15,* 329–365.

Waters, G. S., & Doehring, D. (1990). The nature and role of phonological information in reading acquisition: Insights from congenitally deaf children who communicate orally. In T. Carr & B. A. Levy (Eds.), *Reading and its development: Component skills approaches* (pp. 323–373). New York, Academic Press.

Waters, G. S., Morse, C., & Doehring, D. G. (1984). *An analysis of the beginning reading skills of hearing and orally trained hearing-impaired children.* Paper presented at the annual meeting of the American Speech and Hearing Association, San Fransisco.

5 Subvocalization and Auditory Imagery: Interactions Between the Inner Ear and Inner Voice

J. David Smith
New School for Social Research

Daniel Reisberg
Reed College

Meg Wilson
University of California, Berkeley

Introduction: An Experiment In Auditory Imagery

Consider the following procedure: Subjects are presented with a series of letter/nuumber strings (e.g., "NE1 4 10S"). Visually, this string is unfamiliar to most people, but, when pronounced aloud, it yields a familiar *auditory* stream: "Anyone for tennis?" Subjects are asked to interpret several such strings, without pronouncing them aloud, but instead using auditory imagery.

How might subjects perform this task? One possibility is that they call before the mind's ear an image of someone pronouncing the string, and consult this image to determine what it sounds like. This process would presumably occur in just the same way that we call up a visual image (of a horse, perhaps) and make a judgment about it (how far off the ground is the tip of its tail?). Alternatively, subjects might adopt some form of subvocalization strategy. For example, they might pronounce the string to themselves and "read" the kinesthetic cues resulting from the covert lip and tongue movements. Covertly saying "NE" would *feel* the same as saying "ANY," and subjects could use this (felt) equivalence to decipher the string. As yet another possibility, subjects might covertly pronounce the string and then "listen" with some inner ear to this production by the inner voice. Finally, subjects might use some non-imagery or nonphonological strategy, for example, using prior knowledge or guesswork to construct their interpretation.

To discover how subjects perform this task, we examined performance under four conditions, in a standard selective interference design (2 × 2; between-subjects). Some subjects interpreted strings while hearing auditory input through headphones. Subjects were instructed to ignore this input, and it was, in any event, irrelevant to their task. However, we know from the literature that this manipulation disrupts some aspects of auditory imagery—that is, input from the "outer ear" interferes with the use of the "inner ear" (Baddeley, 1986; Salame & Baddeley, 1982; Segal & Fusella, 1970). Other subjects read the strings while repeating "Tah-Tah-Tah" aloud. Such concurrent articulation is known to disrupt subvocalization—that is, tying up the "outer voice" interferes with use of the "inner voice" (Baddeley, 1986; Besner, Davies & Daniels, 1981; Levy, 1971; Murray, 1968; Slowiaczek & Clifton, 1980). A third group of subjects performed with both the irrelevant auditory input and the concurrent articulation task (both the inner ear and inner voice disrupted); a fourth group received neither type of interference.

This design, with an auditory imagery task performed with either of two kinds of interference, or both, or neither, is the structural frame for many of the experiments reported in this chapter. Figure 5.1 shows the possible results for such an experiment and is the blueprint of possibilities for the experiments we report throughout. If a task requires only the inner voice, then blocking subvocalization will disrupt performance, but an unattended auditory input will not (5.1-A). Conversely, if a task requires only the inner ear, then a concurrent auditory input will be disruptive, but blocking subvocalization will not (5.1-B). If *either* the inner ear or inner voice can support performance of a task, and subjects adopt either strategy as needed, then performance should be undisturbed unless *both* the inner ear and inner voice are blocked by interference tasks (5.1-C). In Fig. 5.1-D, performance suffers if either kind of interference is present, and the combination of both is no worse than either kind of interference alone. This pattern would suggest that subjects need both the inner ear and the inner voice for their task; presumably in this case subjects would be using the inner voice to generate a representation which the inner ear listens to, or scans. Finally, 5.1-E should obtain if neither the inner ear nor the inner voice is required for the task.

The actual result of the letter-string ("NE1 4 10S") experiment was close to that of Fig. 5.1-D. When subjects interpreted strings with no interference (with auditory input absent, and subvocalization possible) they were able to decipher 73% of the strings. But, denied the inner ear or inner voice, performance declined to 40% and 21%, respectively, and to 19% with both forms of interference present simultaneously (both main effects and the interaction were statistically reliable).

The large effect of blocking subvocalization suggests that subjects covertly pronounce these strings to themselves and that this inner speech is blocked by concurrent articulation. This covert articulation could be sufficient to support string interpretation, if subjects used the kinesthetic cues it provided. However, with this kinesthetic strategy the inner ear would not be needed, and so concur-

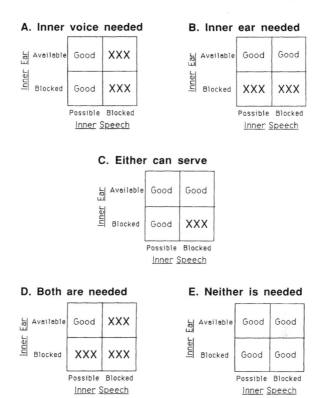

FIG. 5.1. Possible performance patterns resulting from manipulations designed to block use of the inner voice or inner ear.

rent auditory input would not hurt performance. Since it does hurt, the kinesthetic strategy is ruled out in favor of some strategy that requires both the inner ear
and voice. Most likely, subjects produce the strings with the inner voice, "listen"
to themselves with the inner ear, and then make their judgments based on this
auditory image. With this strategy, performance will suffer if either the inner
voice or the inner ear is disrupted. Moreover, if one component of the inner-ear/
inner-voice team is blocked, then there is little further harm from disrupting the
other—having only one available is not much better than having none.

This experiment highlights the empirical and theoretical issues for our chapter. Auditory imagery is a relatively unexplored domain in cognitive psychology,
and one of our purposes (and the purpose of this volume) is to understand the
nature of the auditory representations evoked in imagery—how they are generated, consulted, scanned, etc. Part of what motivates this inquiry is the hope of
ties to imagery in other modalities, allowing broader theories about the relationships of imagery and perception, and the nature of imagery generally.

However, it may turn out that auditory imagery has a rather different profile from other forms of imagery. One important reason for this is that auditory imagery has a potential partner in subvocalization, and this raises several issues. What is the relationship between auditory imagery and subvocalization? Is the partnership found in the letter-string experiment a common one, perhaps a necessary one? Or are there other ways to create auditory images, ways for which subvocalization plays no role? And is the relationship between inner ear and inner voice somehow domain specific, perhaps different for speech imagery than it is for imagery for other classes of sounds? Our chapter is an introduction to these issues.

First, we describe our initial work in this area, a series of studies which drew our attention to the role of subvocalization in auditory imagery (pp. 98–101). Then we summarize the results of other, more recent, experiments which explore the breadth of connection between auditory imagery and the inner voice (pp. 101–104). This exploration is aided by noting the specificity of tasks which interfere with the inner voice and inner ear. This specificity speaks against a "general distraction" hypothesis for interference effects, and has implications for auditory imagery research (pp. 104–106). Next, we discuss the strong convergence between our research on auditory imagery and Baddeley's (and others') work on memory rehearsal and the articulatory loop system. In effect, the rehearsal literature finds exactly the partnership that we do between auditory imagery and subvocalization, implying that this pattern is indeed widespread (pp. 106–108). The partnership is not universal, though, for one can find tasks in which it seems to break down (pp. 108–109). This leads us to consider in more detail subvocalization's role in auditory imagery, both to clarify the theoretical situation, and perhaps to gain predictive control over which imagery tasks will or will not require subvocalization (pp. 109–112). Finally, there appears to be one class of auditory imagery task that requires neither the inner ear nor inner voice as these are usually construed (pp. 112–117). We close with some discussion of an independent phonological store, drawn on by such tasks.

Subvocalization and "Ambiguous Images"

Our early work on auditory imagery was designed simply to test the generality of some claims made about visual images. There has been considerable discussion in the visual imagery literature over how one comes to understand one's own mental images. One possibility is that comprehending an image and perceiving a stimulus are similar acts. On this view, imagery creates some uninterpreted raw material, akin to the proximal stimulus in perception. This depiction is then interpreted by means of a process related to perceiving (cf. Finke, 1980; Finke, Pinker & Farah, 1989; Kosslyn, 1980, 1983).

A rather different view, however, has been suggested by a number of authors (Casey, 1976; Chambers & Reisberg, 1985; Fodor, 1981; Kolers & Smythe,

1984). These authors argue that images have no existence outside of the imager's understanding of them, making the image and its comprehension inseparable. In perception there is a physical stimulus, existing independent of the perceiver, which needs interpretation. In imagery, however, there is no free-standing icon waiting to be interpreted, and no interpretation is needed to learn what the image depicts.

These two views diverge on a number of points (cf. Reisberg & Chambers, 1991; Reisberg & Morris, 1985). The conceptions differ most sharply, though, when we consider the possibility of "ambiguous images." According to the "images are like stimuli" view, the raw material of imagery is inherently ambiguous (cf. Kosslyn, 1983, p. 35). As in perception, the recognition process we apply to our images might be heavily constrained so that the ambiguity is rarely realized. Nonetheless, the potential for reinterpretation would be there, as the raw material, itself indifferent to interpretation, remains on the scene. Imagers could detect the ambiguity of this internal stimulus if "they made an effort to do so" (Kosslyn, 1983, p. 89).

According to the "images are inherently meaningful" view, mental images simply cannot be ambiguous. When an image comes into being, it comes into being as an image of some particular thing. Whether the image was deliberate or unbidden, it arrives in awareness as a depiction of some meaning, so that there is no way to be confused or mistaken about its contents. With no interpretation process and, indeed, with no icon to be interpreted, there is no possibility for reinterpretation, and so no possibility for ambiguity.

Consistent with this latter view, prior studies had indicated that visual images are indeed unambiguous in what they represent (Chambers & Reisberg, 1985; but then see Finke, Pinker & Farah, 1989; also Reisberg & Chambers, 1991). While these data are still the subject of debate, note that the claims at issue should apply across imagery modalities. Therefore, we can obtain converging evidence for these claims from research with image modalities other than vision. Following this logic, Reisberg, Smith, Baxter and Sonenshine (1989) asked whether auditory images are inherently meaningful and, therefore, necessarily unambiguous.

As their ambiguous stimuli, Reisberg et al. (1989) exploited the fact that certain words, if repeated over and over aloud, yield a soundstream compatible with more than one segmentation (Warren, 1961, 1982; Warren & Gregory, 1958). For example, rapid repetitions of the word "life" produce a physical soundstream that is fully compatible with segmentations appropriate to repetitions of "life" or "fly." These repetitions are usually perceived first as one of these words, then the other, then the first, changing in phenomenal form just as the Necker cube or duck/rabbit do. This allows us to ask if *imagined* repetitions produce verbal transformations, just as *heard* repetitions do.

Subjects in these studies were asked to imagine (or, in some conditions, actually heard) a voice repeating the word "stress" over and over. With an actual (perceived) stimulus, 100% of the subjects heard this soundstream transform into repetitions of "dress," a construal fully compatible with the stimulus input. However, this transformation was rarely guessed by a control group, making the transformation a relatively clear indication of bonafide perceptual reversals.

In the Reisberg et al. procedures, subjects who imagined these repetitions often detected the stress-to-dress transformations. This seemed to indicate a sharp contrast with the data from visual imagery (e.g., Chambers & Reisberg, 1985), in which subjects have routinely failed to reinterpret their images. However, subjects' success in "reversing" auditory images turned out to depend on subvocalization. Reisberg et al. (1989, Expt. 1) prevented subjects from subvocalizing by having them chew candy, and this dropped "reversals" (i.e., detections of "dress") from 47% to the level achieved by guessing subjects (25%). Reversals were also reduced (from 73% to 27%) if subvocalization was blocked by having subjects tightly clamp their jaws shut, firmly press their tongue up against the roof of their mouth, and hold their lips firmly shut (Experiment 4; also Wilson, Smith, & Reisberg, unpublished).

The evidence indicates, therefore, that the inner voice is required for this task. Why does the inner voice make image reconstrual possible? Reisberg et al. argued that the inner voice provides an actual (kinesthetic) stimulus for the subject, a stimulus with an existence independent of the subject's understanding of it. Hence the inner voice provides "raw material" to be interpreted and, so, something which can be reinterpreted. Subjects can therefore reconsult the subvocalized speech stimulus and find a different construal.

But whatever the explanation, these results challenged our original purpose— to document the generality of claims about imagery. Instead, they underscored the uniqueness of auditory imagery, given its potential involvement with, and stimulus support by, the inner voice. This led us to consider directly the relation between the inner ear and inner voice in auditory imagery tasks.

The letter-string experiment described at the chapter's start illustrated one possible relation—the partnership. In that experiment subjects needed both inner ear and inner voice to perform, and the disruption of either hurt performance about as much as the disruption of both. Does a similar partnership obtain when subjects try to reconstrue auditory images, as in the stress/dress procedure?

We have already seen that such reconstruals require the inner voice. Is image reconstrual also disrupted if subjects are denied use of the inner ear? Wilson, Smith and Reisberg (unpublished) asked subjects to perform the stress/dress task while hearing an irrelevant message through headphones. This manipulation reduced the number of reversals from 73% to 13%, implying that the inner ear is also necessary for this task. (Blocking either inner voice or inner ear alone reduces performance to guessing levels, or floor, obviating a condition where both kinds of interference are applied simultaneously.)

Thus, the data pattern for the stress/dress task resembles that of the string task described earlier. In both tasks subjects seem to subvocalize the to-be-imagined event, and then listen with the inner ear to what they have themselves produced. Performance suffers if use of either the inner voice or the inner ear is blocked.

This convergence with the string experiment led us to wonder how widespread this pattern is. Is it generally the case that subjects support their imagery with subvocalization, or is this true only for a specific set of tasks? The two tasks described thus far both involve verbal material and speech imagery. Subvocalization might be a particularly salient strategy in such tasks, and so one might believe that our results converge because our deck of tasks is stacked. Therefore, we also explored tasks which required nonspeech images.

The Breadth of the Inner-Ear/Inner-Voice Partnership

Wilson, Smith and Reisberg (unpublished) presented subjects with a list of well-known songs (e.g., "London Bridge is Falling Down," or "Happy Birthday"). Subjects' task was to judge whether the melody rises or falls in pitch from the song's second note to its third. In "Happy Birthday," the third note is higher in pitch than the second, and so "rises" is the correct response. Subjects performed these melody judgments with irrelevant speech input, with subvocalization blocked (subjects repeated "Tah-Tah"), and with both or neither kind of interference.

Consider the possible results of this procedure, as depicted in Fig. 5.1. Subjects might perform this task by singing the song to themselves, and reading the kinesthetic cues (vocal tensions) produced by higher and lower notes. This inner-voice strategy would produce the interference results of Fig. 5.1-A. Alternatively, subjects might imagine a child singing the tune, or an instrument playing it, and consult the image to determine its sequence of up and down pitches. This inner-ear strategy would only be disrupted by irrelevant auditory input, producing the pattern of Fig. 5.1-B. Third, subjects might sing the song to themselves and listen with an inner ear to the production of this inner voice—then the pattern of 5.1-D would be expected (i.e., the pattern we have already observed with the "NE1 4 10S" and stress/dress tasks). Fourth, it might be that neither inner ear nor inner voice is required. For instance, expert musicians could use musical note names, or a visualized musical score, or instrument fingerings, to make the melody judgments abstractly, visually, or motorically. In this case, Fig. 5.1-E would obtain.

The actual result of the experiment was that of Fig. 5.1-D. When subjects performed only the melody judgment task they were correct on 83% of the trials (chance performance would be 50%). With auditory distraction added to disrupt use of the inner ear, performance dropped to 69%. With concurrent articulation added to block subvocalization (but with no auditory distraction), performance was at 66% correct. When both auditory distraction and concurrent articulation were present, there was no further decline; under those conditions subjects were 68% correct. Thus it seems that subjects must produce these strings for themselves, and then "listen" to what they have produced. Once again, the inner voice and ear are used in concert.

Apparently, therefore, the "partnership" data pattern (5.1-D) is not limited to tasks with speech imagery. Even here, though, the stimuli were familiar songs, easily singable and also plausibly subvocalizable. What happens if we examine an auditory imagery task unlikely to rely on subvocalization? Fortunately, the literature contains such a task, and we can apply our selective interference logic to it.

Crowder (1989; Crowder & Pitt, this volume) used a task in which subjects imagine notes played by specific musical instruments. Subjects heard a sine wave and were instructed to imagine this note as played by a flute, guitar or trumpet. Then they heard a second tone, played on one of these three instruments, and they had to judge as quickly as possible whether the imagined and actual tones matched in pitch.

Crowder found reaction times facilitated whenever the relation between real and imaged timbres was congruent with the required pitch comparison. The "same" timbres facilitated "same" pitch trials; "different" timbres facilitated "different" pitch trials. This result strongly implies that instrument timbre is somehow preserved, somehow depicted, in the subjects' auditory image and, moreover, that subjects ignored imaged timbre with great difficulty, because when misleading it actually disrupts performance.

This task is of special interest here because, as Crowder explicitly notes, it seems unlikely that subjects are able to subvocalize the relevant instrument timbres. Thus we would not expect the familiar pattern of Fig. 5.1-D with this task. Blocking subvocalization should not diminish Crowder's facilitation effect, since subvocalization should be irrelevant to timbre imagery. Instead, one expects the pattern of Fig. 5.1-B—a large facilitation effect when concurrent auditory input is absent (i.e., replicating Crowder's own findings), but a much smaller facilitation effect when auditory input is present (to block the use of the inner ear).

To test this hypothesis, Hespos (1989) first replicated the Crowder experiment. Subjects were presented with a sine wave plus a (visual) instruction to imagine a particular instrument playing that frequency; they were then presented with a test tone. For half of the trials, the test tone was the same frequency as the sine wave, for half it was not; for half of the trials, the test tone was the instrument expected, for half it was one of the other two instruments. Figure 5.2-A shows that this baseline condition replicated Crowder's and Crowder and Pitt's findings.

A second group of subjects performed this task in the presence of an irrelevant auditory distractor (a taped voice reading from an anthropology textbook). This irrelevant input was shut off during the presentation of the sine wave and the test tone, but otherwise it was continuously present. This ensured that the auditory distraction was not interfering with the registration of the test stimuli themselves.

A. Crowder replication

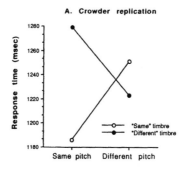

B. Pitch judgments in the presence
of unattended speech

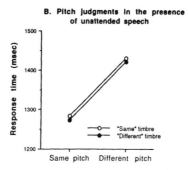

FIG. 5.2.   Reaction time (msec) for subjects to compare the pitch of imaged and actual tones. Panel A shows a replication of Crowder's (1989) findings. Panel B shows results from the same procedure run in the presence of unattended speech.

Figure 5.2-B shows that these conditions eliminated any effect of imagined timbre. That is, the facilitation from imagined timbre was devastated if irrelevant auditory input blocked the inner ear. This is exactly what one would expect if this task does rely on auditory imagery.[1]

Other subjects performed the Crowder task with concurrent articulation to block the inner voice. Subjects in the control group performed while tapping with their fingers. This allowed Hespos to control for any general distraction effects

---

[1]This result addresses a possible concern with the Crowder procedure. One could argue that Crowder's results are not attributable to auditory imagery at all, but reflect some sort of "startle" effect. If subjects are expecting a trumpet tone and hear a trumpet tone, there is no startle, and so response times will be quick. If subjects are expecting a trumpet tone and instead hear a flute, they may be momentarily startled, producing a slight RT disadvantage. The Hespos result seems to rule out this explanation. If startle causes the effect, then the inner ear plays no role in this task, and its disruption by the concurrent auditory input should have no consequences. If instead auditory imagery underlies this result, and not startle, then a concurrent auditory input should eliminate the RT advantage to a timbre match. The result clearly favors the latter account.

from the concurrent task. Summing across these two groups, the data replicate Crowder's findings of a pitch × timbre interaction; that is, the data show the effects of imaged timbre. Critically, this pattern is visible in both the 'tah-tah' and tapping groups—there is no interference type × pitch × timbre interaction. This result implies that the inner voice *is not* needed for timbre imagery, and suggests a sensible boundary to the usefulness of the inner-ear/inner-voice partnership. Perhaps it serves well for sounds which can be subvocalized, but not for others such as timbre.

However, the opposite conclusion was implied by some of Hespos' earlier procedures, when she blocked subvocalization by having subjects sip water through a thin straw. This eliminated the pitch × timbre interaction, and so implies that the inner voice *is* needed for timbre imagery. Since we cannot currently decide between these conflicting sets of data, the possibility remains open that subvocalization may aid in imagining even nonvocalizable sounds. Further studies will resolve the ambiguity attending this important theoretical issue.

The Specificity of Interference Effects

There is a pervasive methodological concern which poses a difficulty in interpreting all our interference data. That is, one must ask which of our manipulations are just generally distracting, and which disrupt specifically the inner ear or inner voice. Fortunately, this issue has received attention, and one can in most cases reject the general distraction hypothesis in both the case of the inner ear and the inner voice.

First, consider the inner ear. Its use is disrupted far more if the concurrent auditory input is phonologically similar to the imagined event. For example, in Salame and Baddeley (1982, 1983; also Baddeley, 1986), subjects were visually presented with digits to recall. During the presentation of the digits, subjects either sat in a quiet room, or heard irrelevant distractors. For some subjects, the distractors were irrelevant digits; others heard nonwords using the same phonemes as the digits (tun, woo, etc.); others heard irrelevant speech that was phonologically dissimilar to the digits (words like jelly, tipple, etc.). The digits and pseudodigits, both phonologically like the to-be-remembered items, caused severe disruption in recall performance; the phonologically dissimilar speech did not. If these inputs were merely distracting, then these results are puzzling: All three messages should have been equally distracting in a general sense; phonology should not have been critical. However, if the irrelevant inputs are specifically disrupting the inner ear (and if the inner ear draws on processes related to those of actual hearing), then it is sensible that the phonological properties of the inputs are critical.

At a practical level, we note that this specificity of interference can guide our choice of interference stimuli in designing imagery experiments. By employing interference that is similar to the to-be-imaged events, one can avoid a weak manipulation and therefore an insensitive design. To see how this matters, consider the following results: Reisberg et al. (1989) reported that reconstrual of speech images (e.g., stress/dress) was not eliminated if use of the inner ear was blocked by presentation of loud white noise. However, Wilson, Smith and Reisberg (unpublished) eliminated image reconstruals using speech heard through headphones as the concurrent auditory input. Superficially, these results conflict, but speech is obviously more similar to the imaged material in this procedure and therefore likely to be a more powerful blocker for the inner ear. Thus the seeming conflict between these two results is easily attributed to the strengths of the particular manipulations employed.

Now consider the case of the inner voice. It is disrupted far more if the articulators are occupied than if a variety of other motor tasks are given to distract the subject. For example, Baddeley (1986) described cases in which the impact of concurrent articulation tasks is compared with that of tapping a finger at a comparable rate. (Baddeley argued that this is the appropriate control since the concurrent articulation is also simple and repetitive—for example, "tah-tah-tah".) Consistently, finger-tapping and related control activities have minimal impact on subjects' performance, while concurrent articulation has considerable impact. Similarly, Reisberg et al. found that stress/dress reversals were eliminated given repetitions of Tah-Tah, but not eliminated given a repetitive tapping task. In an interesting twist on the specificity issue, Bick and Kinsbourne (1986) found that clamping the articulators reduced the hallucinated voices heard by schizophrenics, but a variety of motor controls with hands, eyes, etc., did not (see also Smith, this volume).

Thus we need to distinguish concurrent use of the inner voice from concurrent use of other motor systems. In fact, we may even need a finer distinction. That is, it may be that the inner voice is not a unitary entity that is always suppressed *in toto*. The skill of speaking requires various actions that are usually coordinated into the overall pattern of speech, but these actions can be separated to some extent—we can, for example, hum without moving the articulators, or we can pantomime speech (move the articulators) without voicing, and so forth. Similarly, perhaps different aspects of subvocalization can be isolated and run off separately. Thus the concurrent task of humming, for example, might block the use of covert voicing in subvocalization (or, more precisely, use of the control mechanisms for voicing), but might not block the use of other aspects of inner speech.

Our own research illustrates this point. In Reisberg et al.'s (1989) first experiment, subjects who chewed to block subvocalization showed few stress/dress reversals; subjects who hummed to block subvocalization tended to show more. This makes sense in hindsight, since the stress/dress reconstrual is more a reinterpretation of articulation and its segmentation, and less a judgment about voicing.

By the same reasoning, humming should disrupt imagery judgments that rely on the *voicing* facet of the inner voice, but not on articulation. Wilson, Smith & Reisberg (unpublished) instructed subjects in the difference between voiced and unvoiced consonants. Subjects then received a printed list of 36 one-syllable words, imagined how each would sound if pronounced, and then judged if the initial consonant was voiced or unvoiced. Subjects were 76% correct if this was their only task. Subjects were also somewhat successful if their articulators were clamped tightly shut (68%, not reliably different from 76%). However, performance dropped almost to chance levels if subjects were required to hum aloud while making these judgments (56% correct, reliably different from both 76% and 68%).

Apparently in the stress/dress task, subjects need information about the movement and positions of teeth, tongue and lips; this information is disrupted by chewing, but not by humming. For the voiced/unvoiced task, subjects need information about the vocal cords (or their control mechanism); access to this information is disrupted by humming but not by clamping the articulators. Thus, both of these require subvocalization, and blocking subvocalization disrupts performance in both. However, the subvocalization required in these tasks is quite different and relatively specific, and the interference tasks act in an appropriately specific way.

This pattern makes clear that these concurrent articulation effects are not merely generally distracting; if they were, we would not expect the specificity of these effects. And once again there is a practical consideration: specificity suggests that one might "tune" concurrent articulation tasks to block the relevant aspects of subvocalization, just as one might "tune" unattended auditory inputs to block the use of the inner ear.

Auditory Imagery and Memory Rehearsal

These methodological issues aside, we return now to the data themselves. The experiments described so far seem to show a widespread partnership between the inner ear and inner voice, and the pattern of results shown in Fig. 5.1-D. While these results were all obtained with auditory-imagery tasks, there is another domain in which the identical partnership obtains. That is, our results converge in striking fashion with the theoretical models and empirical results of Baddeley and other memory researchers.

It has long been known that there is a close relationship between short-term memory (or "working memory") and some sort of articulatory coding. For example, subjects in short-term memory tasks frequently err by substituting phonologically similar items for the correct ones (e.g., Conrad, 1964). Recall is also reduced if the to-be-remembered (TBR) items are phonologically similar to each other (e.g., Baddeley, 1966; Conrad & Hull, 1964), even with visually-presented materials. These effects are generally attributed to subvocal rehearsal of the TBR items, a process presumably related to the subvocalization we have been discussing here. This attribution is strengthened by Baddeley, Thomson and Buchanan's (1975) demonstration of the "word-length effect," in which memory span for words that can be pronounced quickly is greater than span for slowly-pronounced words (also Ellis & Henneley, 1980).

To explain these results, Baddeley and others have described a cognitive resource called the "articulatory rehearsal loop." This loop involves two components—subvocal rehearsal and a phonological store (Baddeley, Lewis & Vallar, 1984; Baddeley, 1986). The phonological store (the "inner ear") contains materials recently heard, or materials recently subvocalized (by the "inner voice").

Given this arrangement, consider how ordinary rehearsal would proceed. With a visual presentation, subvocalization is used to load the TBR materials into the phonological store; with auditory presentation, access to this store is automatic. Within a short time (1–2 seconds), the contents of the phonological store will decay, but subvocalization can be used to refresh the store's contents. This renewed presentation will itself soon decay, so that the cycle must be reinitiated.

It should be plain that this conception of working memory relies on a partnership between the inner ear and inner voice, just as does our conception of auditory imagery. (In fact, our conceptions of imagery have been strongly influenced by Baddeley's work. For related proposals, see Campbell, this volume; Caramazza, Berndt, & Basilli, 1983.) And it is this partnership model which successfully captures almost all the data on memory rehearsal outlined earlier.

For example, the word-length effect tells us that pronunciation speed affects memory span; this probably reflects the operation of subvocalization. In contrast, phonologically similar materials are presumably being confused within the phonological buffer. Thus the inner ear is the likely source for subjects' difficulty in remembering phonologically confuseable lists, and for the phonological confusions in the recall itself.

On this proposal, one should eliminate the word-length effect if one prevents the use of subvocalization. This prediction is correct: If subjects must remember word lists while also doing a concurrent articulation task, the word-length effect does not appear in the recall data (Baddeley, 1986; Baddeley et al., 1984; Vallar & Baddeley, 1982). Whether this manipulation also removes phonological confusions depends on how the TBR material is presented. If one *hears* the TBR material, this provides direct access to the phonological buffer. Alternatively, if one initially *sees* the TBR material, the material must enter the inner ear via covert articulation. This leads to two predictions: If phonological confusions occur in the inner ear, and if subvocalization is needed to "load" visually presented materials into the inner ear, then, with visual presentation, a concurrent articulation task should eliminate phonological confusions. Concurrent articulation should not remove phonological confusions with auditory presentation—because items can enter the inner ear directly, and be confused there, with or without subvocalization. Both of these predictions have been confirmed (Baddeley, 1986; Baddeley, Lewis, & Vallar, 1984).

Finally, we know that unattended speech input decreases short term memory span. This is presumably because the unattended inputs have obligatory access to the phonological store, making difficult its use for maintenance rehearsal. Concurrent articulation also decreases span, presumably by blocking subvocalization and so eliminating rehearsal. However, the effects of unattended speech and concurrent articulation are not additive. With either manipulation on the scene, adding the second manipulation has no further effect. This is precisely what one would expect if both the inner voice and the inner ear are required for rehearsal: blocking the use of either is just as bad as blocking the use of both. (Baddeley, 1986, discusses the evidence for these assertions, as well as other evidence relevant to this conception of working memory and of rehearsal. See also Richardson, 1984).

To summarize all of this, subjects' use of the articulatory loop once again fits the pattern depicted in Fig. 5.1-D. That is, memory rehearsal requires both the inner ear and the inner voice.[2] Thus these data provide yet another domain in which subvocalization seems an essential partner of auditory imagery.

"Auditory Imagery" Without the Inner Ear

Not all of the tasks we have explored require the inner voice and inner ear in concert. Timbre imagery may be one case where the inner voice is irrelevant to successful performance. One can also find tasks where the inner ear seems irrelevant. For example, in one of our studies subjects were instructed that "some words that end in 's' sound as if they end in 'z'." Subjects were then given a printed list of words (larks, dogs, halves, cats. . .) and had to judge whether each word, if read aloud, would be pronounced with a final "s" or "z" sound. Different groups of subjects made these judgments with concurrent articulation, with concurrent auditory input, with both, or with neither. The concurrent articulation and the unattended auditory input both involved repetitions of the word "Suzie," pronounced by the subject in the former condition, heard on a tape recorder in the latter. (Given the potential specificity of interference manipulations, as discussed earlier), we made the interference stimuli as similar as possible to the images required for the focal task, to maximize the strength of the manipulations.)

In a related study, subjects were told that "some words that end with 'ed' can be pronounced as if they ended with 't' instead." Subsequently, subjects judged whether each of a list of words (marched, raised, walked. . .) was pronounced with a "t" or "ed" sound. The concurrent articulation and the unattended auditory input in this case both involved repetitions (pronounced by the subject or heard) of the word "Teddy."

---

[2]To put this more precisely, this particular form of memory rehearsal shows this pattern. So-called elaborative rehearsal (e.g., Craik & Watkins, 1973) may show a rather different profile; other forms of "maintenance" rehearsal that don't involve articulation may also be available to subjects.

Figures 5.3-A and 5.3-B show the results from the s/z and d/t tasks, respectively. Concurrent auditory input had no impact on performance. In contrast, concurrent articulation appreciably reduced performance, though not disastrously. In both tasks the data assumed the pattern depicted in Fig. 5.1-A, implying that the inner voice is needed for optimal performance, but not the inner ear.

Subvocalization's Role in Auditory Imagery

The pattern of results in the s/z and d/t procedures clearly contrasts with that in which the inner voice and inner ear cooperate during an auditory imagery task. This implies that subvocalization may play two different roles in tasks involving judgments about sound or pronunciation. In some tasks, subvocalization alone is sufficient for optimal performance. In other tasks, subvocalization acts in concert with the inner ear. For each of these patterns, though, we still need to ask about the *function* of subvocalization. How does subvocalization, acting alone, support the s/z and d/t judgments? And how, in our other tasks, does it "load" (or otherwise interact with) the inner ear? We turn now to both these roles for subvocalization.

One function of subvocalization could simply be to provide kinesthetic cues. This was originally our preferred explanation for the Reisberg et al. (1989) results, in which subjects who subvocalized could reconstrue ambiguous phonological streams (like stress/dress). We believed then that the events of motor production or motor planning gave subjects a kinesthetic stimulus that supported

Performance in judging whether words spelled with "s" are pronounced with "s" or "z"

		Available	90%	78%
Inner				
Ear				
		Blocked	94%	85%

Possible Blocked
Inner Speech

FIG. 5.3.   Selective interference results when subjects judge how the ending of (visually) presented words would be pronounced—whether with an "s" or "z" (top panel), or whether with an "ed" or "t" (bottom panel).

Performance in judging whether words spelled with "ed" are pronounced with "ed" or "t"

		Available	84%	70%
Inner				
Ear				
		Blocked	85%	77%

Possible Blocked
Inner Speech

the reinterpretation process. These kinesthetic cues were neutral, uninterpreted events which could be reconsulted and reconstrued. As it turns out, though, this view was wrong, since we now know that listening to concurrent speech also disrupts this reconstrual process.

However, we can accept a kinesthetic explanation for some tasks, namely those in which subvocalization is sufficient for performance (as in the s/z task). It seems likely that subjects pronounce these stimuli to themselves, and then use the kinesthetic feedback from this pronunciation to make their judgments. This would explain why subjects do not need to listen to this pronunciation with the inner ear, hence the lack of any effect of unattended speech.

Having explained the s/z and d/t tasks in this way, one might even suggest that they are not tasks, or rather need not be tasks, of auditory imagery proper. They are more like judgments about the behavior of one's articulators. Perhaps kinesthesis alone is sufficient for these judgments because they rely on detecting a single simple property of the vocal chords (which is the main difference between pronunciation of the final s and z, or t and d). This is a point however on which further research is needed.

These kinesthetic tasks aside, what is the role of subvocalization in the various "partnership" tasks we have described ("NE1 4 10S;" stress/dress; the melody task, and so on)? In these tasks, as we have seen, kinesthetic cues are not enough. The cost to performance from disruption of the inner ear makes this plain. Instead, it seems that silent speech, or possibly an unrealized motor plan for speech, somehow produces a representation which can be interpreted by mechanisms overlapping with the mechanisms of ordinary hearing. The simple-minded explanation of this is that central mechanisms (neurons, nodes, units) for speech are connected directly to central mechanisms (neurons, nodes, units) for auditory perception. This connection is suggested by several of our experiments and is also made plausible by the substantial evidence implicating covert speech production in speech perception. (Liberman & Mattingly, 1985, provide a recent review of this evidence.)

One can speculate on the exact nature of these central connections. It is believed that the motor plan for a speech act includes a variety of auxiliary representations which will be used to control and check the speech produced (Zivin, 1986). For example, there may be corollary discharge that provides a feedforward signal from motor plans to sensory systems, serving to prepare the latter for the proprioceptive consequences of the movement. A planned speech act could also prime the auditory perceptual system. This acoustic feedforward signal would provide a crucial later check on the auditory correctness of the speech act.

Mechanisms such as these would allow the inner voice to load the inner ear in exactly the sense required by our experimental results. For present purposes, we need not be concerned with the exact form of the connection between speech and hearing, nor with the exact function served by this connection in ordinary speech production. For our purposes, what is critical is that the mechanisms of speech production and speech perception probably rely on each other in diverse ways. In such connections could lie the interaction between inner speech and inner ear that our experiments reveal.

However, these explanations provide a connection between subvocalization and *speech* imagery, not between subvocalization and imagery for other classes of sounds. Yet, as we have seen, subvocalization is also implicated in imagery for pitch (Wilson, 1988; Wilson, Smith & Reisberg, unpublished) and perhaps also in imagery for timbre (Hespos, 1989). In fact, there must be whole classes of sounds which one can imagine but cannot subvocalize, such as the sounds of brakes squealing, or glass breaking. If not subvocalizable, then imagery for these sounds should not be dependent on the inner voice. Yet, as we have noted, it remains possible that subvocalization does aid imagery processes even for these kinds of sounds. We consider briefly the ways in which this might occur, using the example of instrument timbre. This discussion will illuminate several points about the nature and (potential) function of subvocalization.

First, perhaps subjects *can* imitate instrument timbres (and other sounds of this kind), despite claims to the contrary. In this case, subjects could support their imagery with subvocalization, and therefore concurrent articulation should disrupt performance. We do not need to assume here that subjects can vocalize persuasive, realistic instrument imitations. Even mediocre ones might be enough to recreate the reaction-time pattern of perceived timbre. As long as the subvocalized (and so the imaged) trumpet resembled a trumpet tone more than it did other instruments, it might speed comparisons to a perceived trumpet tone, relative to comparisons with other perceived timbres. As a different (but related) possibility, subjects may be able to *plan* these vocalizations, even if they lack the skills or structures to execute the plan. In this case, it would be the motor plan that "loads" the inner ear, and the formation of this plan that is blocked by manipulations of inner speech.

Second, perhaps the subvocalization of the pitch provides a tonal frame, or amplitude envelope, which is then colored to particular timbral specifications by the inner ear. By this view, it might be impossible to hang imagined spectral characteristics onto thin air, but easily possible to assemble them onto an existing, subvocalized pitch. In that event, subvocalization would merely be the carrier wave of the auditory image, and the function of the inner ear would be to modulate that carrier in trumpet-like or flute-like ways. Once again, this claim provides a role for subvocalization and, therefore, an explanation of concurrent articulation's impact.

Our third proposal has a different flavor. Perhaps when the articulators are active (even soundlessly), they have a privileged access in loading the inner ear fairly automatically and obligatorily. As mentioned earlier, Baddeley (1986) has argued that auditory inputs have obligatory access to the inner ear; perhaps the same is true for the products of subvocalization. In this case, our concurrent articulation tasks do not interfere by virtue of preventing subvocalization of the instrument timbres; instead, concurrent articulation loads its own output into the inner ear, and so *displaces* the images of the timbres. Thus, for subjects to create trumpet (and other) timbral images, the requirement may simply be that the articulatory apparatus "shut up" and hold still while the image unfolds. Readers may consult their intuitions on this point. They may notice that in imagining a trumpet tone, an extraordinary stillness descends over the articulators—the mouth may be frozen half-open. (To us this resembles what happens when we listen intently for distant, faint sounds.) Here the idea would be that the auditory imagery system must assume a listening pose to conjure images, and one aspect of this is to still the articulatory mechanism. This discussion calls attention to the fact that there are two distinct classes of explanation for why blocking the inner voice can hurt performance in an auditory imagery task. There is a "Hum-The-First-Few-Bars" explanation, which actually views the subvoice as having a positive role in building the auditory image. The first two of the hypotheses just sketched fall into this category. Then there is the "Shut-Up-I'm-Listening" explanation, in which the inner voice has no positive role, but has the privileged capacity to interrupt processes which would otherwise occur within the inner ear. We hope that further research will allow us to disambiguate these different possibilities.

"Auditory Imagery" Without the Inner Voice or Inner Ear

All of these tasks we have considered thus far have been somehow linked to subvocalization. But this linkage is not universal among tasks involving judgments about sound. Consider the task of deciding if these letter strings would be pronounced like actual English words: "CAYOSS," or "CHARE." Do these pairs of strings sound alike: "raise" and "rays," or "hedge" and "hej"? Decisions like these seem to require judgments about phonology; they presumably cannot be made on the basis of visual information alone. Moreover, subjects have the intuition that they use auditory imagery to answer questions like these— they "hear" in their minds what these strings would sound like if pronounced. This leads us to ask about the role of the inner voice and inner ear in these tasks.

Homophone judgments seem barely to require subvocalization. That is, subjects perform these tasks well even if required to do a concurrent articulation task. In some studies, concurrent articulation has no effect on either speed or accuracy of these judgments (Baddeley & Lewis, 1981; Besner et al., 1981, Exp. 5). In other cases, the suppression of articulation hurts accuracy (never speed) slightly, but leaves subjects still quite accurate (Baddeley & Lewis, 1981; Besner et al., 1981, Exp. 6). In addition, Besner and Davelaar (1982) found a reliable advantage in the recall of pseudohomophones (like phlaim) that persisted despite the suppression of articulation. Even with children, the pattern seems the same: Mitterer (1982) found that young readers classified pseudohomophones as words more than nonword controls. This effect, often attributed to phonological recoding, was not reduced by suppressing subarticulation.

This independence from the inner voice sets homophone judgments apart from all the tasks we have surveyed. One might therefore argue that homophone judgments use "pure" auditory images, closely allied to the inner ear. In essence, subjects may be able to take these visually presented words and create an image of each word's pronunciation by drawing on information already in secondary memory. This information could be a specific memory of a familiar word's pronunciation, or memory for phonological rules (supporting imagery of nonwords). With this (memory) route into the inner ear, subjects would not need to rely on subvocalization. Therefore, we would expect the data pattern shown in Fig. 5.1-B, with performance immune to manipulations of the inner voice, but disrupted by manipulations of the inner ear.

Unfortunately, though, this "inner ear" account does not go through. Baddeley and Salame (1986) asked subjects to make homophone judgments while hearing an unattended auditory input. This manipulation, the classic one for blocking the inner ear, left performance unscathed, implying that the "inner ear" is no more required for these judgments than is the inner voice!

It therefore seems that the phonological representations that afford homophone judgments do not reside in the inner ear. So where are they? One possibility is that the relevant representations "move around," in the following sense. The literature tells us that these homophone tasks are immune to disruption of either the inner voice or inner ear *alone*. Perhaps, though, subjects can make homophone judgments using *either* the inner voice *or* the inner ear, and simply switch strategies depending on which variety of interference is on the scene. Then their pattern would be that of Fig.5.1-C. They would be able to cope with either kind of interference alone. Only in the case of both interference tasks, delivered simultaneously, would performance fall off, because strategy switching would no longer be possible.

Alternatively, perhaps homophone judgments need neither the inner ear nor the inner voice. They might use some other phonological store, one that is not disrupted by the manipulations that affect what we (and many others) call the inner ear. Then subjects would show the pattern of results shown in Fig. 5.1-E: Even with both interference tasks on the scene, performance should stay intact. Obviously the crucial condition for distinguishing 1-C and 1-E is that with both kinds of interference present. To our knowledge, subjects have never been run under this double phonological jeopardy, and so we attempted to clarify this situation.

Subjects made 24 homophone judgments under each of four conditions: while rapidly repeating the digits 1 to 6, while hearing irrelevant speech through headphones, while receiving both interference tasks at once, and while receiving neither. In this within-subject design, the order of conditions was completely counterbalanced across subjects.

As Fig. 5.4-A shows, latency was unaffected by the presence or absence of either interference task. Accuracy was unaffected by irrelevant speech heard, but was decreased slightly (7%) by blocking subvocalization. What is critical for our purposes, however, is that performance stayed robust even given both kinds of interference simultaneously—performance is still fast in that condition, with 82% accuracy, only 7% below subjects' accuracy with no interference.

Given robust performance in all conditions, one wonders whether the homophone task was too easy or the interference manipulations too weak. We know, however, that identical manipulations are strong enough to have clear impact on other imagery tasks. As for task difficulty, note that the subjects were only at 89% accurate with no interference, not at ceiling. Moreover, judgments of rhyme—very similar to homophone judgments and equally easy—are disrupted by interference (Besner, 1987; Wilding & White, 1985).

This confirms that homophone judgments follow the pattern of Fig. 5.1-E, not Figure 5.1-C. Nonetheless, it seems likely that these judgments do require phonological information, which must reside in some store. All of this together implies the availability of a phonological store separate from what we have called the inner ear, and, more important, one that is immune to the kinds of suppression usually taken to disrupt the inner ear and inner voice.

With Besner and others, therefore, we conclude that there are at least two types of phonological representation underlying phenomena such as memory

Time to complete 24 judgments (seconds)

Available	**30.5**	**30.8**
Blocked	**29.8**	**31.6**

Inner Ear (rows); Possible / Blocked Inner Speech (columns)

Percent Correct

Available	**89%**	**83%**
Blocked	**89%**	**82%**

Inner Ear (rows); Possible / Blocked Inner Speech (columns)

FIG. 5.4. Selective interference results with a homophone task. The top panel shows response latencies (sec); the bottom panel shows accuracy data (percent correct).

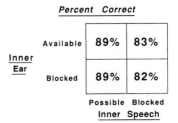

rehearsal, auditory imagery, and related tasks. One of these, the inner ear, is associated with the word length and phonological similarity effects in span, and many of the auditory imagery phenomena we have described here. The inner ear is disrupted by auditory inputs (attended or not) and also appears to be closely tied to the inner voice. That is, articulatory suppression prevents the utilization of this store whenever the relevant stimuli are presented visually. The other form of representation, on the other hand, provides a kind of "lexical ear." It permits lexical access, and these representations can be formed directly from print (or from memory), via some mechanism that does not require subvocalization and the inner voice. (For related findings and discussion, see Baddeley & Salame, 1986; Besner, 1987; Kleiman, 1975; Wilding & White, 1985.)[3] The homophone tasks are the dominant evidence for this second phonological store.

How does this "lexical ear" fit into discussions of auditory imagery? Should we reserve the "imagery" label for the inner-ear/inner-voice team? In this case, we would need to say that the homophone tasks do not draw on auditory imagery, but are accomplished by some other route (e.g., abstract orthographic or pho-nological memory). We note the parallel here to arguments raised by Pylyshyn (e.g., 1981) about visual imagery: Not all tasks concerning visual appearance need draw on visual imagery. In the same spirit, not all tasks concerning sound need draw on auditory imagery. However, we resist simply stipulating that au-ditory imagery requires use of the inner ear, and thus is disrupted by unattended auditory inputs. It seems to us that this is not an issue to be prejudged, and, moreover, we are not certain that much is at stake in deciding to dub this or that store "imagery." For now, we note only that subjects do report that they perform these homophone tasks by covertly "listening" to what the words "sound like." If we use that bit of phenomology as our arbiter, then these tasks do fall within the bounds of imagery.

Whether or not this second phonological store fits one's definition of auditory imagery, there are several interesting issues surrounding it. What is the represen-tational format of this lexical ear? What are the limits on its use? What deter-mines whether a task is served by representations in this store, or by representa-tions in the inner ear? To put the same question in operational terms, what determines whether a task will show the no-interference pattern of Fig. 5.1-E (apparently diagnostic of the lexical ear) or the partnership pattern of Fig. 5.1-D

---

[3]Related data are available from subjects who are unable to speak (anarthric or dysarthric) due to some brain trauma. Despite their lacking overt speech (and perhaps also subvocalization), these subjects are able to do the homophone tasks just described. However, these data are difficult to interpret, given the possibility of an intact capacity in these patients for forming the motor plans for speech, even given the absence of external speech. The interested reader might look at the data in Baddeley and Wilson (1985), Bishop and Robson (1989), or Nebes (1975). For comparison data with *aphasic* patients, see Feinberg, Gonzalez Rothi and Heilman (1986) and Levin, Calvanio and Popovics (1982).

(diagnostic of the inner ear)? We can briefly summarize one current theory on this point.

Besner (1987) argues that the "lexical ear" is sharply limited in several ways. It can access only whole-word phonological units in long term memory. Any operations performed on a phonological code—such as phonemic segmentation and deletion processes, or maintenance in working memory—will not be possible with this whole-word phonological activator. If a task requires these latter operations, then the task will require the inner ear, and not the lexical ear. And, in this case, given the relation between the inner ear and inner voice, performance will be blocked by concurrent articulation.

This proposal explains why, even though homophone judgments survive interference manipulations, closely related tasks do not. Judgments about rhyme, for example, are hurt when articulation is suppressed. These judgments require the post-lexical analysis of phonological representations, in order to ignore word-initial sounds and to compare word endings. Apparently the lexical ear cannot perform these analyses and comparisons; instead, the inner ear is required, and so interference effects surface again.

Given this claim, one might imagine a continuum (or at least an ordered series) of tasks, differing in how much post-lexical analysis they require. At one end of the continuum would be the homophone judgments, requiring only that a whole phonological representation be awakened, with no post-lexical analysis. For such tasks, a representation in the lexical ear would be sufficient, making the tasks immune to our interference manipulations. Judgments of rhyme, on the other hand, would occupy a position closer to the "analysis-needed" end of the continuum, and so demand the services of the inner ear. As a result, these tasks would be vulnerable to interference tasks.

Similar reasoning might apply to our other imagery tasks. The stress/dress task involves reassigning word boundaries; the "NE1 4 10S" task requires building a phonological string from syllables up. Both of these tasks would therefore, on this account, be expected to suffer interference effects; this obviously fits with the data we have reported. One might even speculate that breaking down a familiar tune to determine relative pitches constitutes a segmentation procedure. Given this description, this task also should (and does) show interference effects.

This last point, concerning pitch judgments, raises the possibility that this second phonological store, the lexical ear, is not restricted to the domain of text, or language, or orthography. (Note, in this case, that *lexical* ear would be too narrow a label for this store.) Perhaps this store can carry any representation of sound which can be activated intact and without analysis, from information in long-term memory. Thus, familiar tunes, or any other well-learned auditory sequence, might also have access to this store. Then if tasks drew on this representation (without requirement for further analysis), they would also (like the homophone judgments) be immune to interference effects. This seems a good direction for future research and could greatly enhance the idea that one store consists of "awakened" whole sound representations, while the other store is needed for transformations on, and analysis of, those whole representations.

All of this leaves us, though, with a crucial question: Why is the inner-voice/inner-ear partnership crucial for transforming and analyzing auditory representations? Why is it that subvocalization will support tasks that the lexical ear will not? Our broad suggestion is that certain tasks require "stimulus support" of one sort or another. That is, certain judgments, or certain analyses, require an actual stimulus input. In the absence of some independently occurring stimulus, the subject can *create* a stimulus, via some motoric output (or some motor plan) which then has consequences detectable by the channels of perception. In the particular case of the inner voice (and consistent with our comments on pp. 98–101), subvocalization provides something closely akin to an auditory stimulus for the subject, a stimulus in this case with an existence independent of the subject's understanding of it or operations on it. It is precisely such a stimulus that is needed for tasks requiring that whole representations be transformed or analyzed. We hope, though, that further research will provide more detail about the function of the covert stimulus in auditory imagery.

Summary and Conclusion

In our exploration of auditory imagery, our ideas have evolved considerably. We began with the hope of generalizing visual imagery results into the auditory domain. Then a role for subvocalization emerged as a surprising result for particular tasks. Next the data forced the view that auditory imagery and subvocalization are quite intimately connected, and we have begun to explore the reasons for this partnership and the purpose it serves. We close with the hope that work like ours, and volumes like this one, will bring to auditory imagery greater interest among cognitive psychologists. From our perspective, the issue is no longer one of generalizing theory to visual imagery's poor relation. For we now know that auditory imagery is a rich phenomenon in its own right, especially given its many ties to memory, music, speech and language, to the voices of schizophrenics, and perhaps even to the inner voices of our conscious selves.

REFERENCES

Baddeley, A. D. (1966). Short-term memory for word sequences as a function of acoustic, semantic and formal similarity. *Quarterly Journal of Experimental Psychology, 18,* 362–365.

Baddeley, A. D. (1986). *Working Memory.* Oxford: Clarendon Press.

Baddeley, A. D., & Lewis, V. (1981). Inner active processes in reading: The inner voice, the inner ear and the inner eye. In A. M. Lesgold & C. A. Perfetti (Eds.), *Interactive processes in reading* (pp. 107–129). Hillsdale, NJ: Lawrence Erlbaum Associates.

Baddeley, A. D., Lewis, V., & Vallar, G. (1984). Exploring the articulatory loop. *Quarterly Journal of Experimental Psychology, 36A*, 233–252.

Baddeley, A. D., & Salame, P. (1986). The unattended speech effect: Perception or memory? *Journal of Experimental Psychology: Learning, Memory and Cognition, 12*, 525–529.

Baddeley, A. D., Thomson, N., & Buchanan, M. (1975). Word length and the structure of short-term memory. *Journal of Verbal Learning and Verbal Behavior, 14*, 575–589.

Baddeley, A. D. & Wilson, B. (1985). Phonological coding and short-term memory in patients without speech. *Journal of Memory and Language, 24*, 490–502.

Besner, D. (1987). Phonology, lexical access in reading, and articulatory suppression: A critical review. *Quarterly Journal of Experimental Psychology, 39A*, 467–478.

Besner, D., & Davelaar, E. (1982). Basic processes in reading: Two phonological codes. *Canadian Journal of Psychology, 36*, 701–711.

Besner, D., Davies, J., & Daniels, S. (1981). Reading for meaning: The effects of concurrent articulation. *Quarterly Journal of Experimental Psychology, 33*, 415–437.

Bick, P. & Kinsbourne, M. (1986). Auditory hallucinations and subvocal speech in schizophrenic patients. *American Journal of Psychiatry, 144*, 222–225.

Bishop, D., & Robson, J. (1989). Unimpaired short-term memory and rhyme judgment in congenitally speechless individuals: Implications for the notion of "articulatory coding." *Quarterly Journal of Experimental Psychology, 41A*, 123–140.

Caramazza, A., Berndt, R., & Basilli, A. (1983). The selective impairment of phonological processing: A case study. *Brain and Language, 18*, 128–174.

Casey, E. (1976). *Imagining: A phenomenologial study.* Bloomington, IN: Indiana University Press.

Chambers, D., & Reisberg, D. (1985). Can mental images be ambiguous? *Journal of Experimental Psychology: Human Perception and Performance, 11*, 317–328.

Conrad, R. (1964). Acoustic confusion in immediate memory. *British Journal of Psychology, 55*, 75–84.

Conrad, R., & Hull, A. J. (1964). Information, acoustic confusion and memory span. *British Journal of Psychology, 55*, 429–432.

Craik, F. I. M., & Watkins, M. J. (1973). The role of rehearsal in short-term memory. *Journal of Verbal Learning and Verbal Behavior, 12*, 599–607.

Crowder, R. (1989). Imagery for musical timbre. *Journal of Experimental Psychology: Human Perception and Performance, 15*, 472–478.

Ellis, N. C., & Hennely, R. A. (1980). A bilingual word-length effect: Implications for intelligence testing and the relative ease of mental calculation in Welsh and English. *British Journal of Psychology, 71*, 43–52.

Feinberg, T., Gonzalez Rothi, L., & Heilman, K. (1986). "Inner speech" in conduction aphasia. *Archives of Neurology, 43*, 591–593.

Finke, R. A. (1980). Levels of equivalence in imagery and perception. *Psychological Review, 87*, 113–132.

Finke, R., Pinker, S., & Farah, M. (1989). Reinterpreting visual patterns in mental imagery. *Cognitive Science, 13*, 51–78.

Fodor, J. (1981). Imagistic representation. In N. Block (Ed.), *Imagery* (pp. 63–86). Cambridge, MA: MIT Press.

Hespos, S. (1989). *The characteristics of pitch, timbre and loudness in auditory imagery.* Unpublished bachelor's thesis, Reed College, Portland, OR.

Kleiman, G. (1975). Speech recoding in reading. *Journal of Verbal Learning and Verbal Behavior, 14*, 323–339.

Kolers, P., & Smythe, W. (1984). Symbol manipulation: Alternatives to the computational view of mind. *Journal of Verbal Learning and Verbal Behavior, 23*, 289–314.

Kosslyn, S. M. (1980). *Image and mind.* Cambridge, MA: Harvard University Press.

Kosslyn, S. M. (1983). *Ghosts in the mind's machine.* New York: W. W. Norton.

Levine, D., Calvanio, R., & Popovics, A. (1982). Language in the absence of inner speech. *Neuropsychologia, 20,* 391–409.

Levy, B. (1971). The role of articulation in auditory and visual short-term memory. *Journal of Verbal Learning and Verbal Behavior, 10,* 123–132.

Liberman, A., & Mattingly, I. (1985). The motor theory of speech perception revised. *Cognition, 21,* 1–36.

Mitterer, J. (1982). There are at least two kinds of poor readers: Whole-word poor readers and recoding poor readers. *Canadian Journal of Psychology, 36,* 445–461.

Murray, D. (1968). Articulation and acoustic confusability in short-term memory. *Journal of Experimental Psychology, 78,* 679–684.

Nebes, R. (1975). The nature of internal speech in a patient with aphemia. *Brain and Language, 2,* 489–497.

Pylyshyn, Z. (1981). The imagery debate: Analogue media versus tacit knowledge. *Psychological Review, 88,* 16–45.

Reisberg, D., & Chambers, D. (1991). Neither pictures nor propositions: What can we learn from a mental image? *Canadian Journal of Psychology, 45,* 336–352.

Reisberg, D., & Morris, A. (1985). Images contain what the imager put there: A non-replication of illusions in imagery. *Bulletin of the Psychonomic Society, 23,* 493–496.

Reisberg, D., Smith, J. D., Baxter, D. A., & Sonenshine, M. (1989). "Enacted" auditory images are ambiguous; "Pure" auditory images are not. *The Quarterly Journal of Experimental Psychology, 41A,* 619–641.

Richardson, J. (1984). Developing the theory of working memory. *Memory and Cognition, 12,* 71–83.

Salame, P., & Baddeley, A. D. (1982). Disruption of short-term memory by unattended speech: Implications for the structure of working memory. *Journal of Verbal Learning and Verbal Behavior, 21,* 150–164.

Salame, P., & Baddeley, A. D. (1983). Differential effects of noise and speech on short-term memory. *Proceedings of the Fourth International Congress on Noise as a Public Health Problem* (pp. 751–758). Milam: Centro di Ricerche di Studi Amplifon.

Segal, S. J., & Fusella, V. (1970). Influence of imaged pictures and sounds in detection of visual and auditory signals. *Journal of Experimental Psychology, 83,* 458–474.

Slowiaczek, M., & Clifton, C. (1980). Subvocalization and reading for meaning. *Journal of Verbal Learning and Verbal Behavior, 19,* 573–582.

Vallar, G., & Baddeley, A. D. (1982). Short-term forgetting and the articulatory loop. *Quarterly Journal of Experimental Psychology, 34,* 53–60.

Warren, R. (1961). Illusory changes of distinct speech upon repetition - the verbal transformation effect. *British Journal of Psychology, 52,* 249.

Warren, R. (1982). *Auditory perception.* N.Y.: Pergamon Press.

Warren, R., & Gregory, R. (1958). An auditory analogue of the visual reversible figure. *American Journal of Psychology, 71,* 612–613.

Wilding, J., & White, W. (1985). Impairment of rhyme judgments by silent and overt articulatory suppression. *Quarterly Journal of Experimental Psychology, 37A,* 95–107.

Wilson, M. (1988). *The role of subvocalization in inner speech.* Unpublished bachelor's thesis, Reed College, Portland, OR.

Wilson, M., Smith, J. D., & Reisberg, D. (unpublished). *The role of subvocalized speech in auditory imagery.*

Zivin, G. (1986). Image or neural coding of inner speech and agency? *The Behavioral and Brain Sciences, 9,* 534–535.

6 Constraints on Theories of Inner Speech

Donald G. MacKay
University of California, Los Angeles

Many people report that they can produce speech without moving their lips, and are consciously aware of this internal speech when they solve problems, read, write, or plan their everyday activities (Weisberg, 1980). The experience of inner speech is virtually universal among adults and has played a major role in psychological theory (Dell & Repka, in press). Some psychologists have viewed inner speech as identical to thought (e.g., Watson, 1950), while others have viewed inner speech as a side effect or necessary concommitant of thought (e.g., Sokolov, 1972). Psychologists have also viewed the long-term storage of information as dependent on inner speech or covert rehearsal, as when one silently repeats a telephone number in order to facilitate later recall (Atkinson & Shiffrin, 1968). Few, if any, psychologists probably continue to view the relation between inner speech, memory, and thought in just these ways, but all agree on the importance of inner speech, which, under various names, remains a central construct in psychological theories. For example, units resembling those required for producing inner speech are said to underlie writing (Ellis, 1988), typing (MacKay, in press), and the rehearsal and short-term storage of verbal materials (Baddeley, 1990).

This chapter reviews some fundamental phenomena that must be addressed in theories of inner speech. I begin with the problem of representation: What is the nature of the units underlying the production and experience of inner speech? Three basic representational constraints are addressed:

1. The units involved in inner speech: Internal speech errors, the time to produce sentences internally, and transfer of practice effects indicate that like

overt speech, inner speech involves phonological, morphological, lexical and phrase level units.

2. The nonarticulatory nature of inner speech: Neurolinguistic disorders and experiments on internally produced tongue twisters indicate that movements, however small, of the lips, tongue, velum, and other muscle systems are irrelevant to inner speech. Even the lowest level units for inner speech are highly abstract, representing a range of cognitive activities involving very different muscles (e.g., speech, writing, and typing) or no muscles whatsoever (e.g., language comprehension).

3. The nonauditory nature of inner speech: Theories postulating an auditory code for the "inner ear" must address methodological and theoretical criticisms discussed here, and must explain various differences between internal speech perception and the acoustics of overt speech.

Relations between the perception and production of overt and inner speech pose additional constraints addressed here. An example is: *The irrelevance of motor activity to internal speech:* Viable theories of inner speech must explain why the electromyographic activity that accompanies inner speech is unnecessary for either acquiring or experiencing inner speech. In addition, the theory must explain a set of dissociations between motor abilities and the experience of inner speech. Traditional theoretical approaches to relations between the perception and production of internal speech are discussed with respect to such criteria, and are found wanting.

The role of inner speech in the perception and immediate recall of visual stimuli suggests further constraints for theories of internal speech, as do relations between memory and rehearsed or repeated internal speech. Examples are:

1. *Unrehearsability:* Theories of inner speech must explain why language is sometimes rehearsable, and sometimes not. How, for example, can someone unfamiliar with German accurately rehearse a German word such as /gelb/, but not a German trilled /r/.

2. *Rehearsal and volition:* Theories of inner speech must explain why inner rehearsal is sometimes involuntary and difficult to control.

3. *Effects of overt versus internal rehearsal on speech production:* An interesting set of similarities and differences in the effects of overt versus internal rehearsal on overt speech production provide additional constraints on theories of inner speech.

This chapter begins by reviewing available data bearing on four fundamental issues that theories of inner speech must address: (a) What is the nature or representational character of internal speech?; (b) what is the relation between the perceptual and generative components of internal speech?; (c) how does internal speech relate to overt speech?; (d) and what role does internal speech play in cognitive processes such as the perception of visual stimuli and memory for verbal materials? Although some of these issues are far from resolved, the data reviewed here suggest important constraints that theories of internal speech, present and future, must address.

THE NATURE OF INTERNAL SPEECH

Phenomenal reports of inner speech generally include two components: a "generative" component (i.e., people report selecting the words of inner speech in a way that seems to resemble overt speech production) and an "auditory" component (i.e., people report hearing internally produced words in their "mind's ear"). These "perceptual" and "generative" components may in reality be largely inseparable (see MacKay, 1987, pp. 1–38), but are treated separately here for historic and didactic reasons.

The Generative Component of Internal Speech

As discussed below, direct evidence for the generative component of inner speech comes from the one observable aspect of mental imagery in general, and inner speech in particular: the electromyographic (EMG) activity in the muscles that occurs during mental imagery and covert rehearsal (Jackson, 1930; Sokolov, 1972). A major, as yet unsolved theoretical issue connected with this generative component is how speakers are able to intentionally evoke internal speech.

What Kinds of Units are Involved in Internal Speech?   Evidence on the nature of the units involved in inner speech comes from two sources. One is the errors that speakers detect during internal speech. In preliminary observations, Meringer and Meyer (1895) reported several instances of mental errors detected in their own internal speech and noted that these errors closely resembled those that occur during overt speech. Extending these observations, Dell (1978, 1980) had subjects produce tongue twisters such as "Unique New York" from memory at fixed rates, either aloud or mentally, and report the errors that they detected. The same types of errors were reported during internal speech as during overt speech, usually anticipations, perseverations and reversals of phonological components, but sometimes also anticipations, perseverations or reversals of lexical and morphological components. The recent and more extensive study of Dell & Repka (in press) used the same procedures as Dell's earlier studies and also observed identical types of errors in inner and overt speech. This correspondence of the units underlying inner and overt errors indicates that like overt speech, inner speech involves phonological, morphological and lexical units.

The second source of evidence (MacKay, 1981) indicates that inner and overt speech share additional units at still higher levels. MacKay had subjects practice producing identical sentences as rapidly as possible, either overtly or silently to themselves without moving their lips. The dependent variable was speech rate, and subjects in both conditions timed themselves by pressing one key as they began to say the sentence and another key as they finished. Results of this procedure indicated that both internal and overt speech improved with practice and reached asymptote after about the same number of practice trials.

Then, by adding a transfer paradigm to this procedure and by using German-English bilinguals as subjects, MacKay demonstrated that internal and overt practice caused equivalent improvement in the ability to produce sentential components such as phrases. Specifically, after practicing producing a sentence at maximal rate twelve times in one language, either internally or overtly, the subjects overtly produced a transfer sentence that was either a word-for-word translation or a nontranslation of the practiced sentence in their other language. The results (see Table 6.1) indicated that maximal speech rate was faster when the transfer sentences were translations rather than nontranslations. Moreover, degree of transfer was equivalent for the internal versus overt practice conditions. Because this transfer effect could only be occuring at lexical and phrase levels, and not at the phonological or muscle movement levels (which are completely different for the two languages and provide no basis for transfer), this finding indicates that inner and overt speech involve identical lexical and phrase units. In short, the units for producing inner and overt speech seem to be identical at all levels.

Is the Generative Component Articulatory or Phonological?   A great deal of evidence indicates that the generative component of internal speech and rehearsal involves an underlying code that is phonological rather than articulatory in nature. By standard definition, a generative component with articulatory characteristics represents the activities of particular muscles for the lips, tongue, velum, and other articulatory, laryngeal and respiratory organs, whereas a generative component with phonological characteristics represents not particular muscles,

TABLE 6.1
The Time to Produce a "Transfer" Sentence, Following Production of a Semantically Equivalent Sentence, Either Overtly (Physical Practice) or Internally (Internal Practice), in the Other Language of Bilinguals

| Practice Condition | Nature of the Transfer Sentence | | Facilitation | |
	Nontranslation	Translation	Time Difference	%
Physical practice	2.44 (.26)	2.24 (.23)	.20	8
Internal practice	2.19 (.31)	1.96 (.25)	.23	11

Note. Time in seconds with standard deviations in brackets.

but more abstract units. For example, the same abstract phonological units could and probably do play a role in overt articulation (MacKay, 1987, pp. 7–38), writing (Ellis, 1988) and typing (MacKay, in press), activities that involve completely different sorts of muscles. Indeed, a strong case can be made that the same abstract phonological units also underlie the comprehension of spoken language, an activity that does not involve muscles of any sort (see MacKay, 1987, pp. 62–125).

Studies of internal speech errors (Dell, 1978, 1980; Dell & Repka, in press; Meringer & Meyer, 1895) provide one source of evidence for the phonological rather than articulatory character of the lowest level units for internal speech. As already noted, errors reported during internal speech involve phonological components, but not phonetic, articulatory, or muscle movement components. Strictly articulatory errors (e.g., the slurring of speech sounds commonly seen in the production of overt speech) have never been reported for everyday internal speech.

Moreover, experimental studies (Dell, 1978, 1980) indicate that anticipations, perseverations and reversals occur with the same absolute frequency in overt and inner speech. This additional resemblance suggests that contrary to popular belief, overtly produced tongue twisters result in errors at the phonological level but not at the articulatory or muscle movement level. And because the tongue did not move during the inner speech of Dell's subjects, tongue twister errors must have nothing to do with the tongue. Like the term *auditory imagery* in its current applications to inner speech, "tongue twisters" may be misnamed; they are more accurately described as "phonological twisters."

Patients who are speech-impaired (dysarthric) or congenitally speechless (anarthric) due to brain damage affecting peripheral control of the articulatory musculature provide further evidence for the phonological rather than articulatory nature of internal speech and rehearsal. Wilson & Baddeley (cited in Baddeley, 1990, pp. 86–87) tested the memory of a dysarthric patient who could comprehend language and communicate using a simple keyboard device, and showed that this patient was virtually normal on a wide variety of memory tasks involving inner speech or rehearsal. However, this patient completely lacked the capacity to articulate, indicating that articulatory activity is unnecessary for the normal functioning of internal speech and rehearsal. Nor is articulatory activity necessary in order for children to learn to rehearse subvocally. Bishop & Robson (1989) showed that anarthric children who are incapable of articulation *from birth* are nevertheless virtually normal on a wide variety of memory tasks involving inner speech or rehearsal. On the basis of such evidence, Baddeley (1990) argued that the representation underlying rehearsal and short-term storage of verbal information that he had formerly called the "articulatory loop" was really a "phonological loop," a fundamental theoretical change.

In summary, phenomena that seem to be articulatory in origin, for example, the errors arising during rapid production of phonological twisters, are in fact phonological rather than articulatory. Moreover, available evidence indicates that the generative component of internal speech, which seems on the surface to be articulatory in nature, in fact involves a phonological representation. Finally, activity of the speech musculature is unnecessary for the normal functioning and acquisition of the processes underlying inner speech and rehearsal.

The Perceptual Component of Internal Speech

Phenomenology of the "Inner Ear."   Evidence for the so called auditory aspects of inner speech consists largely of the phenomenal experience of an inner voice without the occurrence of vocal output or of environmental input. The convincing nature of this seemingly auditory experience has led some psychologists to include inner speech within the category of "auditory imagery" and to suppose that an auditory or acoustic representation underlies the perception of inner speech. However, phenomenal experience or introspective report provides a shaky basis for specifying the representational character or theoretical nature of internal speech. The problem is that what seems phenomenally to be auditory often is not. For example, visual events can play a role in determining what people perceive phenomenally as a strictly auditory speech experience, and vice versa.

By way of illustration, consider the McGurk effect. McGurk and MacDonald (1976) seated subjects in front of a video monitor and had them listen to and observe a video recording of a person saying simple CV syllables such as *pa, ba, ta,* or *da.* Their task was simply to verbally identify the syllable that they *heard.* Unbeknownst to the subjects, the auditory syllables had been dubbed-in in synchrony with the speaker's lip movements, and on some trials differed from the speech sounds that these lip movements normally give rise to. For example, the acoustics of a person saying /ta/ might be dubbed in to synchronize with the visual lip movements of a person saying /pa/. This audio-visual conflict condition showed that visual features such as lip closure exerted a strong effect on what syllable the subjects reported hearing. With a conflict between the visual lip movements for /pa/ and the acoustics for /ta/, subjects usually reported hearing the visually based alternative, /pa/, rather than the auditorily based alternative, /ta/. Moreover, these subjects were quite surprised to discover that the /pa/ that they "heard" in this condition changed perceptually to /ta/ whenever they altered the visual input by complying with the experimenter's instructions to close their eyes.

How can a nonauditory event (visual lip movements) unconsciously influence a perception that subjects are convinced on the basis of phenomenal experience has auditory origins? The McGurk effect indicates that the seemingly auditory quality of overt speech perception is not necessarily auditory in origin and cannot be attributed solely to events within auditory or acoustic systems. And what holds for perception of overt speech holds also for perception of internal speech:

The seemingly auditory quality of our internal speech cannot be automatically attributed to events within an auditory or acoustic system, or even, as we will see, to *any* strictly sensory system. Thus, because the term auditory imagery used throughout this volume suggests that general auditory or acoustic representations are involved, a theoretically neutral term such as speech imagery is perhaps more appropriate for describing the seemingly auditory experience that arises during internal speech.

Does an Auditory System Underlie Internal Speech Perception?   It has often been suggested that internal speech is auditory in nature and takes place within the same system that images pure tones, music, and environmental sounds such as a barking dog or a running faucet. For example, Baddeley and Logie (this volume) maintain that environmental sounds automatically access the store for digits, music, and internal speech. One plausible implication of this hypothesis is that normal levels of background music and noise should cause massive interference with speech perception. However, massive interference has never been observed. Even with complex tasks involving the use of verbal memory and reasoning, interference from music and noise has been difficult to demonstrate. Indeed, improvement sometimes occurs (Wilding, Mohindra & Breen-Lewis, 1982); and when interference has been found, the effect has been slight and difficult to replicate rather than massive. For example, Salame and Baddeley (1989) had difficulty replicating their own demonstration that music interferes with the encoding and recall of visually presented digits. Moreover, the music that sometimes did introduce interference was of an especially raucous and distracting sort (e.g., Offenbach's Cancan and Ravel's Bolero). And the weak and difficult to replicate interference effect depended on presenting the music at 75dB *on the average,* much louder than the normal level of speech (about 45–55 dB). There is reason to believe that such music at such levels of amplification could interfere with language comprehension because of effects on timing mechanisms that are shared by the otherwise independent systems for speech, and many other cognitive systems, including those for auditory and musical cognition (MacKay, 1987, pp. 90–111). This being the case, amplified Offenbach may also interfere with tasks that are otherwise unrelated to audition, auditory imagery, or even language (e.g., rotating a mental image of Texas or solving visual analogies). Demonstrating that such interference does not in fact occur is necessary for accepting the hypothesis that interfering effects of music are auditory in nature or specific to a common system for analyzing "pure speech auditory images" and "pure tone auditory images."

In summary, the seemingly auditory quality of inner speech is not necessarily auditory in origin and, without more solid evidence, cannot be attributed to events within systems that are strictly auditory or acoustic in nature. Like producing inner speech, perceiving inner speech may involve a phonological code.

Differences Between Internal Speech and Overt Acoustics.   Many aspects of the acoustics of overt speech are normally absent from our awareness of self-produced internal speech. To illustrate, consider loudness and fundamental frequency, integral characteristics of the acoustics of overt speech. Unlike overt speech perception, awareness of the loudness and fundamental pitch of words produced internally is normally absent. Moreover, speakers normally fail to note the absence of these omnipresent characteristics of overt speech. If forced to characterize their own internal voice on these dimensions, they might say that their internal speech has neutral loudness and fundamental pitch. Consistent with such introspections, Intons-Peterson (this volume) presents experimental evidence suggesting that loudness is an attribute of sounds that is not specified in auditory imagery.

Such observations suggest that there exists a separate system for analyzing concepts related to acoustic aspects of speech such as loudness, intonation, sex of speaker, and speaker emotion or mood, and that this "auditory concept system" can operate in parallel with systems representing the phonological and sentential components of inner speech. Figure 6.1 illustrates the relations between these sytems for everyday language perception, which can be conceptualized as follows: An acoustic analysis system (see Fig. 6.1) feeds an initial analysis of speech in parallel to a phonological system and to an auditory concept system that categorically codes, for example, emotional content, intonational

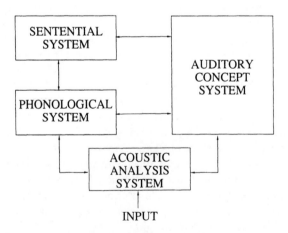

INPUT

FIG. 6.1. Possible relations between the systems analyzing the acoustics, phonology, syntax and auditory concepts related to speech (e.g., loudness, sex of speaker, speaker identity, emotional content, and intonation). These same acoustic analyses and auditory concept systems may or may not analyze the acoustics for environmental concepts such as a barking dog and a car's horn.

category, loudness, sex of speaker, and speaker identity, including the distinction between self-produced versus other-produced speech.

Representations in the auditory concept system are hierarchically related to, but fundamentally different from, those in the acoustic analysis system. For example, whereas the auditory concept system would represent speaker sex directly and categorically (as male vs. female), the acoustic analysis system would represent speaker sex in terms of a variety of acoustic properties, one of which is the speaker's average fundamental frequency. And whereas the auditory concept system would represent intonation directly and categorically (e.g., as interrogative vs. declarative), the acoustic analysis system would represent intonation in terms of a variety of acoustic properties, one of which is the relative rise or fall in fundamental frequency during the final word or syllable of an utterance (see Levelt, 1989, pp. 312–317). Similarly, whereas the auditory concept system would represent the emotional attitude of a speaker directly and categorically (e.g., as excited vs. calm), the acoustic analysis system would represent emotional attitude via many acoustic properties, one of which is the relatively high pitched or shrieky voice quality of an excited speaker (see Levelt, pp. 102).

Representations in the auditory concept system are also fundamentally different from those in the phonological and sentential/syntactic systems. The phonological system represents syllables and speech sounds and their order of occurence in words, while those in the sentential/syntactic system can generate language-specific propositions to represent any information whatsoever. Unlike auditory concepts, however, propositions are noncategorical. Thus, whereas the auditory concept system would represent speaker identity categorically (e.g., familiar vs. unfamiliar), the sentential/syntactic system would represent speaker identity in terms of propositions such as "My son is talking to me," or, "Kenny MacKay is talking to me."

Unlike the phonological and sentential/syntactic systems, the internal structure of the auditory concept system in Fig. 6.1 is relatively unexplored, and its exact limits remain to be determined. For example, the auditory concept system may or may not also analyze the concepts underlying identification of environmental sounds such as a barking dog or a car's horn, and may or may not also analyze musical concepts. If not, then the auditory concept system in Fig. 6.1 requires a more specific label, say, "speech concept" system, to distinguish it from, say, "music concept" systems. For musicians, the complexity of these music concept systems might rival those for language itself.

Perhaps there are even separate, parallel systems for more specific *speech* concepts such as speaker identity, intonation, and emotional attitude. And perhaps the acoustic analysis system also has a complex internal structure with separate and parallel subsystems for representing phonetics as opposed to, say, the acoustics of music or of environmental sounds. Figure 6.1 captures none of these yet to be explored possibilities.

However, the analysis in Fig. 6.1 is consistent with observations indicating that internal speech produced in one's own voice behaves differently from internal speech produced in the voice of someone else, as when imagining the voice of a friend or of a famous figure such as Margaret Thatcher or John Kennedy. Geiselman and Glenny (1977) had subjects rehearse words either in their own voice or in a familiar but imagined male or female voice. A surprise recognition test for these words was then presented, and, as might be expected, recognition was superior when the voice used during rehearsal and recognition matched in sex. Interestingly, however, no such interaction was observed for words that subjects had rehearsed in their own voice: Recognition performance was no better when the words to be recognized were spoken by someone of same sex as the subject. This finding suggests that one's own inner voice is neutral with respect to sex (see Geiselman & Glenny), and the as yet unanswered theoretical question is why. The reason within the present analysis is that one's own inner speech is generated within the phonological and sentential systems of Fig. 6.1, and both of these systems are neutral with respect to loudness and fundamental frequency. However, imagining the sound of another person's voice requires both of these systems, *plus* the auditory concept system, operating in parallel (see Fig. 6.1). For as we have seen, the auditory concept system is required to represent speaker sex and loudness, and this added information can help speakers discriminate the traces for internally generated versus overtly perceived speech (but not always; see, e.g., Johnson & Raye, 1981; R. E. Anderson, 1984).

Such observations contradict the common assumption (see e.g., Baddeley & Logie, this volume) that there exists a single seat or locus for the inner ear, and that this locus is the same for all imagery with phenomenally auditory origins. Different aspects of the same speech signal such as phonology, loudness, fundamental frequency and intonation may come together in lower level systems such as the acoustic analysis and muscle movement systems for producing speech (MacKay, 1987, p. 16) but may be analyzed within parallel but separate higher level systems that represent self-produced and imagined inner speech differently. Although boundaries of these higher level systems remain to be explored, it currently seems unwise to assume that auditory events for speech, music, and environmental sounds are analyzed at all levels within a common system.

RELATIONS BETWEEN INTERNAL AND OVERT
SPEECH PERCEPTION AND PRODUCTION

Relations between the perception and production of internal and overt speech have been the focus of a great deal of research. Five examples from this research tradition are discussed here, from both contemporary literature and classical literature of the 1920s and 1930s.

Processing Differences Between Internal and Overt Speech

Just as internal speech lacks characteristics of the overt speech signal, internal and overt speech differ in their processing characteristics, in both perception and production. For example, the generation of internal speech takes much longer than the perception of otherwise identical overt speech (MacKay, 1987, p. 114). Similarly, it takes longer to generate an image of, say, a letter (about 2 sec) than to recognize the corresponding visually presented letter (about 500 msec; Cocude & Dennis, 1986). Finally, the maximal rate of internal speech is much faster than the maximal rate of overt speech, all other factors being equal. Although an early comparision of the rate of internal and overt speech using data from a single subject (Landauer, 1962) failed to obtain a statistically reliable difference, subsequent and more systematic tests by R. A. Anderson (1982), MacKay (1981), Marshall and Cartwright (1978, 1980), and Weber and Castleman (1970) have uniformly found that internal speech procedes more rapidly than overt speech. Faster rates for internal versus overt production have also been observed for other highly practiced skills, for example, imagining oneself tying a shoelace versus actually tying a shoelace (Annett, 1988). The more rapid rate of internal speech suggests a possible benefit of internal rehearsal relative to overt rehearsal (see MacKay, 1981 for others) and requires explanation in theories of internal and overt speech.

Effects of Internal and Overt Speech Production on Perception

The issue of whether and how internal and overt speech production influences ongoing speech perception is currently rather controversial. To illustrate, consider the current, apparently unrecognized conflict between the findings of Lackner (1974) and Reisberg, Smith, Baxter & Sonenshine (1989) on the verbal transformation effect (VTE). The VTE refers to the fact that perception changes when an acoustically presented word is repeated via tape loop for prolonged periods (5 sec to several minutes). After hearing the word *pace* repeated for 3 minutes, for example, subjects report hearing words such as *face, paste, base, taste,* or *case,* and the number of perceptual forms and the rate of perceptual change from one form to another increases systematically as a function of time or repetitions (Warren, 1968).

The conflict between Lackner and Reisberg et al. arises from a variant of the standard VTE experiment discussed above. The variant involves repeated production of a word that results in a phenomenon known as the missing feedback effect: In a very well controlled experiment, Lackner found that the perceptual changes that occur when listening to a repeating word *fail to occur* when the subjects themselves are producing the repeated word; the auditory feedback that accompanies repeated *production* of a word fails to trigger verbal transformations. Lackner's subjects repeated a word every 500 msec for several minutes and later listened to a tape recording of their own output over earphones in a sound-proof booth. The subjects experienced the usual transformations when *listening* to the tape recording of their own output, but, for some reason, experienced almost no perceptual transformations when *producing* the word.

This missing feedback effect is empirically interesting because the acoustic events at the ear are identical when hearing the input during versus after production. The missing feedback effect is also theoretically interesting because it bears on theories of the relation between speech perception and speech production. Lackner (1974) attributed the missing feedback effect to a corollary discharge or efference-copy that accompanies the motor command to produce a word. This corollary discharge cancels or inhibits the external (proprioceptive and auditory) feedback resulting from producing the word, so that the on-line auditory input during production fails to bring about the fatigue induced perceptual changes that are the hallmark of the VTE. An unsolved problem in Lackner's account is why no *production errors* resembling the perceptual errors occurred when subjects actively repeated a word: Why doesn't fatigue also induce production errors?

The recent work of Reisberg et al. (1989) on the VTE also bears on these issues but has received empirical and theoretical interpretations that are quite different from those of Lackner. For example, Reisberg et al. claimed that VTEs do not differ for the standard perception procedure versus production procedures resembling those discussed above, although aspects of their data seem to contradict this empirical claim and support the findings of Lackner: In one experiment using the standard VTE perceptual procedure, 98% of Reisberg et al.'s subjects perceived a particular transform (e.g., *dress* for the repeating word *stress*) during 2 minutes or less of repetition, whereas 20% fewer subjects (i.e., 78%) perceived this transform when they repeatedly produced the word *stress*. In another similar experiment, 100% of the subjects hearing *stress* in the perception condition reported the transform *dress,* and 100% of the subjects in the production condition reported perceiving *dress* while repeatedly producing *stress*. Thus, a major difference remains in the results of the production condition in Lackner (few transforms of any type) versus Reisberg et al. (100% and 78% transforms of a particular type). Whereas Reisberg et al.'s perception subjects reported only 1.0 to 1.28 times as many transforms as their production subjects, Lackner's perception subjects reported about 15 times as many transforms as his production subjects.

The low probability of transforms in Lackner's (1974) production condition is almost certainly not attributable to reduced subject expectations of transforms. Because Lackner's subjects were instructed to monitor for and report deviations in perceived vowel quality, however small, as they repeatedly produced a word, the instructions surely led them to expect changes in their repeated productions.

Nor is the difference attributable to the procedure in Reisberg et al.'s (1989) perception condition of having an experimenter produce the words repeatedly and perhaps variably from one production to the next. In a pilot study, Reisberg et al. found no difference between conditions where an experimenter said the word repeatedly, where the subject said the word repeatedly, and where the word was generated repeatedly via computer (not unlike Lackner's tape loop procedure). Nor is the difference between the two studies readily attributable to differences in scoring procedures. Reisberg et al.'s scoring procedure was, if anything, more stringent than Lackner's so that, arguably, their production condition should have resulted in fewer rather than more transformations. In short, reasons for the differing results in these two studies are currently unknown and difficult to imagine, and the issue of the effects of language production on language perception in the verbal transformation task remains unresolved.

However, in an additional experiment, Reisberg et al. found a systematic relation between the VTE and "degree of enactment" on the part of subjects who themselves produced a word or phrase repeatedly either aloud (overtly), whispering, or silently (mouthing). Overtly articulated repetitions were said to be highly enacted, whispered repetitions less enacted, and silently mouthed repetitions still less enacted. Thus, progressively fewer subjects reported perceiving the preselected transform when they repeatedly spoke (85%), whispered (68%), or silently mouthed (53%) the word or phrase. Reisberg et al. concluded that the verbal transformation effect reflects an interpretive process that varies in direct proportion with the degree of enactment that accompanies a repeating stimulus originating via auditory input or via feedback from production. Other conditions in Reisberg et al. suggested that this repeating stimulus need not originate externally, via sensory channels, but could also originate internally, as when subjects imagine hearing themselves or a friend saying a word repeatedly.

Is Motor Activity Necessary
for Perception of Internal Speech?

The classical hypothesis that motor activity is necessary for perceiving internal speech and other forms of imagery has been extensively examined and conclusively rejected. Early experiments showed that microscopic muscular movements, invisible to the naked eye, occurred during internal speech and other forms of imagery, and interestingly, this same EMG activity invariably precedes by a few milliseconds the full blown muscle activity that occurs during normal movements (e.g., Schmidt, 1982). From these observations it was hypothesized that EMG activity triggers sensory feedback that once was deemed essential for thinking and imagery (see e.g., Weisberg, 1980).

Consistent with the hypothesis that EMG activity triggers feedback necessary for centrally generated imagery, EMG responses were initially found to be localized or specific to the type of images experienced, rather than general or nonspecific in nature (Jacobson, 1930, 1931; Max, 1937): The pattern of EMG activity during imagery and during overt performance of the same action seemed to be identical. However, other studies reviewed by Feltz and Landers (1983) have raised questions about whether the EMG innervations associated with imaging occur more generally throughout the body than do corresponding overtly produced movements.

Even more damaging to the EMG-feedback hypothesis, a large number of early studies indicated that EMG activity was not necessary for internal imagery, and specifically not for the seemingly auditory imagery that often accompanies internal speech (Sokolov, 1972), silent reading (Pintner, 1913), and problem solving (Weisberg, 1980). For example, paralysis (Smith, Brown, Tolman & Goodman, 1947) and anesthetization of the lips and tongue (Dodge, 1896, as cited in Weisberg), and other forms of interference with EMG activity in speech muscles leave the ability to generate internal speech unimpaired (Sokolov, 1972). Such findings are inconsistent with the original hypothesis that low level motor activity and sensory feedback are necessary for perception of internal speech.

Also contrary to the feedback hypothesis, and to the more general hypothesis that EMG activity is essential for imagery, are the data on congenital and acquired dysarthria discussed above. If control of inner speech is fundamentally phonological rather than articulatory, and does not depend on peripheral musculature, as the data of Wilson and Baddeley (in Baddeley, 1990) suggest, then peripheral feedback from the musculature is also irrelevant to the control of inner speech and rehearsal. Similarly, if inner speech can be learned without use of the peripheral musculature, as the data of Bishop and Robson (1989) suggest, then feedback from peripheral musculature is also irrelevant to the acquisition of inner speech and rehearsal.

Dissociations Between Motor Activity and Perceptual Experience

Motor activity and perceptual experience can be dissociated because the production and perceptual experience of internal speech is unimpaired when the ability to move the corresponding muscles is prevented, for example, by motor paralysis or brain damage. The "fis phenomenon" (Smith, 1973) represents another such dissociation. Young children often have difficulty producing the muscle movements for a speech sound in certain phonetic environments even though they can perceive and presumably imagine these speech sounds perfectly well. For example, a child might say fis instead of fish but nevertheless be able to perceive the distinction between fis and fish: Thus, if an adult imitates the child by saying "O.K., here's your fis," the child will strenuously object, "No, no: FIS, FIS," indirectly indicating perception of the fis-fish distinction. Moreover, if a tape recording of the child saying the word "fis" (instead of "fish") in isolation is later played to the child, the child will perceive "fis" rather than "fish" with high probability.

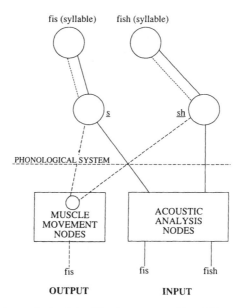

FIG. 6.2. An analysis of the "fis phenomenon" in children. Solid lines represent bottom-up connections. Broken lines represent top-down connections.

Figure 6.2 illustrates a general framework for explaining the "fis phenomenon" and other dissociations between motor abilities and perceptual experience. The input, either "fish" or "fis," is accurately analyzed in an acoustic analysis system and in a phonological system that plays a role in both perceiving and producing the distinction between these sounds. The problem arises in a subordinate system that represents the muscle movements for producing /s/ and /sh/ in this context: The phonological units for both /sh/ and /s/ have been mapped onto the units for producing /s/ within this muscle movement system, so that the child produces "fis" instead of "fish," the correctly intended and executed output *at the phonological level.*

A phenomenon that resembles the *fis* phenomenon in certain respects can be observed in the internal speech of adults who speak with a foreign accent or in a dialect that differs from the speech that they hear on a daily basis. For example, I speak a standard Canadian dialect with a distinctive "clipped" pronounciation of words containing the dipthong "ou" (e.g., *out, about, south,* etc). Despite having lived in California for two and a half decades, I fail to produce the standard American versions of these "ou" words in normal, everyday language production. Even with slow and deliberate attempts, I am unable to adequately produce an American "ou." Moreover, I normally fail to distinguish between the Canadian and American versions of "ou" in my everyday perception of spoken American, or in my internal and external speech, I automatically produce the

Canadian "ou" and perceive the American "ou" without becoming aware of the acoustic difference between the two. Here, then, is another aspect of speech acoustics (Canadian "ou") that is absent from internal speech *and overt perception,* as if acoustic characteristics of the American "ou" have been mapped onto a single abstract phonological unit that represents both (see Fig. 6.3). As a result, both perception and internal speech are neutral with respect to these acoustic properties. However, this single abstract "Canamerican ou" unit has been mapped onto a single pattern of muscle movements that correspond to the Canadian rather than the American "ou" (see Fig. 6.3), so that only the Canadian "ou" is overtly produced.

This accent phenomenon further illustrates how internal speech perception (the neutral "ou") can differ from acoustics of overt speech. Such differences between internal and overt speech are not limited to special dialects or accents, but are quite general in nature: As we have seen, many aspects of overt speech perception are absent during self-produced internal speech, as if inner speech involves the phonological system but not the acoustic analysis and/or muscle movement systems (see Fig. 6.1–6.3).

Are Perceptual Systems Completely Independent from Output Systems?

Within the framework (Fig. 6.2–6.3) for explaining dissociations between motor abilities and perceptual experience, some of the systems for perception and

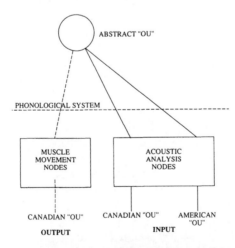

FIG. 6.3. An analysis of an "accent phenomenon" in the internal speech of an adult Canadian preceiving and producing American "ou" in words such as *out, south, house,* etc. Solid lines represent bottom-up connections. Broken lines represent top-down connections.

production of speech are shared rather than separate. MacKay (1987) reviewed a wide range of data for such shared perception/production systems. This evidence suggests that language perception and production, including the inner ear and inner voice, share the same phonological and sentential systems. However, the idea of a shared perception/production system for phonology has not gone unchallenged. Baddeley (1990) and Baddeley and Salame (1986) argued from dual task performance that input systems are separate from output systems at the phonological level. Their simultaneous tasks were comprehension of visually presented sentences and repeated internal or overt articulation of a word or syllable such as *the, the, the, the, the*. . . . The results indicated very little interference between these two tasks: Sentences were understood almost as well when subjects were repeating the syllable as when they were not. On the basis of this relative lack of interference, Baddeley concluded the following:

1. Input systems for analyzing the sentences must be separate from output systems for producing words or syllables;

2. An articulatory loop for rehearsing a word such as *the* must be separate from the systems for analyzing visually presented sentences resembling "moast peepul seemd tue bee aybul tue heer thuh werds eevan wen thay wurr seying thuh";

3. The inner voice must be separate from the inner ear because saying *the* repeatedly had little effect on the task of deciding whether visually presented nonwords are or are not phonologically compatible with real words, as is the case for the words "moast peepul seemd tue bee aybul tue heer thuh wirds internully."

However, all of these conclusions are open to question on several grounds. One is that repeating a syllable such as *the* may occupy only a small subcomponent of the phonological and other systems for comprehending sentences (see MacKay, 1987, pp. 52–55). This being the case, little interference would be expected in these tasks, even if (a) input systems for analyzing sentences and output systems for producing the word *the* are shared; (b) there is no articulatory loop that is separate from the phonological units for producing or repeating a word such as *the;* and (c) the inner voice is not completely separable from the inner ear.

TRADITIONAL ACCOUNTS OF RELATIONS BETWEEN INTERNAL AND OVERT SPEECH

The traditional theoretical approach to the perception of internal speech incorporates the idea of a "double agent," an internal speaker who speaks and an internal listener who listens. This "double agent assumption" is so common and accepted as to have become built into the everyday meaning of terms such as "speak" and "talk" in English and many other languages: The term "speech" implies talking to someone, so that internal speech must refer to talking to oneself, a hypothetical duplicate of the self who is listening rather than talking.

Many examples of the double agent assumption could be cited from the recent literature. Baddeley's (1986, 1990) articulatory/phonological loop theory represents an example that has addressed the issue of imagery during covert rehearsal, but it has so far failed to address the issues related to language production and perception that are of interest here. I therefore examine Levelt's (1989) recently proposed Perceptual Loop theory of how we generate and comprehend internal speech as an illustration of the "double agent" view.

Levelt argued that language production proceeds top down through a hierarchy of semantic nodes and phonological nodes. The lowest level nodes in this phonological production system are linked to the phonological perceptual system via two pathways: an internal "loop" that is used for perceiving internal speech, and an external "loop" that includes the muscle movement system, the auditory system, and a separate phonological system for perceiving both overt and internal speech. Under the double agent assumption, then, systems for producing speech are separate from comprehension systems, which also monitor internally and externally generated versions of the output for errors. How this second agent (the language comprehension system) "knows" that the production system has made an error, substituting *table* for *chair*, for example, is unspecified in Levelt's theory.

Reisberg et al. (1989) raised the double agent problem to another level by assuming that the internal listener (Levelt's language perception system) is capable of becoming an internal producer of auditory images: That is, Reisberg et al. proposed that auditory images for verbal materials can be generated internally using mechanisms that are independent of the usual mechanisms for producing language. Why we need such a listener-production system as well as the traditional production-production system, and how this duplicate listener-production system differs from the normal production system for language and speech pose additional problems that this view must solve. The answer of Reisberg et al. that a duplicate production system is needed for imagining and anticipating strictly auditory sounds that we cannot produce (say, the honking of a goose) may apply to "pure auditory imagery" but runs into difficulties when applied to inner speech because, as we have seen, the production of inner speech is fundamentally phonological rather than auditory in nature.

Levelt's support for his so-called Perceptual Loop theory is weak and open to alternate interpretations that apply also to other versions of the double agent assumption. The main source of support for Levelt's theory is an effect of auditory masking on the detection of a particular type of experimentally induced speech error in a study by Lackner and Tuller (1979). Lackner and Tuller had subjects repeat experimentally constructed phonological twisters such as pi-di-ti-gi at a controled rate for 30 sec and push a button every time they noticed making an error. In one (nonmasking) condition the subjects produced the phonological twisters without masking, and in another (auditory masking) condition, they heard white noise that masked their auditory feedback. Subjects detected errors involving substitutions of the place of articulation feature (e.g., ti-di-ti-gi instead of pi-di-ti-gi) no more often in the masking than in the nonmasking conditions (116 vs. 98). However, they detected errors involving substitutions of the voicing feature (e.g., di-di-ti-gi instead of pi-di-ti-gi) more often in the masking than in the non-masking conditions (252 vs. 175). To explain why voicing errors are easier to detect in the masking condition, Levelt argued that masking suppresses use of the external (auditory) loop, leaving only the internal loop (from the phonological production system to the phonological perceptual system). To explain why the masking effect was specific to voicing errors, Levelt argued that voicing (unlike place of articulation) depends on a small production difference that translates into large acoustic effects. Levelt then argued that the large acoustic effects in voicing errors are easiest to pick up using the external loop (acoustic analysis system) that happens to be suppressed in the masking condition, thereby making voicing errors more difficult to detect.

These arguments seem tenuous on several counts: One is that contrary to Levelt's assumption, there are as many production differences between voiced and unvoiced speech sounds as there are perceptual differences (Lisker, 1978). Moreover, comparing the "size" of articulatory and acoustic differences for different phonological features or for different values of the same phonological feature is like comparing eggs to chickens: To make sense, the comparison requires a theory of the relation between the two, and if such a theory were available, the notion of "size" would almost certainly be irrelevant (as is the case for the theory relating eggs and chickens).

Another problem is that important aspects of Lackner and Tuller's (1979) data find no explanation in Levelt's theory. For example, voicing errors were not only detected more often in Lackner and Tuler's masking condition, they also *occurred* much more often than place of articulation errors (427 vs. 214) in both the masking and nonmasking conditions. This additional finding is difficult to explain in Levelt's theory.

Another implication of Levelt's Perceptual Loop theory is that self-produced phonological errors should be detected more quickly and easily than word errors (all other factors being equal). The reason is that word errors involve units that are higher in the output hierarchy and thus further from the perceptual monitor for detecting them; thus, more time would be needed to reach the monitor for detecting word errors than for detecting phonological errors. Although further data are required for resolving this issue, available data do not support this prediction: Nooteboom (1980) reported that lexical errors are as easy to detect as phonological errors. This finding is difficult to explain without further assumptions in Levelt's theory.

Another problem for Levelt's Perceptual Loop theory concerns the nature of mental errors, that is, errors that occur during internal speech. Under the Perceptual Loop theory, overt speech should enable superior error detection (all other factors being equal) because the external loop in overt speech allows a second opportunity for detecting errors that is absent during internal speech. However, Dell's (1978, 1980) data do not support this prediction and are difficult to explain without further assumptions in Levelt's theory.

In conclusion, the traditional concept of an internal listener that monitors self-produced outputs derives from a figure of speech that may represent a poor foundation for building a theory of the structures and mechanisms underlying language perception and error monitoring. Moreover, the internal listener concept is functionally questionable: The "double agent" approach to comprehension of internal speech must address the fundamental issue of why speakers must independently "listen to" the meaning and sound of what they are saying internally when they know all along the meaning and sound of what they are saying.

THE ROLE OF INTERNAL SPEECH
IN VISUAL WORD PERCEPTION

Just as nonauditory events can influence a seemingly auditory experience, as in the McGurk effect, nonvisual events can influence a seemingly visual experience. In particular, phonological processes that are involved in internal speech can influence the perception of visual stimuli. Unlike the McGurk effect, effects of internal phonology on visual perception are not new. One of the earliest themes of research in cognitive psychology was to show that a phonological code resembling inner speech contributes to tasks that involve visual stimuli, for example, silent reading (Pintner, 1913), visual word and letter detection (MacKay, 1972), and immediate recall of visual letter strings (Sperling, 1960). For example, MacKay demonstrated that phonological factors play a role in the ability to detect letter strings presented briefly via tachistoscope. Neither the stimulus nor the response was auditory, phonetic, or phonological in nature: Subjects were instructed simply to write down exactly what they saw.

Subjects were informed that the letter strings would consist of either correctly or incorrectly spelled words, and on half the trials they were told what word would be presented (correctly or incorrectly spelled). Two types of misspellings were presented: phonologically compatible misspellings, which can be pronounced in the same way as the original word (e.g., *werk* for *work*), and phonologically incompatible misspellings, which require a different pronunciation from the original word (e.g., *wark* for *work*). The data showed that phonologically incompatible misspellings were easier to detect than phonologically compatible ones, indicating that a phonological code must play a role in detecting visually presented letter strings under these conditions. This same effect had been observed earlier (MacKay, 1969) for subjects attempting to detect misspellings embedded in briefly presented sentences such as "Nobody knew thet the werk was compleated on the new buildung." Interestingly, however, it was shown (MacKay, 1972) that with tachistoscopic presentation of individual words, the difference between phonologically compatible and incompatible misspellings only emerges when subjects are verbally warned of what word will be presented. With no advance warning, the same phonologically incompatible strings are no easier to detect than phonologically compatible ones. This finding indicates that like inner speech, the phonological processes that underlie detection of visual letter strings are neither simple nor completely automatic in nature.

THE ROLE OF INTERNAL SPEECH
IN IMMEDIATE RECALL OF VISUAL INPUTS

Sperling (1960) and Conrad (1964) have provided widely cited evidence that the code underlying immediate recall of visual letter strings is not visual but acoustic or phonological in nature and resembles inner speech. For example, Conrad showed that the pattern of errors that subjects make in immediate recall of visually presented consonant sequences resembled the pattern of perceptual errors that they make in identifying the same syllables presented auditorily against a background of white noise. Conrad and Hull (1964) extended this finding by showing that sequences of "acoustically similar" consonants (e.g., D, V, T, P, C) are harder to recall than sequences of "acoustically different" consonants (e.g., F, Y, D, R, K). Interestingly, however, Wickelgren (1965) and others have demonstrated that "acoustic similarity" only disrupts ability to recall the *order* of the letters and, if anything, tends to *facilitate* recall of the letters themselves. This finding presents a challenge for the hypothesis of Baddeley (1990) and Baddeley and Logie (chapter 8, this volume) that "acoustic similarity" reduces recall by impairing our ability to discriminate between similar traces. Impaired trace discrimination might reduce recall of the letters themselves and perhaps also their order (exactly how remains to be specified by Baddeley & Logie). But without additional assumptions, the trace discrimination hypothesis cannot explain why short-term recall is impaired for order but *not* items in strings of phonologically similar leters. Again, the exact nature of phonological processes underlying cognitive acts such as the recall of visual letter strings is not simple, not strictly visual, and not yet explained.

In summary, aspects of the code underlying perception and immediate recall of visual letter strings is not visual, and like inner speech, may be phonological in nature.

MEMORY, REHEARSAL AND INTERNAL SPEECH

The topics of memory, rehearsal and internal speech are closely related because the covert rehearsal that occurs, for example, when one silently repeats a telephone number for later recall, seems indistinguishable from internal speech (see also Baddeley and Logie, this volume). Indeed, rehearsal and its effects on memory may represent one of the main functions of internal speech. Accounts of the relation between memory, rehearsal, and internal speech are of course available (see e.g., Baddeley and Logie, this volume), and to review here the evidence that is consistent with these theories would be redundant. However, it is worth noting that we are a long way from theoretical consensus on relations between memory, rehearsal, and internal speech. For example, as Baddeley (1990, p. 72) notes, the well known data advanced in support of his own theory are "capable of being explained in several other ways."

What follows are some additional and less widely recognized constraints on extant and future theories of memory, rehearsal and internal speech.

Unrehearsability

Certain types of information, such as a particular smell, seem difficult to call up and rehearse or imagine in detail. Why are some types of information rehearsable, for example, familiar words or sentences, whereas other types of information are unamenable to rehearsal without extensive training, for example, isolated pure tones (Wickelgren, 1966)? It is not that phonology per se is easily rehearsed: For example, sentences heard in a foreign language are unrehearsable even if the phonology of these sentences is compatible with English phonology. Nor does rehearsability depend critically on storage capacity or stimulus complexity per se: Relatively simple stimuli, for example, a single phoneme such as a German trilled /r/, cannot be accurately rehearsed by someone unfamiliar with German.

Perhaps the main determinant of rehearsability is prior practice. If a behavior such as a trilled /r/ is so unfamiliar that the appropriate muscle movements have not been learned, internal rehearsal will be of little help in the overt expression of the behavior (see MacKay, 1981). The language memory literature has been able to overlook this limitation of internal rehearsal because the internally rehearsed behavior at issue (skilled language production) is a special case: Over the course of a lifetime the muscle movements for producing familiar words and syllables in one's native language have become highly practiced (see MacKay, 1981, 1982). In general, however, internal rehearsal tends mainly to benefit either simple skills that have been practiced since early childhood, or the complex skills of virtuoso performers, for example, professional musicians and sports players who have extensively practiced all levels of the skill (MacKay, 1981). Conversely, as

Feltz and Landers (1983) pointed out, unless subjects have some prior experience in a task, little or no effect of internal rehearsal is found.

Rehearsal, Volition and Awareness

As Baddeley and Logie (this volume) point out, conscious experience is one of the defining characeristics of inner speech and auditory imagery in general. However, like consciousness itself, the inner speech that occurs during rehearsal does not require conscious or intentional initiation. Although rehearsal can be and often is voluntary, it is not *necessarily* voluntary. For example, speakers are often unable to voluntarily remove an internally recurring phrase from awareness (Bargh, 1990; Reisberg, 1989): The phrase continues to repeat as if it were being rehearsed involuntarily. The partially involuntary nature of inner rehearsal may have contributed to Parkin's (1987, p. 11–12) observation that, "it is a perverse fact about human memory that we often remember things we would rather forget and forget things we want to remember." The involuntary repetitions seen in compulsive behaviors likewise suggest that repetition is not always under voluntary control.

Effects of Overt and Internal Rehearsal on Behavior

Studies of overt and internal rehearsal have focussed mainly on long-term memory tasks. However, interesting effects of overt versus internal rehearsal have also been observed for aspects of behavior such as errors and the maximal rate of speech. As reviewed here, these effects provide important new constraints on theories of inner speech.

Improvement Following Internal Versus Overt Rehearsal.   Effects of internal and overt rehearsal differ in interesting and counterintuitive ways. When subjects (MacKay, 1981) practiced producing identical sentences either overtly or internally at maximal rate, internal speech initially improved faster with practice, but reached asymptote after about the same number of practice trials as overt speech. These results are shown in Fig. 6.4 (right panel), where the average production time (in secs per sentence) is plotted on log-log coordinates. As can be seen, both internal and overt speech improved as a function of practice, which in itself is interesting because the subjects were trying to speak at their maximum rate throughout. The regularity of the functions in Fig. 6.4 is also noteworthy. The practice function for the overt rehearsal condition is completely linear, as would be expected under the power law that describes most learning curves.

However, an important irregularity distinguished the results for internal versus overt rehearsal: Learning resulting from internal rehearsal was more rapid than

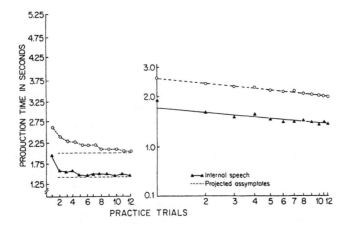

FIG. 6.4.   Left panel: Time to produce identical sentences (in seconds) overtly (circles) versus internally (triangles) as a function of practice. Adapted from MacKay (1982). Right Panel: Log-log replot of the left panel data.

could be expected from log-log linearity on the initial practice trial (see Fig. 6.4). This "upward deviation" from log-log linearity indicates that internal speech improved faster than did overt speech following that initial trial.

Such upward deviations from log-log linearity are not limited to inner speech, but have been observed in other cognitive skills as well. For example, Snoddy (1926) reported an initial upward deviation from log-log linearity in the practice function for a mirror tracing task. Subjects watched their actions reversed in a mirror as they used a pencil to trace the outline of a visual pattern such as a star. The time per pattern (corrected for errors) is shown in Fig. 6.5 (as replotted in Newell & Rosenbloom, 1981). As can be seen there, production times improved rapidly with practice over the first four trials and then settled into log-log linearity for the remaining 55 trials. Explaining such deviations are a major challenge for theories of internal and overt rehearsal involving a wide range of cognitive skills (see MacKay, 1982).

Correlated Rates for Internal and Overt Rehearsal.   As can be seen in Fig. 6.4, internal speech proceeded more rapidly than overt speech across all 12 practice trials in MacKay (1981) (see also Anderson, 1982; Marshall & Cartwright, 1978, 1980; and Weber & Castleman, 1970). However, for a given subject, maximal rates of internal and overt rehearsal were highly correlated. Subjects who produced sentences quickly during overt rehearsal (MacKay, 1981) also produced them quickly during internal rehearsal, as might be expected if internal and overt rehearsal involved many of the same components (i.e., the Phonological and Sentential systems in Fig. 6.1–6.3).

Transfer Effects from Internal to Overt Speech. By adding a transfer paradigm to the procedure discussed above and by using German-English bilinguals as subjects, MacKay (1981) demonstrated that internal and overt rehearsal cause equivalent improvement in the ability to produce the phonological and sentential components of a sentence. Specifically, the subjects practiced producing a sentence in one language at maximal rate either internally or overtly and then produced a transfer sentence that was either a word for word translation or a nontranslation of the practiced sentence in their other language. The results (see Table 6.1) indicated that the maximal rate of speech was faster when the transfer sentences were translations rather than nontranslations. Moreover, the degree of transfer following internal and overt practice was equivalent.

Differing Effects of Overt Versus Internal Rehearsal on Errors. Dell (1978, 1980) reported that various types of errors (anticipations, perseverations, and reversals) occurred with identical absolute frequency in inner and overt speech. However, Dell and Repka's (in press) more recent study of effects of internally and overtly rehearsing phonological twisters gave a slightly different pattern of results. Dell and Repka's subjects reported inner slips less frequently, and more often in syllable-, word-, and phrase-initial positions, relative to overt slips. Moreover, overt rehearsal or repetitions of a phonological twister reduced the probability of errors during subsequent overt production of the twister, but inner rehearsal failed to reduce errors when a twister subsequently was articulated overtly.

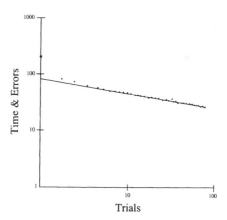

FIG. 6.5. Production times (corrected for errors) as a function of practice (log-log coordinates) in a mirror tracing task (from Snoddy, 1926, modified from the replot of Newell and Rosenbloom, 1980). Filled circles represent the "upward deviation" from log-log linearity (see text for explanation).

To explain these new results, Dell and Repka invoked an earlier suggestion of Vygotsky and others that speakers are capable of abbreviating their inner speech by omitting noninitial segments in syllables and words, especially words occupying noninitial positions in a phrase. Dell and Repka then explained the differences between their results and those of Dell (1978, 1980) in terms of individual differences in this hypothesized process of phonological abbreviation. Whereas subjects in Dell and Repka were all undergraduates, most of the subjects in Dell were psychology graduate students engaged in the study of short-term memory. Unlike undergraduates, these graduate students would have been quite knowledgeable about internal speech and its theoretical importance, and so may have been less likely to abbreviate their internal speech than the undergraduates in Dell and Repka. However, further research on these issues is clearly needed.

SUMMARY AND CONCLUSIONS

This chapter has reviewed a number of fundamental constraints or requirements that theories of inner speech must address. The present list of constraints is undoubtably incomplete, and will surely grow as the field progresses. Contained within the list, however, are *sine qua non* requirements for a viable theory: Theories of inner speech which fail to capture these constraints can be considered incomplete or inadaquate, and the traditional "double agent" approach to explaining relations between perception and production of internal speech seems to fall within this category.

What sort of theory will be needed for explaining the fundamental phenomena of inner speech? The theory must postulate a hierarchy of units, including units representing phrases, words, morphemes, and above all, phonological components. In producing inner speech, these units must be activated in sequence, but without activating muscle movement units for overt articulation.

The theory of inner speech must explain why some aspects of language are impossible to generate internally, why inner speech is sometimes involuntary and difficult to control, and why effects of overt and internal rehearsal on speech production are similar in some respects and different in others. However, the theory of inner speech must not give a central role to articulatory units or abilities, or to electromyographic activity within articulatory, laryngeal and other speech muscles. Nor is it necessary for the theory of inner speech to postulate a strictly *auditory* code for the "inner ear."

In addition to providing a standard against which to evaluate current theories, the criteria outlined here can be used to develop new and more adequate theories. Indeed, I myself hope to use these criteria in extending my own theory of language perception/production (MacKay, 1987) to cover inner speech. A final question concerns the generality of the present criteria. If they apply to other inner skills besides language production/perception, the present chapter may provide a rough outline for what a general theory of imaging must eventually explain.

ACKNOWLEDGMENTS

The author thanks D. Reisberg, D. Burke, and two anonymous reviewers for valuable comments on an earlier version of this chapter.

REFERENCES

Anderson, R. A. (1982). Speech imagery is not always faster than visual imagery. *Memory and Cognition, 10,* 371–80.

Anderson, R. E. (1984). Did I do it or only imagine it? *Journal of Experimental Psychology: General, 113,* 594–613.

Annett, J. (1988). Motor learning and retention. In M. M. Gruneberg, P. E. Morris, & R. N. Sykes (Eds.), *Practical aspects of memory: Volume II* (434–440). Chichester, England: Wiley.

Atkinson, R. C., & Shiffrin, R. M. (1968). Human memory: A proposed system and its control processes. In K. W. Spence (Ed.), *The psychology of learning and motivation: Advances in research and theory* (Vol. 2, pp. 89–195). New York: Academic Press.

Baddeley, A. (1986). *Working memory.* Oxford University Press.

Baddeley, A. (1990). *Human memory: Theory and practice.* Boston: Allyn & Bacon.

Baddeley, A., & Salame, P. (1986). The unattended speech effect: Perception or memory. *Journal of Experimental Psychology: Learning, Memory, & Cognition, 12*(4), 525–529.

Bargh, J. A. (1990). Conditional automaticity: Varieties of automatic influence in social perception and cognition. In J. S. Ulleman & J. A. Bargh (Eds.), *Unintended thought* (pp. 3–51). New York: Guilford.

Bishop, D. V. M., & Robson, J. (1989). Unimpaired short-term memory and rhyme judgement in congenitally speechless individuals: Implications for the notion of "articulatory coding." *Quarterly Journal of Experimental Psychology, 41a,* 123–141.

Cocude, J., & Dennis, R. W. (1986). The time course of mental imagery: Latency and duration of mental images. In D. G. Russel & D. F. Marks (Eds.), *Imagery 2.* Dunedin, New Zealand: Human Performance.

Conrad, R. (1964). Acoustic confusion in immediate memory. *British Journal of Psychology, 55,* 75–84.

Conrad, R., & Hull, A. J. (1964). Information, acoustic confusion and memory span. *British Journal of Psychology, 55,* 429–432.

Dell, G. S. (1978). Slips of the mind. In M. Paradis, (Ed.), *The Fourth LACUS Forum.* (pp. 69–75). Columbia, SC: Hornbeam Press.

Dell, G. S. (1980). *Phonological and lexical encoding in speech production: An analysis of naturally occurring and experimentally elicited speech errors.* Unpublished doctoral dissertation, University of Toronto, Toronto, Canada.

Dell, G. S., & Repka, R. J. (in press). Errors in inner speech. In B. Baars (Ed.), *Experimental slips and human error: Exploring the architecture of volition.* New York: Plenum.

Dodge, R. (1896). Motoric speech production. Cited in Weisberg, R. W. (1980). *Memory, thought and behavior.* New York: Oxford University Press.

Ellis, A. W. (1988). Normal writing processes and peripheral acquired dysgraphias. *Language and Cognitive Processes, 3*(2), pp. 99–127.

Feltz, D., & Landers, D. (1983). The effects of mental practice on motor skill learning and performance: A meta-analysis. *Journal of Sport Psychology, 5,* 211–220.

Geiselman, R. E., & Glenny, J. (1977). Effects of imagining speakers' voices on the retention of words presented visually. *Memory & Cognition, 5,* 499–504.

Jacobson, E. (1930). Imagination of movement involving the skelatal muscles. *American Journal of Physiology, 91,* 567–608.

Jacobson, E. (1931). Imagination, recollection, and abstract thinking involving the speech musculature. *American Journal of Physiology, 97,* 200–209.

Johnson, M. K., & Raye, C. L. (1981). Reality monitioring. *Psychological Review, 88,* 67–85.

Lackner, J. (1974). Speech production: Evidence for corollary discharge stabilization of perceptual mechanisms. *Perceptual and Motor Skills, 39,* 899–902.

Lackner, J. R., & Tuller, B. H. (1979). The role of efference monitoring in the detection of self-produced speech errors. In W. E. Cooper & E. C. T. Walker (Eds.), *Sentence processing: Psycholinguistic studies presented to Merrill Garrett* (pp. 281–294). Hillsdale, NJ: Lawrence Erlbaum Associates.

Landauer, T. K. (1962). Rate of implicit speech. *Perceptual and Motor Skills, 15,* 646.

Levelt, W. J. M. (1989). *Speaking: From intention to articulation.* Cambridge, MA: M.I.T. Press.

Lisker, L. (1978). *Rapid* vs. *rabid:* A catalogue of acoustic features that may cue the distinction. *Haskins Laboratories Status Report on Speech Research, 54,* 127–132.

MacKay, D. G. (1969). Phonetic factors in the perception and recall of spelling errors. *Neuropsychologia, 6,* 321–325.

MacKay, D. G. (1972). Input testing in the detection of misspellings. *American Journal of Psychology, 85,* 121–128.

MacKay, D. G. (1981). The problem of rehearsal or mental practice. *Journal of Motor Behavior, 13,* 274–285.

MacKay, D. G. (1982). The problems of flexibility, fluency, and speed-accuracy trade-off in skilled behavior. *Psychological Review, 89,* 483–506.

MacKay, D. G. (1987). *The organization of perception and action: A theory for language and other cognitive skills.* New York: Springer-Verlag.

MacKay, D. G. (in press). Spontaneous and evoked slips of the pen, tongue, and typewriter. In G. Blanken, J. Dittmann, H. Grimm, J. C. Marshall, & C. W. Wallesch (Eds.), *Linguistic Disorders and Pathologies.* Berlin: Walter de Gruyter & Co.

Marshall, P. H., & Cartwright, S. A. (1978). Failure to replicate a reported implicit/explicit speech equivalence. *Perceptual and Motor Skills, 46,* 1197–1198.

Marshall, P. H., & Cartwright, S. A. (1980). A final (?) note on implicit/explicit speech equivalence. *Bulletin of the Psychonomic Society, 15,* 409.

Max, L. (1937). An experimental study of the motor theory of consciousness IV: Action current responses in the deaf during awakening, kinesthetic imagery and abstract thinking. *Journal of Comparative Psychology, 24,* 301–344.

Meringer, R., & Meyer, K. (1895). *Versprechen und verlesen.* Stuttgart: Behrs Verlag.

McGurk, H., & MacDonald, J. (1976). Hearing lips and seeing voices. *Nature, 264,* 746–748.

Newell, A., & Rosenbloom, P. S. (1981). Mechanisms of skill acquisition and the law of practice. In J. R. Anderson (Ed.), *Cognitive skills and their acquisition* (pp. 1–56). Hillsdale, NJ: Lawrence Erlbaum Associates.

Nooteboom, S. G. (1980). Speaking and unspeaking: Detection and correction of phonological and lexical errors in spontaneous speech. In V. A. Fromkin (Ed.), *Errors in linguistic performance. Slips of the tongue, ear, pen and hand* (pp. 87–95). New York: Academic Press.

Parkin, A. J. (1987). *Memory and amnesia: An introduction.* New York: Basil Blackwell.

Pintner, R. (1913). Inner speech during silent reading. *Psychological Review, 30,* 129–153.

Reisberg, D. (Nov., 1989). *Anticipations and after-thoughts: How far does the "present" extend?* Paper presented at the 30th Annual Meeting of the Psychonomics Society, Atlanta, GA.

Reisberg, D., Smith, D., Baxter, D., & Sonenshine, M. (1989). Enacted auditory images are ambiguous; Pure auditory images are not. *Quarterly Journal of Experimental Psychology, 41A,* 619–181.

Salame, P., & Baddeley, A. (1989). Effects of background music on short-term memory. *Quarterly Journal of Experimental Psychology, 41A,* 107–122.

Schmidt, R. A. (1982). *Motor control and learning: A behavioral emphasis.* Champaign, Ill.: Human Kinetics.

Smith, N. V. (1973). *The acquisition of phonology: A case study.* New York: Cambridge University Press.

Smith, S. M., Brown, H. O., Tolman, J. E. P., & Goodman, L. S. (1947). Lack of cerebral effects of D-tubocurarine. *Anesthesiology, 8,* 1–14.

Snoddy, G. S. (1926). Learning and stability. *Journal of Applied Psychology, 10,* 1–36.

Sokolov, Y. N. (1972). *Inner speech and thought.* New York: Plenum.

Sperling, G. (1960). The information available in brief visual presentations. *Psychological Monographs: General and Applied, 74,* 1–29.

Warren, R. M. (1968). Verbal transformation effect and auditory perceptual mechanisms. *Psychological Bulletin, 70,* 261–270.

Watson, J. B. (1950). *Behaviorism.* New York: Norton.

Weber, R. J., & Castleman, J. (1970). The time it takes to imagine. *Perception & Psychophysics, 8,* 165–168.

Weisberg, R. W. (1980). *Memory, thought and behavior.* New York: Oxford University Press.

Wickelgren, W. A. (1965). Short-term memory for phonemically similar lists. *American Journal of Psychology, 78,* 567–574.

Wickelgren, W. A. (1966). Associative strength theory of recognition memory for pitch. *Journal of Mathematical Psychology, 6,* 13–61.

Wilding, J., Mohindra, N., & Breen-Lewis, K. (1982). Noise effects in free recall with various orienting tasks. *British Journal of Psychology, 73,* 479–486.

7 The Auditory Hallucinations of Schizophrenia

J. David Smith
New School for Social Research

Auditory hallucinations figure prominently in many schizophrenic episodes (Lehmann & Cancro, 1985; Sartorius, Shapiro, & Jablonsky, 1974). As a result, hallucinatory phenomena, (such as audible thoughts or voices) are first-rank symptoms of schizophrenia in the principle diagnostic systems (Schneider, 1959; see also American Psychiatric Association, 1980; Mellor, 1970). The voices are often obscene, insulting and accusing. They intrude and command attention; and can compel response—even if self-destructive (Kolb, 1977; Lehmann & Cancro, 1985).

What are these auditory hallucinations—phantom sensations, vivid mental images, just thoughts mis-taken for percepts, or something else? In this chapter I explore the cognitive processes underlying voices, because I believe that explaining them will help explain psychosis and aid in its treatment. To illustrate this possibility, contrast two theories of madness.

In one theory, the patient's sensory world shatters. Perhaps there is a breakdown of selective attention, flooding consciousness with chaotic sensory inputs that "sweep away the stable constructs of a former reality" (McGhie & Chapman, 1961, p. 112; see also Chapman, 1966; Freedman & Chapman, 1973; Neale & Oltmanns, 1980; Schwartz, 1982). Or perhaps an endogenous hallucinogen produces ghost sensations (Kolb, 1977; Shapiro, 1981). In these accounts, hallucinations are taken as sensed, or received, mental phenomena, and along with other sensory aberrations they lead the dance to psychosis. Other symptoms (delusions, etc.) accrete around this perceptual core, as secondary attempts to explain the voices or the sensory overload (George & Neufeld, 1985; Hoffman, 1986; McGhie & Chapman, 1961; Winters & Neale, 1983).

In a second theory, psychosis arises from unconscious conflicts too terrifying to express or admit. As they erupt, perhaps under extreme stress, the patient tries to deny or disown them. Delusions are one means to accomplish this, since thoughts controlled or thoughts inserted are not properly yours. But the most distant, safest expression is possible if the thoughts are externalized, believed perceived, "hallucinated." In this case, hallucinations begin just as thoughts, not as disturbed perceptual processing. Thus psychosis leads in the dance to hallucinations. Voices are the final, efficient crystallization of a delusional system evolved to express forbidden contents without owning them.

Arieti (1974) was one who believed that patients began with feelings of self-condemnation or self-hate and then concretized these into hallucinations—"the rotten personality becomes the rotten body that smells" (p. 268). Sechehaye (1951) also described hallucinations as sophisticated delusions. Early on, "the ego is overpowered; it casts out what horrifies it and is shocked at the exteriorized unconscious feelings. . . . The ego has no time to elaborate these feelings, these unconscious tendencies, into a bearable, verbally symbolic form, into the thematic auditory hallucination with its familiar characteristics of spatial and sensory localization." Only later will the patient "hear the voices in a truly sensory way" (pp. 117–118).

Are hallucinations perceptual, causal symptoms of mental illness, or secondary adjustments to mental illness? Are they a false perceptual itch that delusions scratch, or the perceptual frost that forms on cold psychoticism already in place? This contrast illustrates how the cognitive status of hallucinations matters for understanding psychosis, and motivates this analysis of their production and the mental representations that underlie them. I begin by describing the two classes of theory which have dominated the literature on hallucination.

SENSORY-RECEPTIVE THEORIES
OF HALLUCINATION

Most theories of hallucinations begin with a *Continuity Hypothesis* (cf. Horowitz, 1975; Savage, 1975). The idea is that mental experiences such as sensations, perceptions, dreams, images, fantasies, delusions and thoughts—in approximately that order—are not sharply distinct but are arrayed along some continuum. They differ in their vivacity, concreteness, coherence, in our volitional control of them, and in their reality insistence. There are sensations (vivid, unbidden, real), thoughts (vague, willed, abstract), and images somewhere between.

The Empiricist philosophers sired this continuum. They made sensations the primary stuff of mental life. As one scaled cognition towards ideas, the mental events became pale remnants of sensations—only in sleep, fever, and madness did ideas recover the force and liveliness to deceive the mind (Hume, 1739/1888, pp. 1–2). Hobbes said, "Imagination therefore is nothing but decaying sense" (Hobbes, 1651/1958, ch. 1–3). This idea passed directly to the early neurophysiologists. Jackson (1958) summed it up: "The idea is a faint percept, the percept is a vivid idea" (p. 211).

Now consider hallucinations, first as a general phenomenon (in schizophrenia, organic brain syndromes, delirium, alcohohol psychosis, etc.). Almost all definitions place hallucinations far toward the sensory end of the continuum. For example:

"Hallucinations are deviations in sensory and perceptual experience . . . A hallucination is the registration of a perception in the absence of a stimulus" (Reed, 1985, p. 15).

Hallucinations are "perceptions experienced without recognizably relevant sensory stimulation" (Wells, 1985, p. 840).

A hallucination is the "apparent perception of an external object when no such object is present" (Arieti, 1974, p. 266).

A hallucination is "a perceptual-like event that occurs in the absence of a specific external stimulus" (Crider, 1979, p. 39).

"Hallucinations are sensory experiences or perceptions without corresponding external stimuli" (Lehmann & Cancro, 1985, p. 683).

A hallucination is "a sensory perception without external stimulation of the relevant sensory organ." (American Psychiatric Association, 1980, p. 359).

This sense of hallucinations descended from Esquirol (1838/1845) and was dominant in the 19th and early 20th centuries (Arieti, 1974). The hallucination was believed to be "the transformation of a thought into a sensation" (Lelut, 1846, cited in Arieti, p. 269) or an idea that comes from where memories are stored that goes back to the perceptual centers and becomes a hallucination (Tanzi, 1909).

Jackson (1958) also perceptualized hallucinations. They were release phenomena which occurred when higher brain centers were lost and inhibition waned. Madness was one releaser. Hallucinations resulted "from irritations propagated up to the highest centres, that is, to the uncontrolled, and thus overready-to-act, nervous arrangements left in these centres" (p. 25). Thus Jackson took hallucinations to depend on some perceptual seed or nidus—an irritation of eyes or ears, or of the sensory centers one step higher (p. 25; see also Horowitz, 1978).

Other theories link hallucinations to sensory deprivation (Arieti, 1974; Horowitz, 1975; Solomon & Kleeman, 1985; West, 1962). This idea is that reduced input into the central nervous system allows a "release into awareness of previously recorded perceptions, through the disinhibition of brain circuits that represent them" (West, p. 281). West depicts this idea quite beautifully. A man in a room with a fire looks out a window as the sun sets. As dark falls, the input from the outside world decreases, but the window more and more reflects the scene inside the room back to the man's eye. So when "the daylight (sensory input) is reduced . . . images originating within the rooms of our brains may be perceived as though they came from outside the windows of our senses" (West, p. 281; see also Feder, 1982).

Now consider schizophrenic hallucinations in particular. Not suprisingly, the theories that explain voices often have the same sensory ring to them (see George & Neufeld, 1985). For Arieti (1974), schizophrenic hallucinations appeared when a higher mental representation regressed to a lower perceptual level— "phylogenetically and ontogenetically lower than the levels of verbal thought, and lower even than the level of images." Hallucinations "were originally thoughts or images that have changed into perceptions." Hallucinations were *not* simply intense images. "Images, stored in our memory, may be used by hallucinations, but they are reproduced with the modalities of perception" (p. 269).

There are also sensory deprivation hypotheses about schizophrenia. Perhaps schizophrenics withdraw socially, and this deprivation produces compensatory hallucinations. Or perhaps patients withdraw autistically to avoid chaotic perceptual worlds, then hallucinate in response to this self-induced sensory deprivation (McReynolds, 1960).

Finally, a variety of LSD theories have linked schizophrenic hallucinations to some endogenous hallucinogen that alters sensory experience and brings on psychedelic states (Hoffer, Osmond & Smythies, 1954; Kety, 1969; Shapiro, 1981). The fortunes of the mescaline, methylation, and related hypotheses have waxed, then waned since the early studies (McKinney, 1985). Still, mescaline hallucinations feel quite perceptual to subjects. Their attractiveness as a model for schizophrenic hallucinations shows once again the dominant sensory metaphor.

IMAGERY THEORIES OF HALLUCINATIONS

The theories just described place hallucinations far down the mental continuum, towards sensation and perception. Other theories move up the continuum one step and describe hallucinations as some abnormality of mental imagery. There are two opposing theories.

In one theory, an individual experiences few auditory images, making the rare exceptions surprising and compelling by contrast. Cohen (1938) found that auditory hallucinators had less vivid auditory imagery than visual imagery. Visual hallucinators had less vivid visual imagery than auditory imagery. Seitz and Molholm (1947) replicated this result and concluded that "one of the factors on which auditory hallucinations may depend is a relatively low percentage of auditory imagery" (p. 479). Starker and Jolin's (1982) hallucinating schizophrenics also reported their auditory imagery to be impoverished. Heilbrun, Blum, and Haas (1983) explored the choices patients made for visual or auditory imagery, using target images (e.g., hands clapping) that would support imagery in either modality. Schizophrenics with auditory hallucinations used less auditory imagery than schizophrenics without hallucinations.

In the opposing theory, hallucinations arise from peculiarly vivid imagery. For example, Horowitz (1975, 1978) suggested that more vivid internal images would seem more external, "real," and disturbing; hence vividness of imagery was a significant clinical issue for him. In support of the vividness hypothesis, Mintz and Alpert (1972) found that hallucinating schizophrenics, more than normal controls, rated auditory images as vivid and believed actual auditory stimuli had occurred.

Against the vividness hypothesis, Brett and Starker (1977) failed to replicate the Mintz and Alpert finding. If anything, their schizophrenics had impoverished imagery when the content of the images was emotional or interpersonal (see also Bentall & Slade, 1985).

Finally, against either imagery hypothesis, Heilbrun, Blum, and Haas (1983) found that hallucinators and nonhallucinators had equally vivid auditory imagery when the imagery task required them to use it. Roman and Landis (1945) found no link between auditory hallucinations and the strength or weakness of either auditory or visual imagery; nor did Catts, Armstrong, Norcross, and McConaghy (1980). And Slade (1976) reported enhanced imagery vividness for both hallucinating and nonhallucinating psychotics compared to normals, but no differences between the first two groups.

Clearly neither imagery hypothesis—that hallucinations are rare and surprising images, or especially vivid images—finds consistent support. Bentall and Slade (1985) concluded that "generally speaking, the hypothesis that hallucinators suffer from an abnormality of mental imagery has not been a fruitful one" (p. 160).

Unfortunately, all these studies tap *self-reports* of imagery vividness and preference. Consequently, they risk demand characteristics, failures of introspection, social desirability, and validly differing criteria of vividness across groups and individuals. Schizophrenics lack insight generally, and their hallucinations could easily produce a peculiar vividness criterion. And even among normals, *general* self-report measures of imagery (like those used in these studies) do not always predict interesting, functional differences in actual performance on imagery tasks. So perhaps it is unsurprising that such measures do not distinguish hallucinators and nonhallucinators.

Given this failure of self-reports, another research strategy seems indicated. One might explore the functional equivalences between auditory hallucinations and imagery, on the one hand, and auditory hallucinations and perception, on the other. A persistent idea is that auditory hallucinations are farther down the mental continuum than ordinary auditory images. If so, then auditory hallucinations should "behave" more perceptually than images. To show this, one could use the auditory analogues of well known visual imagery studies—scanning studies, zooming studies, etc.—which have explored the functional parallels between imagery and perception. This research is now becoming possible, as recent research and the present volume break the silence on auditory imagery in the cognitive literature. Such research could aid a serious demonstration that auditory hallucinations do occur towards the sensory end of mental life. And after all, this demonstration is key, because as I discuss now, the imagery theories of hallucinations still accept that hallucinations are sensory/receptive phenomena.

THE SENSORY/RECEPTIVE SLANT
OF IMAGERY THEORIES

In the cognitive literature, most theories of mental imagery accept that imagery and perception share some common processing space. Kosslyn (1980, 1983) took the image as some uninterpreted raw material in a visuo-spatial buffer, akin to the proximal stimulus in perception, which is later interpreted by a process related to perceiving. Farah (1985) also pointed to the representational medium shared by imagery and perceptual inputs (see also Finke, 1980; and a review in Finke, 1985).

Given a shared representational medium, one predicts that imagery processes and perceptual processes could be confused. In fact, as early as 1910, Perky found that faint stimuli seemed like mental images to subjects. Conversely, Johnson, Raye, Wang, and Taylor (1979) found that subjects remembered the *imagining* of objects as *actual presentations* of the objects, and vivid imagers made this mistake more often. Johnson et al. suggested that vivid imagers built more accurate or more pictorial representations of the object, making their former images feel more like former perceptions. Similarly, Johnson and Raye (1981) argued that remembered images might be confused for remembered perceptual experiences if the images had many sensory features encoded with them.

Now consider hallucinations again. The shared imagery–perceptual register is a perfect theoretical backdrop if one believes that hallucinations are mental images confused for actual percepts. The potential for confusion exists because of the shared medium. Now one is only left to explain why hallucinations are "special" images, so that they are confused as percepts. Are they more sensory, vivid, surprising, emotionally riveting? Or perhaps images seem more compelling because verbal thought is simultaneously impaired. Then the images will remain poorly encoded, free-floating in the imagery–perceptual buffer; hence like percepts not yet translated into other meanings (Horowitz, 1975, 1978).

Not surprisingly, imagery theories of hallucinations adopt the idea of the shared register. For Horowitz, hallucinations were represented in buffers that also received input from external sensations. Kass (1968) also mapped hallucinations onto the nervous centers involved in waking perception. This idea about hallucinations has a distinguished pedigree. As James (1950) said it: The physiological process underlying hallucinations "must consist of an excitement from within of those centres which are active in normal perception, identical in kind and degree with that which real external objects are usually needed to induce" (v. 2, p. 122–131).

Doubtless the shared medium is a perfect, and plausible, mental model for imagery theories of hallucinations to adopt. But for present purposes the crucial point is the theoretical commitment this entails. By adopting that model, one naturally retains an externalist, stimulus, perceptual sense of the hallucination.

In fact, some imagery theories of hallucinations are just too sensory. For example, Horowitz (1975) takes hallucinations to represent increased internal input to the imagery system. He models such increased input by electrically or chemically stimulating the optical tract, the visual cortex, or points in between. The result is perceptual images, more complex for "higher" centers stimulated (cf. Horowitz & Adams, 1970). However, the stimulation Horowitz describes is not internal, the resulting mental events are not images, at least not in any sense required to explain spontaneous hallucinatory experiences. The central nervous system knows only transduction—such artificial stimulation will create unbidden, passively received, external sensations in every relevant cognitive or brain sense. One cannot just excite sensory pathways and hope to study hallucinations, or images. This "imagery" description of hallucinations is indistinct from earlier, sensory descriptions.

Savage (1975) also criticizes the dogged attempts of neuropsychologists to provide "stimulus" explanations for hallucinations. "Like his externalist predecessor, he assumes that perception, veridical and nonveridical, can be understood in terms of what stimuli do to the organism. What in fact is required is an understanding of what the organism does to the stimuli. Perception and hallucination should not be thought of as passive, receptive processes, but as active, constructive processes. To explain hallucinations as effects of brain stimulation is as unsatisfactory as to explain them as effects of physical stimulation. Instead we must come to understand the internal activity of hallucination (and perception) production" (p. 280).

In the end, sensory and imagery theories are close kin in explaining auditory hallucinations. Early theories placed ideas into the perceptual system, so that they "arrived" through the senses. Imagists place ideas into a shared imagery–perceptual register so that they seem perceived. Both explanations proceed by placing the phenomenon of hallucinations *well toward the receptive machinery of the cognitive system* (see also Alpert, Rubenstein & Kesselman, 1976). Both keep the feel of the hallucination as received and sensory. Yet, for several reasons, these basic assumptions may not be justified for the case of schizophrenic hallucinations.

CONCERNS ABOUT THE SENSORY/RECEPTIVE
HYPOTHESIS

Sensory explanations of schizophrenic hallucinations have always failed to address several basic questions about hallucinations: Why do auditory hallucinations predominate? Why voices? Why language? Visual hallucinations are relatively uncommon in schizophrenia; auditory hallucinations predominate in ratios of 2:1 (Jansson, 1968), 5:1 (George & Neufeld, 1985; Malitz, Wilkens, & Esecover, 1962) or 10:1 or more (Feinberg, 1962; Horowitz, 1978; Mintz & Alpert, 1972; Roman & Landis, 1945). By contrast, organic brain states and affective disorders bring mainly visual hallucinations (Brown, 1977), perhaps distinguishing schizophrenia from other hallucinogenic dysfunctions (George & Neufeld, 1985). But a sensory view does not allow such distinctions—without important additional assumptions that have not been forthcoming.

In addition, the sensory view implies a particular phenomenology to hallucinations. The voices should feel external—from outside the head, not inside the mind. In fact, the internal/external distinction is an old one. Baillarger (1846) distinguished psych-sensorial hallucinations, those which seem to strike on the outward ears, from psychical hallucinations, those produced in the interior of the soul. It is also an old belief that "sicker" patients should have more sensory/external hallucinations (Junginger & Frame, 1985).

However, in Judkins and Slade (1981), one third of hallucinating schizophrenics experienced mostly internal voices, the same proportion as in Alpert and Silvers (1970). Mott, Small, & Anderson (1965) also found that only schizophrenic hallucinators (among other hallucinating groups such as alcoholics) experienced internal voices to any extent, and there was no evidence that more externally perceived hallucinations seemed more real. According to Semrad (1938), "the patient often found himself handicapped by inadequate word facilities to describe his experience and in formulating it would oscillate between having heard a voice and having had a thought" (pp. 58–59). Some subjects did describe the voices as "perceptual." However, even here, the voices were not perceived as through the ears or clearly external ". . . I do not hear them in my ear . . . they talk inside of me . . . they are talking through my head . . . it is inner voices, voices in the mind, the voice of conscience" (pp. 59–60).

Even when external, voices are seldom localized spatially (one fourth of the time in Alpert & Silvers, 1970). Junginger and Frame (1985) also found schizophrenics mixed on this point. Semrad's patients felt the voices all around them in the atmosphere, and coming through the air. Junginger and Frame concluded that "the notion that voices perceived as originating outside the head are characteristic of schizophrenia should probably be abandoned" (p. 153).

Nor are voices loud and clear to the schizophrenic: Their sensory clarity is questionable. Semrad's (1938) hallucinating psychotics (32 were schizophrenic) heard whispers, mumblings, possible voices, sounds like muffled microphones, etc. In Junginger and Frame (1985; see also Junginger, 1986), patients found their verbal hallucinations soft, not loud, and judged their reality with difficulty. In Junginger and Rauscher (1987), patients judged a headphone voice louder and clearer than their recent verbal hallucinations (see also Hoffman, 1986).

Here it is useful to juxtapose the hallucinations of schizophrenia and alcoholism, which contrast sharply. Auditory hallucinations also figure prominently in alcohol hallucinosis. These experiences are a paradigm of external, sensory hallucinations, unlike schizophrenic voices.

As Semrad (1938) described alcohol hallucinations, their sensory vividness was very marked, and experienced usually in both ears. Patients would look around to reply to them, or try to see where they were coming from. Some patients had tinnitus, or sensations of buzzing noises.

In Gross, Halpert, Sabot, and Polizos (1963; see also Saravay & Pardes, 1967, 1970), hallucinating alcoholics heard voices nearby, but in a realistic, possible location, one where the patient could not see them—behind a wall, around a corner, in the next apartment. The alcoholic frequently searched for those making the voices, or tried to join them. The schizophrenic never does this (Strauss, 1962; see also Parker & Schilder, 1935).

In Alpert and Silvers (1970), alcohol hallucinations included noises, music, and unintelligible voices; schizophrenics heard intelligible voices almost exclusively. Alcohol hallucinations were clearly external and spatially localized; these in schizophrenia were internal or external and vaguely localized (e.g., from the sky). They concluded that alcohol hallucinations were sensory, spatially placed, and emergent from a background of noises and unintelligible voices. As they say, localization, filtering and masking effects, etc. are dependent on relatively peripheral auditory structures. The sensory feel of these hallucinations may explain their attention-demanding quality—the alcoholic is distracted with difficulty from his voices. By contrast, schizophrenic voices are more cognitive, like audible thoughts, have greater intelligibility, poorer localization, and are less attention demanding.

Why these differences? One possible explanation is that alcohol hallucinations are elaborations of a sensory seed, and this explains their sensory properties. Semrad (1938) found substantial toxic deafness in his alcohol psychosis group (14 of 38), suggesting that alcohol directly targets hearing centers and the sensory acuity for high tones. Saravay and Pardes (1967, 1970) also found many elementary hallucinations (brief sounds and noises) in alcohol hallucinosis, and attributed these sounds to middle ear pathology which was heard as ringing, clicks, etc. Hallucinations could be built on these, or could emerge from within a texture of such sounds.

Thus sensory/receptive theory easily explains the alcoholic's sensory hallucinations. The theory fares much less well in describing the schizophrenic's ethereal voices—soft and mumbled, in the body, or vaguely in the air, arriving on beams, rays, or signals.

There is one last difficulty with a receptive theory of schizophrenic hallucinations. Such a theory most naturally sugests a dysfunction of brain centers involved in speech *reception* and analysis (cf. Green & Preston, 1981). Yet brain stimulation here fails to produce the coherent, language hallucinations of schizophrenia. It mainly produces nonauditory hallucinations, nonverbal sounds or repetitive sequences of words recalled from memory (Bazhin, Wasserman, & Tonkonogii, 1975; Green & Preston, 1981; Halgren, Walter, Cherlow, & Crandall, 1978; Penfield & Perot, 1963; Weingarten, Cherlow, & Holmgren, 1977), not the didactic, clever, piquant comments of the voices. Thus Green and Preston (1981) suggest that one might have to stimulate more frontal areas, involved in speech *production,* to reproduce voices such as those heard by schizophrenics. In fact, they link auditory hallucinations to the mechanism of actively produced inner speech, not to the mechanism of passively received auditory sensation (see also Bazhin et al., 1975).

So one must be troubled about a sensory/receptive theory of schizophrenic voices. Yet this theory has acquired substantial historical momentum, which is difficult to check. Moreover, since the sensory view of hallucinations generally works as a diagnostic tool in schizphrenia, there is a temptation to be pragmatic and leave the matter at that. However, the cautions in this section suggest that historical inertia and diagnostic convenience may need resisting in this case.

It is possible to outline the kind of alternative theory one might wish for. It would move hallucinations up the mental continuum, away from sensation and perception, and *toward the productive machinery of the cognitive system.* It would focus on the domains of speech and language to capture schizophrenic hallucinations more precisely. These two considerations might focus attention on inner speech, just as Bazhin et al. (1975) and Green and Preston (1981) suggested. And of course the theory would be tailored to the phenomenology of schizophrenic voices. It should explain how voices feel real and frightening, like actual stimuli in some respects. But—though it seems almost contradictory—the theory should also predict that voices would be poorly externalized and localized.

One can solve this theoretical problem. A growing literature finds an intimate connection between inner speech and auditory imagery, to which several chapters in the present volume attest. In this connection lies the alternative theory. My research on auditory imagery, with Dan Reisberg and Meg Wilson, led me to the alternative, and this is the departure point I choose for entering into it. However, I soon realized that what was at issue was an older, "orphaned" idea about schizophrenic hallucinations.

AUDITORY HALLUCINATIONS, AUDITORY IMAGERY AND INNER SPEECH

Imagery theories of hallucinations, as discussed above, adopt a particular view of mental imagery. It is that mental images begin with some neutral raw material, like a proximal stimulus in a perceptual buffer, that is then interpreted by a process related to perceiving (Horowitz, 1975, 1978; see also Finke, 1980; Kosslyn, 1980, 1983). In this view images are like stimuli—they might even surprise, frighten, and seem like a sensory visitation. By this view images would also have the potential to be ambiguous—imagined reversible figures like Necker Cubes, Duck/Rabbits, or their auditory analogues should reverse. This potential exists because the imagery raw material, itself indifferent to interpretation, could be reconsulted and reconstrued (see also Reisberg & Chambers, 1986).

Reisberg, Smith, Baxter and Sonenshine (1989) asked if auditory images are like stimuli by this criterion of neutrality, ambiguity, and reversibility. To do so, we exploited the fact that certain words, if repeated, yield a soundstream which is fully compatible with more than one segmentation (Warren, 1961; Warren & Gregory, 1958). Rapid repetition of the word "life," for example, produces a physical soundstream which can be heard as repetitions of "life," or "fly." These repetitions undergo phenomenal shifts for the listener, just as the Necker Cube or duck/rabbit figures do for the seer. We asked if imagined, not heard, repetitions of these stimuli also shift.

Many subjects do reconstrue these auditory images. Thus these images are stimulus-like by one criterion—they apparently involve some freestanding icon that can be reapproached and reconstrued. However, this result obtains because subjects throw the imagined speechstream into their articulators and subvocalize it, perhaps with movements of the tongue, lips, and teeth. We believe this subarticulation provides the "stimulus" that affords reconstrual. If this subvocalization is eliminated, for example, by blocking subarticulation, the auditory images remaining do not support reconstrual—they are unambiguous. This result led us to distinguish subvocalized auditory images, which do act like stimuli in supporting reconstrual, from auditory images that are not subvocalized and do not act like stimuli in this way.

In other research, we find that subjects subvocalize in making judgments about melodies and in other tasks of auditory imagery. It seems quite natural for them to subvocalize the auditory image, to make it as robust and accessible as possible.

Possibly the alternative account of schizophrenic voices is now plain. Suppose schizophrenics hallucinated voices by subvocalizing them, so that hallucinations were subvocalized speech images. Then hallucinations would be actively produced inner speech, not "received" auditory percepts. Of course language and voices would predominate. Moreover, some stimulus properties of voices would be explained. The subvocalized images would involve a freestanding icon which could be reapproached and reinterpreted, but which might also surprise and frighten. Yet despite these stimulus properties, we would expect hallucinated voices not to feel spatially localized, and not to be well externalized.

One evening, I told a Baltimore psychiatrist how, with ordinary undergraduates, blocking the articulators (immobilizing the teeth, tongue, and lips) eliminated the stimulus qualities of the subvocalized auditory image. His response stunned me. He described a colleague who used identical blocking procedures to *stop the auditory hallucinations of schizophrenics.* My research soon revealed that a subvocalization hypothesis of voices has surfaced occasionally, so that there is scattered prior evidence on this point.

THE SUBVOCALIZATION THEORY
OF SCHIZOPHRENIC HALLUCINATIONS

Early on, Maudsley (1886) pointed out that the insane hear interior voices in their heads, not distinct, articulated utterances in their ears. Parish (1897) went one step farther, taking auditory hallucinations to be automatic speech—the un-noticed, audible articulation of one's own thoughts. Seglas (1914) acknowledged this as one possible class of verbal hallucination. LaGache (1935) also suggested that verbal hallucinations are distorted self-produced speech. Evidence awaited the research of Gould.

Evidence from Electromyography

For Gould (1948, p. 371), hallucinations were the automatic activity of thought and its motor expression as covert language. He thought that the tonic muscle tension of schizophrenics should make covert speech more overt. As he said,

> Since it is in many a habitual accompaniment to thought, the now augmented subvocal speech happens automatically, and murmured speech or intensified sub-vocal speech is produced. The patient, usually unaware of self-production, misin-terprets his own speech as an intrusion of alien speech or "voices." He is not repeating his verbal hallucinations; he is either hearing his own automatic whisper-ing or is experiencing the auditory representation of speech produced by intensified motor impulses arising from hyperactivity of his vocal musculature during think-ing. (1950, p. 116)

This general idea was supported in Cerny (1964, 1965) and Lindsley (e.g., 1963).

But Gould's evidence was weak. He took brief EMG readings from resting schizophrenics and normals, in the areas of eye, jaw, larynx, biceps. Eighty percent of hallucinating schizophrenics showed increased muscle tension of the articulators, compared to 10–20% of other patients and normals. Unfortunately, we don't know whether patients were hallucinating during muscle recording—hallucinating status was determined afterwards—or whether readings from other muscle groups were also elevated. General muscle tension, including artic-ulators, would occur if only hallucinating schizophrenics were sicker, more stressed, or more afraid, as well as they might be.

Roberts, Greenblatt, and Solomon (1952) supported a general arousal in-terpretation of these results. They confirmed occasional increased subvocal activity in hallucinating schizophrenics. However, this abnormal activity infrequently coincided with an auditory hallucination.

McGuigan (1966) did find a link between EMG activity and hallucinations in one schizophrenic patient. Articulatory activity and breathing increased just prior to reported hallucinations. And noticeable whispering accompanied them. In two cases the whisperings were audible and matched the hallucination's content. Arm muscle activity did not rise in synchrony with hallucinations, indicating that the relevant EMG activity was restricted to the speech system.

This correlative finding leaves open the question of whether the subvocal activity *is the hallucination*. It might instead be the epiphenomenon indicating more central processes. Or the subject might be shadowing the hallucinated voice. And N = 1 is not ideal. Still, McGuigan suggested that covert oral language behavior may be necessary to create a hallucination, and that the "hallucinatory" experience is initiated when a person talks to himself.

Inouye and Shimizu (1970) studied nine schizophrenics, using electromyographic techniques. Patients delimited auditory hallucinations with switch presses, and these corresponded with bursts of vocal activity in 47.6% of cases. In another condition, subjects were told to press the switches at random times but when no voices were present. These presses were accompanied by bursts of vocal activity in only 8.3% of cases. The switch pressing usually began shortly after the EMG activity began to be recorded. The durations of switch pressing and EMG activity were well correlated. And subjectively "louder" hallucinations tended to be accompanied by EMG bursts; subjectively "softer" hallucinations not.

Junginger and Rauscher (1987) compared 19 hallucinating and 22 nonhallucinating psychotic patients. Hallucinators did show higher vocal potentials. Potentials from other muscle groups were only slightly raised, but enough to render unreliable the crucial interaction between hallucinating/nonhallucinating and speech musculature/other musculature. Junginger and Rauscher also evaluated the vocal activity before and after 402 hallucinations. Vocal activity was not significantly higher in the three seconds prior to a report of a hallucination than in the 3 sec following, as it should be if vocal activity caused the hallucination. Similarly, vocal activity was not higher in the two seconds prior to a hallucination than in the 7th and 8th seconds prior. Across all subjects, the percentage of reported hallucinations that was coincident with higher vocal EMG (46%) was no greater than when subjects just listened to tape recorded statements (49%). Thus Junginger and Rauscher failed to support the hypothesis "that verbal hallucinations become 'audible' through muscle activity" (p. 108).

Unfortunately, two cautions attend this study. First, Junginger and Rauscher's subjects showed diverse psychotic patterns (schizophrenic, schizoaffective, depressive, or bipolar disorders), so this study was not properly about schizophrenic hallucinations, which may be unique. Second, it is unclear that the proper control for EMG activity during voices is EMG activity during listening to statements (where shadowing, commenting, and responding may be likely). In fact, Innouye and Shimuzu's subjects showed EMG bursts co-ocurring with hallucinations 47% of the time, just the 46% Junginger and Frame found. However, Innouye and Shimuzu's subjects showed EMG bursts between hallucinations only 8.3% of the time, much lower than Junginger and Frame's 49% during listening. It seems that subjects may subvocalize during hallucinations and also during listening—this is a different conclusion than that they do not subvocalize during hallucinations. Consistent with this, Gould (1949) found that audible speech increased subvocal speech in a schizophrenic patient.

Evidence from Blocked Subarticulation

Recently, a New York therapist provided me with an illustrative "blocked articulation" anecdote. He described a woman patient who had wandered her ward for years, with her mouth clamped wide open. She resisted all efforts to help her stop this behavior, saying that when she clamped her mouth open it stopped her voices.

Like this patient and the psychiatrist described earlier, some researchers have blocked subarticulation in a therapeutic intervention to stop the voices. Evenson (1987) found that when subjects hummed it controlled their voices. For one woman, this explained why her voices never visited her in her garden—she hummed while working there. Erickson and Gustafson (1968) stopped voices in their patients with humming and gargling. Green's (1978) patients combatted hallucinations by naming objects around them (see also Green, Glass, & O'Callaghan, 1980; Green & Preston, 1981; James, 1983). Green and Preston (1981) also suggested that auditory hallucinations represent abnormal speech production, not abnormal sensation and perception.

Unfortunately, all these studies were quite small, with no controls over placebo or expectancy effects. And none of these studies distinguished general distraction from specific articulatory disruption. That is, it might be that any distracting activity (foot tapping, finger drumming, etc.)—not just articulatory activity—would have the same benefit for patients. If so, then general distraction would presumably be the cause of the reduced voices, not specific articulatory interference with the voices.

Bick and Kinsbourne (1987) carried out the most sophisticated study in this area. They studied 18 hallucinating schizophrenics. Patients closed eyes tight, opened mouths wide, made fists and squeezed, etc., and reported for each action whether the voices got worse, better, or neither. Mouth opening abolished voices, other actions did not.

As Bick and Kinsbourne pointed out, previous correlational work did not address cause and effect. The patient could have been shadowing the voices. But then freezing the articulators would not have inhibited the perceptual experience. In addition, this study helps rule out general distraction and placebo effects by including other actions besides mouth opening. Thus Bick and Kinsbourne infer the following sequence of events: "The patient subvocalizes, listens to his or her covert speech, and attributes it to another" (p. 223).

Bick and Kinsbourne (exp. 2) also hypnotized 21 normals to "hear voices." The subjects heard low-volume, barely intelligible murmuring similar to schizophrenic hallucinations. They showed responses of amusement or bewilderment. And mouth opening, more than other actions, also abolished voices for these hypnotized normals. Apparently these subjects also found subvocalization a natural strategy to externalize and perceptualize an auditory image. Reisberg et al.'s (1988) subjects responded identically when needing stimulus-tinged auditory images that could be reinterpreted—that is, they spontaneously subvocalized the required speech images. Why should schizophrenics be different regarding this natural strategy?

A related result emerged in Slade (1974), who administered various cognitive tasks to schizophrenics. He found voices reduced while naming letters, but not while copying them. Note that this is one manipulation a researcher might use to evaluate the inner voice's role in auditory hallucinations. Hallucinations and copying as concurrent tasks do not mutually interfere. Hallucinations and letter naming do—suggesting they compete for the same limited pool of articulatory resources.

Evidence from Case Studies

Gould (1949) presented the case of a woman who muttered to herself almost nonstop. She reported a snapping sound, perhaps made by a telegraph station, and heard two different voices, which she listened to and chuckled at.

EMG recordings and amplification of all speech sounds showed that subvocalization and hallucinations coincided in onset and duration. When intelligible, the subvocal speech was the same in content as the voices. When the subvocal speech was indistinct, the patient had trouble "hearing the voices." Observers rated the speed of her subvocalized speech at about 130 w.p.m., exactly as fast as she estimated her voices talked, and twice as fast as her normal whispering. The snapping sound she reported was clearly made by her tongue. And of the patient's two voices, one spoke on breathing in, the other on breathing out.

Green and Preston (1981) strongly amplified all a patient's vocalizations, for the patient also, and found that this increased the clarity and volume of the patient's subvocalizations. (This maneuver also threatened the study's interpretability, since these amplified whisperings and mutterings were audible to the patient too, and might have changed his speech behavior.) Nonetheless, extraordinary exchanges were then recorded, between the patient's normal speaking voice, and a whisper that was the patient's "hallucinated" voice. For example, the experimenter suggested that the patient talked to himself. The patient replied, "No I don't (normal voice) . . . What is it (low whisper) . . . Mind your own business, darling, I don't want him to know what I was doing (medium whisper) . . . See that, I spoke to ask her what she was doing and she said mind your own business (normal voice)" (p. 206).

Evidence from Self-Report Data

Patient descriptions of hallucinations can also suggest the mode of their production (Gould, 1950). Sometimes the patient is lucid and the description coherent. For example:

> M. L.: "I thought they were really voices but it was really myself thinking to myself. At first I thought it was somebody talking to me . . . I had been so nervous I could think I could hear it . . . I was talking out loud, but to myself instead of thinking . . . just loud enough to hear myself say it—not real loud—just out loud; kind of whispering-like to myself." (p. 111)

> W. K.: "It's something inside my head, maybe just my memory. It seems like someone is talking to me or I am talking to myself." (p. 111)

However, even delusional, incoherent descriptions agree. Some patients feel the voices in their throats, diaphragms, mouths, and tongues (p. 112).

> K. N.: "They use a broadcast voice that is more an expressed thought broadcast than an actual voice. It is the vibration from the larynx and when you receive them you almost seem to feel them as much as hear them . . . My tongue seems to be beating out messages."

> E. B.: "It affects your ears, and comes out of your mouth all the time."

> J. A.: "I feel the vibration like from the words just above the tongue. Sometimes inside where the brain is, sometimes over here (larynx), sometimes where the heart is, but mostly inside the mouth. It's in the mouth and then I hear it in the head part; after it was said I heard it in the ear."

> G. R.: "Two of them down the river talking inside of me. Down here along the voice nerve." (Points along the front of his neck). "It's the same as you talk to yourself. You can feel it inside, same action . . . I hear a woman's voice coming right through me. It felt as though it was coming out of my mouth. I could feel it through the air passages, I could hear it through my mouth . . . Somebody is attacking me and my lips move."

> L. M.: "The sound seems to strike out of my neck, and sometimes, there is a pulling of the muscles. I'm not doing it—pulling it back and forth. It's being done by something unseen . . . It seems funny how the voices come out of your throat. It seems to ooze through one's skin. Unless it is an invisible current that comes through my neck" (p. 423) . . . "I'm hearing the voices again—they're coming right through the voice box." (p. 424)

Finally, some patients even note that the voices usurp the apparatus they (the patient) would like to use for talking (Gould, 1950, p. 112).

> G. R.: "They bear down on my nerves in front and interfere with my talking."

> L. M.: "Sometimes when I talk someone else is on the wire; the words hit together. When I go to talk someone else is there to talk. It seems as though there are two people trying to talk from the same voice box."

From these lines of evidence, subvocalization proponents conclude that auditory hallucinations represent inner speech enacted (cf. Johnson, 1958, 1967, 1978). A recent textbook of clinical psychiatry addressed the subvocalization hypothesis as follows: "Auditory hallucinatory experiences are often associated with movement of the laryngeal musculature, suggesting that the patient is uttering subvocally the words he perceives in his hallucination, just as a child does as he learns to read silently" (Kolb, 1977, p. 138). Flor-Henry (1986) concluded:

> During verbal hallucinosis there is myogenic activation of the vocal system triggered by disorganized inner speech . . . Auditory hallucinations are reflections of altered neural structures responsible for verbal-linguistic expression. Abnormal activation of these neural sets produces subliminal subvocalization, "hallucinations of inner speech," which because unintended are perceived subjectively as foreign to the self. (p. 523)

CONCERNS ABOUT THE SUBVOCALIZATION HYPOTHESIS

Yet evidence for the subvocalization hypothesis is less than ideal. The introspective reports are compelling, but introspections can mislead, and Gould doubtlessly reported patient descriptions selectively to buttress the subvocalization claim. Other data come from clinical interventions that lack appropriate controls. Still other studies link auditory hallucinations with high vocal activity, without also ruling out activity in other muscle groups. Nonetheless, of the most sophisticated studies in this area, three do show a close link between subvocalization and auditory hallucinations (Bick & Kinsbourne, 1987, Exp. 1; Inouye & Shimizu, 1970; Slade, 1974). One study (Junginger & Frame, 1985) does not support that link, though unfortunately it was not properly a comparison between hallucinating and nonhallucinating schizophrenics. Overall the situation regarding the subvocalization idea is promising, though further research is clearly needed regarding this neglected hypothesis. Important reviews of cognition in schizophrenia still ignore subvocalization entirely (cf. George & Neufeld, 1985).

A second problem is that even if subvocalization of voices sometimes occur, it could represent only a subset of schizophrenic auditory hallucinations. Baillarger

(1846) distinguished psychosensory hallucinations (perceived through the ears) and psychic hallucinations (produced in the soul). Maudsley (1886) also distinguished hallucinations that were more sensory or more internal. Lang (1938, 1940), who described his own battle with schizophrenia, emphasized that schizophrenics hear voices proper that are different from the "thoughts out loud." Rund's (1986) opinion was that one should maintain this distinction between self-generated voices inside one's head and "true" hallucinations (voices originating from the outside).

Actually, this problem is not really so difficult for a subvocalization view. For one thing, there seem to be no data at present that directly support or force such a distinction. For another thing, there are different degrees and levels of subvocalization and enactment which could easily span the range of mental events from thoughts, to "thoughts out loud," to full-fledged voices. We have already encountered two cases where subjectively loud and clear hallucinations tended to be accompanied by EMG bursts; subjectively softer hallucinations not (Gould, 1949; Inouye and Shimizu, 1970).

But this range of effects points to a third problem for subvocalization accounts. They are plagued by a certain vagueness, because they do not specify the level of involvement by the speech system. Sometimes the subvocalized hallucination seems audible, to patient and experimenter, suggesting that schizophrenics hear but misattribute their own speech. Other times, the stimulus provided by the covert enactment seems only kinesthetic, produced by the soundless activity of the articulators.

This kinesthetic interpretation is defensible. Much evidence implicates speech production in speech perception (Liberman & Mattingly, 1985; Richardson, 1984; Salame & Baddeley, 1982). So tacit articulation could provide a nonacoustic speech stimulus, which is then interpreted through the usual channels for speech processing. Actually, the enactment could even stop at motor planning for speech, short of articulator movement. Motor plans for speech probably include a variety of auxiliary representations that will be used to control and check the speech produced. For example, there may be corollary discharge, a feedforward signal from motor plans to sensory systems that prepare the latter for the proprioceptive consequences of the movement. An efferent copy of the planned movement may also be laid down and later used to check the actual speech act for correctness (Zivin, 1986). It is easy to imagine that a planned speech act could also prime the auditory perceptual system. This acoustic feedforward signal would provide a check on the auditory correctness of the speech act.

The point is that the mechanisms of speech production and speech perception probably interact in diverse ways, involving several different representations of verbal images as they become accomplished speech acts, and therefore giving rise to several different sources of imagery-speech confusions (or hallucinations). The implication is that subvocalization theories should strive for greater clarity— do they rest on audibility, kinesthesia, motor planning, or what?

There is a fourth problem with the subvocalization hypothesis. It suggests that hallucinations represent the uncoupling of inner speech and broader thought. Somehow there develops a failure of recognition of the subvocalization system that makes the kinds of inner speech streams you and I have, as the stock in trade of our daily cognitive lives, feel inserted, alien, and terrifying. But if so, one must explain how and why the subvocalization system could split off from the rest of mental life, so that subvocalized verbal images grew to be foreign to the ego, instead of being part of the internal dialogue of thought (see Smith, 1991).

CONCLUSIONS

Neither the sense, image, nor subvoice theory comes with a knockdown punch for its peers. Each raises theoretical questions, offers a mixed data base, and therefore needs further study and refinement.

From a cognitive perspective, this drift between theories represents an unacceptable weakness in the literature on psychosis. To see just one instance of this, consider how research in schizophrenia would be changed simply by taking a sensory or subvoice stance.

Cognitive Predispositions

Many researchers seek cognitive risk factors for psychosis. Most hypothesized deficits are sensory or attentional—in attentional filtering, sensory habituation, slowness of sensory encoding, or excessive stimulus uptake (cf. Kietzman, Spring, & Zubin, 1985). These theories fit comfortably with a sensory idea about auditory hallucinations.

But under a subvoice hypothesis, one might ask if children prone to psychosis are delayed in acquiring inner speech, if it stays more overt or externalized (perhaps because these children are loners from an early age), if it is more in the second or third person, or if it is more freely borrowed by imaginary companions, so that it never becomes fully self-owned. In short, one would seek habits of (inner) speech that risked its breaking off from the ego; instead of the operating characteristics of perceptual systems that risked their being overwhelmed.

Environmental Triggers

Stress and aloneness are known to bring on psychosis in those predisposed (Birley & Brown, 1970; Brown & Birley, 1968; Brown, Harris, & Peto, 1973). A sensory interpretation of these precipitating factors might be that stress and extreme arousal threaten sensory overload, crumbling perceptual filters, etc. Or perhaps extreme aloneness brings sensory deprivation and compensatory hallucinations in its wake.

A subvoice perspective would evaluate how these life changes target the systems of language and inner speech, not those of attention and perception. In fact, both loneliness and stress likely do change our use of the inner voice. We encourage, comfort, instruct outselves in an internal dialogue that becomes more frequent, salient, and overt—one can become sick of one's own voice. As one patient said of his auditory hallucinations, "I am quite positive it is caused by a lack of conversation—opportunities to speak to people. If a person doesn't have the opportunity to speak to someone he will speak to himself. To speak is a natural desire; when that desire is suppressed it must come out some way or another" (Gould, 1950, p. 111).

Early Warning Signs

Patients entering psychosis report many peculiar symptoms. Most discussions of these focus on the sensory and perceptual changes—brighter colors, more grating, harsher sounds, difficulty focusing or sustaining attention, the loss of perceptual constancies, and a sense of perceptual chaos and surreality (Freedman & Chapman, 1973; McGhie & Chapman, 1961).

The subvoice hypothesis would highlight other potential danger signs. There could be increased talking to oneself. There could be talking in accents for variety's sake, as self-talk became tiresome. One of Gould's (1950) patients said, "I was thinking and inwardly expressing my thoughts with an Italian accent . . . (I) sometimes use a French accent or English accent just for fun and especially since I know my own thoughts are being lifted and checked" (p. 112). Another patient said, "They have influenced my thoughts to make them seem Scotch or Irish" (p. 112). Another possibility would be a deadly switch in inner speech to the second or third person at some point. Or self-hate and loathing could come more and more to reside in inner speech so it became less friend, more foe. Finally, there could be a satiation effect, where one's voice lost meaning and meness because one got satiated with it, and perhaps sick of it, so that it seemed surreal and tiresome. In fact, schizophrenics do often report that their voices begin to sound quite strange to them—metallic, faraway, harsh, hollow—early in the progression to psychosis (Freedman, 1974).

Performance Deficits

Schizophrenics show many cognitive deficits. Theories that try to assimilate these deficit findings, and thus describe more generally schizophrenic thought and cognition, usually focus on the patient's perceptual or attentional difficulties, or the patient's conceptual/language disorder.

However, note that inner speech is a basic tool in human thought and problem solving—blocking subarticulation impairs memory, learning, and reasoning (Baddeley, 1986). The subvoice hypothesis implies that the patient may lose touch with, or control over, the inner voice—perhaps including its use in thinking. In addition, the hallucinating patient may be performing a concurrent articulatory task (making voices) at some points during laboratory performance. So one might ask if the attention, reasoning, and learning deficits schizophrenics show are predicted by the loss of inner speech as a useful guide, sequencer and planner in problem solving.

The point in the last several paragraphs is not that the subvoice hypothesis is true. The point is that the sensory and subvoice views of hallucinations suggest broadly different research strategies in almost every area. This highlights the importance of making the high-level theoretical choice between them. Even beyond affecting research in schizophrenia, this theoretical difference cuts to our central metaphors about psychosis.

Where Will the Mind Break?

In the dominant metaphor for madness there is some "break" within the mind. It is understood, variously, as a breakdown of ego defenses, releasing horrors into consciousness; as ruptured ego boundaries, with the loss of the self/other distinction and the dissolution of mature object relations; as a break with reality, so that internal and external realities are confused; as a split in the will, causing confusion, indecision, and even catatonia; or as a breakdown of the perceptual/attentional walls and filters that hold the world's sensory chaos at bay.

These interpretations disagree sharply on where in the mind, where in the cognitive system, the psychotic break occurs. Cognitive theories usually describe a rupture close to the sensorium, at the interface between self and world, with perceptual/attentional walls caving in (Chapman, 1966; Corbett, 1976; Freedman & Chapman, 1973; George & Neufeld, 1985; McGhie & Chapman, 1961; Neale & Oltmanns, 1980; Schwartz, 1982). McGhie and Chapman concluded that the "fundamental disorder in schizophrenia was a cognitive one, most clearly evident in the fields of attention and perception, and that other aspects of the patient's symptomatology could be interpreted as his reactions to this basic disorder" (p. 103). In this description of madness, an intact self is overwhelmed by perceptual chaos. The sensory and imagery theories of auditory hallucinations fit best with this perceptual sense of the psychotic break, and have allied themselves with it.

In other theories of psychosis, the failure of the cognitive system is not at the sensorium, but much deeper, and the problem is not that an intact self is overwhelmed. Instead, in these theories, the self, itself, has shattered. For example, Bleuler (1950) believed that psychosis split the will into several equipotential forces. Freud (1933) suggested that the schizophrenic's voices were a regressive splitting off of an observer function (the superego) from the rest of the ego, when the voice of conscience, formerly well-integrated in the function of the ego, broke apart from the self, and reemerged as the voices of former object ties (p. 85 and ff.). Modell (1958, 1960, 1962) followed Freud's line in his studies of the phenomenology of voices. They were most often the voices of parents and caretakers, and their role was to guide, instruct, criticize, allow and prohibit, reward and punish, help and scorn. They sometimes conversed with a patient "in a manner reminiscent of the internal conversation a normal individual has with himself" (1962, p. 169).

Freud relied on a curious image to convey the cognitive architecture that allowed such a split. It captures just the swirl of auditory imagery and inner speech that the subvoice hypothesis depends on. Where once the child heard the auditory or verbal prohibitions emanating from parental objects, the adult's ego must now respond to similar demands internalized within the superego's structure. To do so, the ego is "wearing an auditory lobe" (p. 170).

This overseeing-superego function that Freud and Modell described is, quite likely, closely allied to our inner voice or internal dialogue. In almost all descriptions of the cognitive-emotional system (Deffenbacher, 1980; Meichenbaum, 1977; Meichenbaum & Butler, 1980; Sarason, 1980; Vygotsky, 1962), the inner voice is our executive function in guiding behavior, our evaluator, self-regulator, rewarder and punisher. It is our meta-look at ourselves, a superego to the ego, it is the mind's "I." If this overseer function split off from the cognitive system, the split could easily be tied to a failure of recognition of the inner voice, and to auditory hallucinations of exactly the kind schizophrenics experience. Consequently, the subvocalization hypothesis about hallucinations is extraordinarily comfortable with theories of psychosis such as Bleuler's, Freud's, or Modell's (see also Smith, 1991).

Thus, one returns to the observation that began the chapter. Alternative theories of hallucinations do point toward contrasting interpretations of the psychotic break. By turns, they depict a surface rupture in the attentional skin, or the deep self divided against itself. These metaphors for psychosis are profoundly different. Schizophrenic voices are rarely loud and clear—they whisper, mumble, mutter at the patient, vaguely in the air or in the head. But the phenomenon of voices is loud and clear on one point. While their cognitive psychology hangs confused in two such different theoretical worlds, we sorely miss an important clue in the riddle of psychosis.

REFERENCES

Alpert, M., Rubenstein, H., & Kesselman, M. (1976). Asymmetry of information processing in hallucinators and nonhallucinators. *The Journal of Nervous and Mental Disease, 162,* 258–265.

Alpert, M., & Silvers, K. N. (1970). Perceptual characteristics distinguishing auditory hallucinations in schizophrenia and acute alcoholic psychoses. *American Journal of Psychiatry, 127,* 74–78.

American Psychiatric Association. (1980). *Diagnostic and statistical manual of mental disorders* (3rd ed.). Washington DC: Author.

Arieti, S. (1974). *Interpretation of schizophrenia.* New York: Basic Books.

Baddeley, A. (1986). *Working memory.* Oxford, UK: Clarendon Press.

Baddeley, A., & Hitch, G. J. (1974). Working memory. In G. Bower (Ed.), *Recent advances in learning and motivation*, Vol. 9, (pp. 47–90). New York: Academic Press.

Baddeley, A., & Lewis, V. J. (1981). Interactive processes in reading: The inner voice, the inner ear and the inner eye. In A. M. Lesgold and C. A. Perfetti, (Eds.), *Interactive processes in reading* (pp. 107–129). Hillsdale, NJ: Lawrence Erlbaum Associates.

Baillarger, J. (1846). *Des hallucinations*. Paris: Bailliere.

Bazhin, E. F., Wasserman, L. I., & Tonkonogii, I. M. (1975). Auditory hallucinations and left temporal lobe pathology. *Neuropsychologia, 13*, 481–487.

Bentall, R. P., & Slade, P. D. (1985). Reality testing and auditory hallucinations: A signal detection analysis. *British Journal of Clinical Psychology, 24*, 159–169.

Bick, P. A., & Kinsbourne, M. (1987). Auditory hallucinations and subvocal speech in schizophrenic patients. *American Journal of Psychiatry, 144*, 222–225.

Birley, J. L. T., & Brown, G. W. (1970). Crises and life changes preceding the onset or relapse of acute schizophrenia: Clinical aspects. *British Journal of Psychiatry, 116*, 327–333.

Bleuler, E. (1950). *Dementia Praecox or the group of schizophrenias*. New York: International Universities Press.

Brett, E. A., & Starker, S. (1977). Auditory imagery and hallucinations. *The Journal of Nervous and Mental Disease, 164*, 394–400.

Brown, J. (1977). *Mind, brain, and consciousness: The neuropsychology of cognition*. New York: Academic.

Brown, G. W., & Birley, J. L. T. (1968). Crises and life changes and the onset of schizophrenia. *Journal of Health and Social Behavior, 9*, 203–214.

Brown, G. W., Harris, T. O., & Peto, J. (1973). Life events and psychiatric disorders: 2. Nature of the causal link. *Psychological Medicine, 3*, 159–176.

Catts, S. V., Armstrong, M. S., Norcross, K., & McConaghy, N. (1980). Auditory hallucinations and the verbal transformation effect. *Psychological Medicine, 10*, 139–144.

Cerny, M. (1964). Electrophysiological study of verbal hallucinations. *Activitas Nervosa Superior, 6*, 94–95.

Cerny, M. (1965). On neurophysiological mechanisms in verbal hallucinations: An electrophysiological study. *Activitas Nervosa Superior, 7*, 197–198.

Chapman, J. (1966). The early symptoms of schizophrenia. *British Journal of Psychiatry, 112*, 225–251.

Cohen, L. H. (1938). Imagery and its relation to the schizophrenia symptoms. *Journal of Mental Science, 84*, 284–346.

Corbett, L. (1976). Perceptual dyscontrol: A possible organizing principle for schizophrenia research. *Schizophrenia Bulletin, 2*, 249–265.

Crider, A. (1979). *Schizophrenia: A biopsychological perspective*. Hillsdale, NJ: Lawrence Erlbaum Associates.

Deffenbacher, J. L. (1980). Worry and emotionality in test anxiety. In I. G. Sarason (Ed.), *Test anxiety: Theory, research, and applications* (pp. 111–128). Hillsdale, NJ: Lawrence Erlbaum Associates.

Erickson, G. D., & Gustafson, G. J. (1968). Controlling auditory hallucinations. *Hospital Community Psychiatry, 19*, 327–329.

Esquirol, J. E. D. (1845). *Mental maladies: A treatise on insanity* (E. K. Hunt, trans.). Philadelphia: Lee and Blanchard. (Original work published 1838).

Evenson, R. C. (1987). Auditory hallucinations and subvocal speech. *American Journal of Psychiatry, 144*(10), 1364–1365.

Farah, M. (1985). Psychophysical evidence for a shared representational medium for mental images and percepts. *Journal of Experimental Psychology: General, 114*, 91–103.

Feder, R. (1982). Auditory hallucinations treated by radio headphones. *American Journal of Psychiatry, 139*(9), 1188–1190.

Feinberg, I. (1962). A comparison of the visual hallucinations in schizophrenia with those induced by mescaline and LSD-25. In L. J. West (Ed.), *Hallucinations* (pp. 64–76). New York: Grune and Stratton.

Finke, R. A. (1980). Levels of equivalence in imagery and perception. *Psychological Review, 87,* 113–132.

Fink, R. A. (1985). Theories relating mental imagery to perception. *Psychological Bulletin, 98*(2), 236–259.

Flor-Henry, P. (1986). Auditory hallucinations, inner speech, and the dominant hemisphere. *The Behavioral and Brain Sciences, 9,* 523–524.

Freedman, B., & Chapman, L. J. (1973). Early subjective experience in schizophrenic episodes. *Journal of Abnormal Psychology, 82,* 46–54.

Freedman, B. J. (1974). The subjective experience of perceptual and cognitive disturbances in schizophrenia. *Archives of General Psychiatry, 30,* 333–340.

Freud, S. (1933). *New introductory lectures on psychoanalysis* (W. J. H. Sprott, Trans.). New York: Norton.

George, L., & Neufeld, R. W. J. (1985). Cognition and symptomatology in schizophrenia. *Schizophrenia Bulletin, 11*(2), 264–284.

Gould, L. N. (1948). Verbal hallucinations and activity of vocal musculature: An electromyographic study. *American Journal of Psychiatry, 105,* 367–372.

Gould, L. N. (1949). Auditory hallucinations and subvocal speech: Objective study in a case of schizophrenia. *Journal of Mental Disease, 109,* 418–427.

Gould, L. N. (1950). Verbal hallucinations as automatic speech: The reactivation of dormant speech habit. *American Journal of Psychiatry, 107,* 110–119.

Green, P. (1978). Interhemispheric transfer in schizophrenia: Recent developments. *Behavioural Psychotherapy, 6,* 105–110.

Green, P., Glass, A., & O'Callaghan, M. A. J. (1980). Some implications of abnormal hemisphere interaction in schizophrenia. In J. H. Gruzelier and P. Flor-Henry (Eds.), *Hemisphere asymmetries and psychopathology.* London, MacMillan.

Green, P., & Preston, M. (1981). Reinforcement of vocal correlates of auditory hallucinations by auditory feedback: A case study. *British Journal of Psychiatry, 139,* 204–208.

Gross, M. M., Halpert, E., Sabot, L., & Polizos, P. (1963). Hearing disturbances and auditory hallucinations in the acute alcoholic psychoses. I: Tinnitus: Incidence and significance. *Journal of Nervous and Mental Disease, 137*(5), 455–465.

Halgren, E., Walter, R. D., Cherlow, D. G., & Crandall, P. H. (1978). Mental phenomena evoked by electrical stimulation of the human hippocampal formation and amygdala. *Brain, 101,* 83–117.

Heilbrun, A., Blum, M., & Haas, M. (1983). Cognitive vulnerability to auditory hallucination: Preferred imagery mode and spatial location of sounds. *British Journal of Psychiatry, 143,* 294–299.

Hobbes, T. (1958). *Leviathan:* Parts I and II. H. W. Schneider (Ed.), Indianapolis: Bobbs-Merrill. (Original work 1651)

Hoffer, A., Osmond, H., & Smythies, J. (1954). Schizophrenia: New approach; result of year's research. *Journal of Mental Science, 100,* 29–45.

Hoffman, R. E. (1986). Verbal hallucinations and language production processes in schizophrenia. *The Behavioral and Brain Sciences, 9,* 503–548.

Horowitz, M. J. (1975). Hallucinations: An information processing approach. In R. K. Siegel & L. J. West (Eds.), *Hallucinations* (pp. 163–195). New York: Wiley.

Horowitz, M. J. (1978). *Image formation and cognition.* New York: Appleton-Century Crofts.

Horowitz, M. J., & Adams, J. (1970). Hallucinations on brain stimulation: Evidence for a revision of the Penfield hypothesis. In W. Keup (Ed.), *Origin and mechanisms of hallucinations* (pp. 13–22). New York: Plenum.

Hume, D. (1888). *Treatise of Human Nature*. L. A. Selby-Bigge (Ed.), Oxford: Clarendon Press. (Original publication 1739)

Inouye, T., & Shimizu, A. (1970). The electromyographic study of verbal hallucinations. *Psychophysiology, 3,* 73–80.

Jackson, J. H. (1958). In J. Taylor, G. Holmes, & F. M. R. Walshe (Eds.), *Selected writings of John Hughlings Jackson*. London: Staples Press.

James, D. A. E. (1983). The experimental treatment of two cases of auditory hallucinations. *British Journal of Psychiatry, 143,* 515–516.

James, W. (1950). *Principles of psychology*. New York: Dover.

Jansson, B. (1968). The prognostic significance of various types of hallucinations in young people. *Acta Psychiatrica Scandinavia, 44,* 401.

Johnson, F. H. (1958). Auditory hallucinations as interpreted by means of recorders. *Anatomical Record, 130,* 321.

Johnson, F. H. (1967). Neurophysiological disuse of inner speech as used in thinking in schizophrenia. *Anatomical Record, 157,* 366.

Johnson, F. H. (1978). *The anatomy of hallucinations*. New York: Nelson-Hall.

Johnson, M. K., & Raye, C. L. (1981). Reality monitoring. *Psychological Review, 88,* 67–85.

Johnson, M. K., Raye, C. L., Wang, A. Y., & Taylor, T. H. (1979). Fact and fantasy: The roles of accuracy and variability in confusing imaginations with perceptual experiences. *Journal of Experimental Psychology: Human Learning and Memory, 5,* 229–240.

Judkins, M., & Slade, P. (1981). A questionnaire study of hostility in persistent auditory hallucinators. *British Journal of Medical Psychology, 34,* 243–250.

Junginger, J. (1986). Distinctiveness, unintendedness, location, and nonself attribution of verbal hallucinations. *The Behavioral and Brain Sciences, 9,* 527–528.

Junginger, J., & Frame, C. L. (1985). Self-report of the frequency and phenomenology of verbal hallucinations. *The Journal of Nervous and Mental Disease, 173,* 149–155.

Junginger, J., & Rauscher, F. P. (1987). Vocal activity in verbal hallucinations. *Journal of Psychiatric Research, 21,* 101–109.

Kass, W. (1968). The experience of spontaneous hallucination. *Bulletin of the Menninger Clinic, 32,* 67–85.

Kety, S. S. (1969). Biochemical hypotheses and studies. In L. Bellak & L. Loeb (Eds.), *The schizophrenic syndrome* (pp. 155–171). New York: Grune and Stratton.

Kietzman, M. L., Spring, B., & Zubin, J. (1985). Perception, cognition, and information processing. In H. I. Kaplan & B. J. Sadock (Eds.), *Comprehensive textbood of psychiatry/IV* (pp. 157–179). Baltimore, MD: Williams and Wilkins.

Kolb, L. C. (1977). *Modern Clinical Psychiatry*. Philadelphia: Saunders.

Kosslyn, S. (1980). *Image and mind*. Cambridge, MA: Harvard University Press.

Kosslyn, S. (1983). *Ghosts in the mind's machine: Creating and using images in the brain*. New York: Norton.

Lang, J. (1938). The other side of hallucinations. *American Journal of Psychiatry, 94,* 1089–1097.

Lang, J. (1940). The other side of hallucinations. *American Journal of Psychiatry, 96,* 423–430.

LaGache, D. (1935). Les hallucinations verbales et le parole. *Psychological Abstracts, 9,* 529.

Lehmann, H. E., & Cancro, R. (1985). Schizophrenia: Clinical features. In H. I. Kaplan and B. J. Sadock (Eds.), *Comprehensive textbood of psychiatry/IV* (pp. 680–713). Baltimore: Williams and Wilkins.

Liberman, A., & Mattingly, I. (1985). The motor theory of speech perception revised. *Cognition, 21,* 1–35.

Lindsley, O. R. (1963). Direct measurement and functional definition of vocal hallucinatory symptoms. *Journal of Nervous and Mental Disease, 136,* 293–297.

Malitz, S., Wilkens, B., & Esecover, H. (1962). A comparison of drug induced hallucinations with those seen in spontaneously occurring psychoses. In J. West (Ed.), *Hallucinations* (pp. 50–63). New York: Grune and Stratton.

Maudsley, H. (1886). *Natural causes and supernatural seemings*. London: Kegan Paul, Trench and Co.

McGhie, S., & Chapman, J. (1961). Disorders of attention and perception in early schizophrenia. *British Journal of Medical Psychology, 34,* 103–116.

McGuigan, F. J. (1966). Covert oral behavior and auditory hallucinations. *Psychophysiology, 3,* 73–80.

McKinney, W. T. (1985). Animal models for psychosis. In H. I. Kaplan and B. J. Sadock (Eds.), *Comprehensive textbood of psychiatry/IV* (312–320). Baltimore, MD: Williams and Wilkins.

McReynolds, P. (1960). Anxiety, perception and schizophrenia. In D. D. Jackson (Ed.), *The etiology of schizophrenia* (pp. 248–292). New York: Basic Books.

Meichenbaum, D. (1977). *Cognitive behavior modification: An integrative approach*. New York: Plenum.

Meichenbaum, D., & Butler, L. (1980). Toward a conceptual model for the treatment of test anxiety: Implications for research and treatment. In I. G. Sarason (Ed.), *Test anxiety: Theory, research, and applications* (pp. 187–208). Hillsdale, NJ: Lawrence Erlbaum Associates.

Mellor, C. S. (1970). First rank symptoms of schizophrenia. *British Journal of Psychiatry, 117,* 15–23.

Mintz, S., & Alpert, M. (1972). Imagery vividness, reality testing, and schizophrenic hallucinations. *Journal of Abnormal Psychology, 79,* 310–316.

Modell, A. H. (1958). The theoretical implications of hallucinatory experiences in schizophrenia. *Journal of American Psychoanalytical Association, 6,* 442–480.

Modell, A. H. (1960). An approach to the nature of auditory hallucinations in schizophrenia. *Archives of General Psychiatry, 3,* 63–70.

Modell, A. H. (1962). Hallucinations in schizophrenic patients and their relation to psychic structure. In L. J. West (Ed.), *Hallucinations* (pp. 166–173). New York: Grune and Stratton.

Mott, R., Small, I., & Anderson, J. (1965). Comparative study of hallucinations. *Archives of General Psychiatry, 12,* 595–601.

Neale, J. M., & Oltmanns, T. F. (1980). *Schizophrenia*. New York: Wiley.

Parish, E. (1897). *Hallucinations and illusions*. London: Walter Scott.

Parker, S., & Schilder, P. (1935). Acoustic imagination and acoustic hallucination. *Archives of Neurology and Psychiatry, 34,* 744–757.

Penfield, W., & Perot, P. (1963). The brain's record of auditory and visual experience. *Brain, 86,* 595–696.

Perky, C. W. (1910). An experimental study of imagination. *American Journal of Psychology, 21,* 422–452.

Reed, K. (1985). *Lectures in psychiatry*. St. Louis, MO: W. H. Green.

Reisberg, D., & Chambers, D. (1986). Neither pictures nor propositions: The intensionality of mental images. In C. Clifton (Ed.), *The eighth annual conference of the cognitive science society* (pp. 208–222). Hillsdale, NJ: Lawrence Erlbaum Associates.

Reisberg, D., Smith, J. D., Baxter, D. A., & Sonenshine, M. (1989). "Enacted" auditory images are ambiguous; "Pure" auditory images are not. *Quarterly Journal of Experimental Psychology, 41*(3), 619–641.

Richardson, J. (1984). Developing the theory of working memory. *Memory and Cognition, 12,* 71–83.

Roberts, B. H., Greenblatt, M., & Solomon, H. C. (1952). Movements of the vocal apparatus during auditory hallucinations. *American Journal of Psychiatry, 108,* 912–914.

Roman, R., & Landis, C. (1945). Hallucinations and mental imagery. *Journal of Nervous and Mental Disease, 102,* 327–331.

Rund, B. R. (1986). Verbal hallucinations and information processing. Commentary on R. E. Hoffman, Verbal hallucinations and language production processes in schizophrenia. *Behavioral and Brain Sciences, 9,* 531–532.

Salame, P., & Baddeley, A. (1982). Disruption of short-term memory by unattended speech: Implication for the structure of working memory. *Journal of Verbal Learning and Verbal Behavior, 21,* 150–164.

Sarason, I. G. (1980). *Test Anxiety: Theory, research, and applications.* Hillsdale, NJ: Lawrence Erlbaum Associates.

Saravay, S. M., & Pardes, H. (1967). Auditory elementary hallucinations in alcohol withdrawal psychosis. *Archives of General Psychiatry, 16,* 652–658.

Saravay, S. M., & Pardes, H. (1970). Auditory "elementary hallucinations" in alcohol withdrawal psychoses. In W. Keup (Ed.), *Origin and mechanism of hallucinations* (237–244), New York: Plenum.

Sartorius, N., Shapiro, R., & Jablonsky, A. (1974). The international pilot study of schizophrenia. *Schizophrenia Bulletin, 1,* 21–35.

Savage, C. W. (1975). The continuity of perceptual and cognitive experiences. In R. K. Siegel & L. J. West (Eds.), *Hallucinations* (p. 257–286). New York: Wiley.

Schneider, K. (1959). *Clinical psychopathology.* New York: Grune and Stratton.

Schwartz, S. (1982). Is there a schizophrenic language? *Behavioral and Brain Sciences, 5,* 579–626.

Sechehaye, M. (1951). *Autobiography of a schizophrenic girl.* New York: Grune and Stratton.

Seglas, J. (1914). Hallucinations psychiques et pseudohallucinations verbales. *Journal de Psychologie, 11,* 299.

Seitz, P., & Molholm, H. B. (1947). Relation of mental imagery to hallucinations. *Archives of Neurology and Psychiatry, 57,* 469–480.

Semrad, E. V. (1938). Study of the auditory apparatus in patients experiencing auditory hallucinations. *American Journal of Psychiatry, 95,* 53–63.

Shapiro, S. A. (1981). *Contemporary Theories of Schizophrenia.* New York: McGraw Hill.

Slade, P. D. (1974). The external control of auditory hallucinations: An information theory analysis. *British Journal of Social and Clinical Psychology, 13,* 73–79.

Slade, P. D. (1976). An investigation of psychological factors involved in the predisposition to auditory hallucinations. *Psychological Medicine, 6,* 123–132.

Smith, J. D. (1991). The cognitive architecture of psychosis. Manuscript in preparation.

Solomon, P., & Kleeman, S. T. (1985). Sensory deprivation. In H. I. Kaplan & B. J. Sadock (Eds.), *Comprehensive textbook of psychiatry/IV* (838–851). Baltimore: Williams and Wilkins.

Starker, S., & Jolin, A. (1982). Imagery and hallucination in schizophrenic patients. *The Journal of Nervous and Mental Disease, 170,* 448–451.

Strauss, E. W. (1962). Phenomenology of hallucinations. In L. J. West (Ed.), *Hallucinations* (pp. 220–232). New York: Grune and Stratton.

Tanzi, E. (1909). *A textbook of mental diseases.* New York: Rebman.

Vygotsky, L. S. (1962). *Language and Thought.* Boston: MIT Press.

Warren, R. (1961). Illusory changes of distinct speech upon repetition—the verbal transformation effect. *British Journal of Psychology, 52,* 249.

Warren, R., & Gregory, R. (1958). An auditory analogue of the visual reversible figure. *American Journal of Psychology, 71,* 612–613.

Weingarten, S. M., Cherlow, D. G., & Holmgrem, E. (1977). The relationship of hallucinations to the depth structures of the temporal lobe. *Acta Neurochirurgica Suppl., 24,* 199–216.

Wells, C. E. (1985). Organic syndromes: Delirium. In H. I. Kaplan & B. J. Sadock (Eds.), *Comprehensive textbook of psychiatry/IV* (pp. 838–851). Baltimore: Williams and Wilkins.

West, L. J. (Ed.). (1962). *Hallucinations.* New York: Grune and Stratton.

Winters, K. C., & Neale, J. M. (1983). Delusions and delusional thinking in psychotics: A review of the literature. *Clinical Psychology Review, 3,* 227–253.

World Health Organization. (1973). *Report of the International Pilot Study of Schizophrenia.* Geneva: Author.

Zivin, G. (1986). Image or neural coding of inner speech and agency? *The Behavioral and Brain Sciences, 9,* 534–535.

8 Auditory Imagery and Working Memory

Alan Baddeley
MRC Applied Psychology Unit, Cambridge, England

Robert Logie
University of Aberdeen, Scotland

Most of us appear to be able to conjure up from memory the recollection of auditory events that seem to have at least some of the characteristics of the initial acoustic experience. The recollections of the particular voice of a friend, or of a famous statesman such as Winston Churchill, the opening bars of "Beethoven's Fifth Symphony," or the sound made by a creaking door are all instances of auditory imagery. In a survey of 500 non-student adults, McKellar (1965) noted that 93% of respondents reported experiencing some form of auditory imagery. This gives some indication of its ubiquitous nature, but what are the defining characteristics of such imagery?

For the purpose of this discussion, we make the following assumptions: (a) that an auditory image involves a conscious experience, (b) that this resembles in certain, as yet unspecified ways the experience of hearing the sound in question directly, but (c) the image can be present in the absence of any auditory signal, and (d) it can be evoked intentionally by the subject.

It is perhaps worth commenting in detail on our first two assumptions, both of which have a somewhat checkered history of application to the problems of visual imagery. In opting to include conscious awareness as one component of our definition of auditory imagery, we do not wish to suggest that there is a simple mapping between the information contained in an image and the reported experience. There is abundant evidence from studies of visual imagery to indicate that rated vividness does not predict the capacity of subjects to store and manipulate visuo-spatial information (Kosslyn, Brunn, Cave, & Wallach, 1985; Richardson, 1980), and we would be unwise to assume a more straightforward relationship in the case of auditory imagery. Nevertheless, we believe that the subjective experience of imagery, regardless of its validity as an indicator of the underlying processes, is a phenomenon that needs to be explained by any complete model of the imagery process. That does not mean, of course, that a model that can not yet account for this is therefore without interest.

Our second assumption, namely that auditory imagery and auditory perception show certain resemblances is again analogous to earlier developments in visual imagery, which as a study has been criticized on occasion as being too preoccupied with attempting to demonstrate similarities between imagery and vision (e.g., Baddeley, 1990). Our assumption here is that auditory imagery and hearing will have some features in common and some differences, and exploring the differences is at least as important as attempting to list similarities. It may of course prove to be the case that auditory imagery and audition are totally separate systems, but we regard this as inherently unlikely.

In contrast to visual imagery, which has been extensively explored in recent years, auditory imagery has been largely neglected. We ourselves are as guilty as anyone of ignoring this intriguing field, and consequently what follows is not a well worked-out and empirically supported theory of auditory imagery, but rather, a series of speculations that might form the basis for a subsequent program of research. The speculations are based on the extensively explored area of short-term phonological memory, and suggest as a hypothesis that the phonological short-term storage component of the working memory model originally developed by Baddeley and Hitch (1974) may represent the seat of auditory imagery. A parallel case has been made for the role of the visuo-spatial sketchpad in visual imagery (Baddeley, 1986; Logie, 1989, 1991).

We begin by outlining the articulatory or phonological loop component of working memory, after which we explore the evidence in support of a view that the short-term phonological store may play a crucial role in auditory imagery. We first discuss the attempts to produce measures of phonological awareness in connection with both normal subjects and brain-damaged patients. Then we consider evidence for the disruption of short-term phonological memory by irrelevant or unattended sounds. This is followed by a discussion of the role of short-term phonological memory in processing music.

Unfortunately, virtually none of this work has directly tackled the issue of conscious awareness, with the result that any conclusions about auditory imagery are inevitably indirect. The chapter concludes with some brief suggestions for ways in which this could be remedied.

THE WORKING MEMORY MODEL

The concept of working memory refers to the assumption that some form of temporary storage is necessary for the performance of many cognitive skills. Initially, working memory was assumed to be synonymous with short-term memory, a limited capacity store that was widely assumed to rely principally on verbal coding. The concept of a simple unitary store ran into major problems however, inducing Baddeley and Hitch (1974) to replace it with the concept of a multi-component working memory.

The model was assumed to have three principal components, namely an attentional control system known as the Central Executive aided by two slave systems, both of which were capable of actively maintaining material in short-term storage. One of these, the Visuo-spatial Sketchpad is assumed to be responsible for setting up and maintaining visual images, while the other, the Articulatory or Phonological Loop, is assumed to be capable of temporarily storing and rehearsing verbal information. The system is also assumed to have access to long-term memory and to utilize more passive modes of temporary storage that typically involve the temporary priming of representations in memory. The recency effect in long- and short-term memory is assumed to be the result of applying a particular retrieval strategy to such primed representations (Baddeley, 1986). For the present purposes, the Articulatory or Phonological Loop is assumed to be of particular relevance, and hence will be described in more detail.

The Phonological Loop

The Phonological Loop is assumed to comprise two components, namely a temporary phonological store linked in with an articulatory rehearsal process. Its strength lies in its simplicity, in that making only minimal assumptions, it can account for a very broad range of findings from within the laboratory, as well as accounting for neuropsychological evidence and evidence from the development of language in children.

The store is assumed to be capable of holding memory traces of phonologically encoded material, with the underlying trace decaying within about two seconds to a point at which it is no longer retrievable. Such traces may be set up either by the direct auditory presentation of speech-like material or through the subvocalization of visually presented material by the subject. The process of overt or covert subvocalization is also assumed to be capable of maintaining the memory trace by reactivating it. This simple two-component model can explain a wide range of phenomena, including the effects on short-term recall of the phonological similarity or the length of the items to be retained, of concurrent irrelevant presented speech, and of concurrent vocalization of an irrelevant word. These are described below.

FACTORS INFLUENCING MEMORY SPAN

Phonological Similarity

Immediate memory span for sequences of similar items (e.g., the word sequence *MAN CAN MAD MAP CAT*) is consistently poorer than for phonologically dissimilar sequences (e.g., *PIT DAY SUP COW PEN*) (Baddeley, 1966; Conrad & Hull, 1964).

Word-Length Effect

Immediate memory span is poorer for sequences comprising long words (e.g., *OPPORTUNITY UNIVERSITY ALUMINIUM,* etc.) than for short words (e.g., *SUM HATE WIT,* etc.) (Baddeley, Thomson, & Buchanan, 1975).

The Irrelevant Speech Effect

Immediate memory for sequences of visually-presented items such as digits is impaired by the simultaneous presentation of spoken material which the subject is instructed to ignore. The effect, which is also referred to as the *unattended speech effect,* does not depend on the intensity of the irrelevant sound and is just as strong when the irrelevant auditory material is in an unfamiliar foreign language (Colle, 1980; Colle & Welsh, 1976; Salamé & Baddeley, 1982).

Articulatory Suppression

Memory span for verbal materials is reduced when the subject has to suppress rehearsal by continuously articulating some irrelevant sound such as the word "the" (Murray, 1965). Articulatory suppression interacts in a coherent way with the other listed variables. When material is presented visually, then articulatory suppression removes the phonological similarity effect (Murray, 1968), it obliterates the word length effect, whether presentation is visual or auditory (Baddeley, Lewis, & Vallar, 1984), and it removes the irrelevant speech effect (Salamé & Baddeley, 1982). This complex pattern of results can not readily be explained in terms of simple distraction or cognitive overload but does fit neatly into the phonological loop model.

Theoretical Interpretation

The Articulatory or Phonological Loop model explains this pattern of results as follows. Phonological similarity impairs performance because the store operates using a phonological code. Similar items are less discriminable, and hence more liable to error at retrieval. Articulatory suppression interacts with similarity when material is presented visually, since it prevents the visual material being translated into a phonological code. If the material is not phonologically coded, then the similarity along this dimension is irrelevant since memory must rely on some other form of code, possibly visual or semantic.

The word-length effect is assumed to occur because the subvocal rehearsal process operates in real time. Consequently, long words take longer to rehearse, allowing more trace decay to occur and hence leading to poorer performance. If the subject is suppressing articulation, then he or she is unable to rehearse, with the result that the effect of word length ceases to be relevant. This occurs whether presentation is auditory or visual, because it influences the process of rehearsal, but not storage.

The irrelevant speech effect is assumed to occur because spoken material gains obligatory access to the phonological store, and hence is able to corrupt the store with irrelevant material.[1] The store is normally used to enhance retention of visually presented material, but this is only possible if the subject is able to re-code the material through the articulatory control process. If this is prevented by articulatory suppression, then the phonological store cannot be used, and the presence or absence of irrelevant material becomes irrelevant.

Neuropsychological Evidence

Shallice and Warrington (1970) reported a patient, KF, who had a digit span of only two items but nevertheless showed normal long-term memory performance. Such patients presented problems for the view current at the time, which was that the only way long-term learning could occur was through the unitary limited capacity short-term memory store (Atkinson & Shiffrin, 1968). The working memory model is able to deal with this problem by assuming that such patients have a deficit in the Phonological Loop system. A detailed study of one such patient indicated that her deficit could plausibly be interpreted as one of short-term phonological storage (Vallar & Baddeley, 1984). Subsequent research has indicated that this system is important for long-term learning, but only of pho-nological material, whereas most studies of long-term verbal memory have al-lowed the patient to code semantically or visually (Baddeley, Papagno, & Vallar, 1988).

Other studies have been concerned with the nature of the subvocal rehearsal process. Baddeley and Wilson (1985) tested a patient who had become totally unable to speak as a result of brain-stem damage that had nevertheless left his language capacities intact. This patient showed a digit span within the normal range, together with clear phonological similarity and word-length effects, indi-cating that the Phonological Loop was operating comparatively normally. Subse-quent studies have revealed a number of similar cases, although differences occur. Some anarthric patients reliably fail to show clear effects of phonological similarity or word length. This is most likely due to damage to parts of the system other than, or in addition to, overt output (Logie, Cubelli, Della Sala, Nichelli, & Alberoni, 1989; Vallar & Cappa, 1987). A study by Bishop and Robson (1989) has shown that even children who have never been able to speak may nevertheless show a comparatively normal pattern of phonological sim-ilarity and word length effects, suggesting the possibility that the system may develop relatively normally without at any point involving overt speech.

One way of interpreting the presence of these phenomena in the absence of an ability to produce overt speech is to argue that the process of subvocal rehearsal operates at a relatively deep level that involves some automatic process of echo-

---

[1]While we believe that the assumption of obligatory access gives the best account of available data, it is not universally accepted; for an alternative interpretation see Morris and Jones (1990).

ing back the incoming speech. It is this process that may be impaired in some, but by no means all, anarthric patients (Logie et al., 1989). There is good evidence to suggest that the repetition of spoken material by normal adults is a highly compatible response for which reaction time is not influenced by number of alternatives (Davis, Moray, & Treisman, 1961), and which does not interfere with other concurrent attention demanding activities (McLeod & Posner, 1984). It is plausible to assume that such a mechanism might form a crucial component of the acquisition of language. Work on the acquisition of lip-reading skills in children suggests that the association between the visual pattern of movements and phonological information is acquired within the first few months of life relatively automatically, and it seems not unreasonable to assume that the link between audition and speech could also be acquired automatically at a similar period as part of a complex multi-modal language processing system (Campbell & Wright, 1989).

Whether or not we accept this interpretation, however, it seems clear that overt or, one suspects, even relatively covert articulation is not essential for the operation of the loop; for that reason, it is perhaps less misleading to refer to it as the *Phonological* Loop rather than the *Articulatory* Loop. This leaves more open the nature of the rehearsal process.

Normal Language Acquisition

There is a very marked and systematic tendency for memory span to increase with age. A range of studies have suggested that much, if not all, of this steady increase can be attributed to rate of subvocal articulation. Memory span of children of varying ages and of adults can be predicted rather accurately simply on the basis of the rate at which they are able to articulate the relevant material (Hitch, Halliday, & Littler, 1989; Hulme, Thomson, Muir, & Lawrence, 1984; Nicholson, 1981). Young children appear to show phonological similarity and word length effects from a very young age when presentation is auditory, although these effects do not appear until the age of approximately 8 when material is presented visually, for example, as pictures of objects that must be recalled by name (Hitch, Halliday, Dodd & Littler, 1989).

Although it seems unlikely that increased rate of the articulatory control process is the only determinant of increased span with age, it does appear to offer a surprisingly good account of the data, and one that appears to be rather stronger than alternative views such as an age related increase in general processing capacity of the type postulated by Pascual-Leone (1970) or Case, Kurland, and Goldberg (1982), when these views are directly compared (Hitch, Halliday, Schaafstal, & Schraagen, 1988).

Recent evidence suggests that the Phonological Loop may play an important role in normal language development, as well as in the development of memory span. Gathercole and Baddeley (1989) have shown that the capacity to hear and repeat back nonwords is highly correlated with vocabulary at age 4, and continues to be a better predictor of vocabulary than nonverbal intelligence or any of the other variables measured. It has also been found that children who are selected as having delayed or impaired language development, coupled with normal intelligence, show a very striking impairment in the capacity to echo back nonwords (Gathercole & Baddeley, in press). The group of 8-year-old children studied were performing at the level of 4-year-olds on this task, while their general language development as measured by vocabulary and reading was only two years behind their age, suggesting that the deficit in short-term phonological memory may well be primary, with the reading and vocabulary deficits being a consequence of this impairment.

WORKING MEMORY AND AUDITORY IMAGERY

We have described the Phonological Loop component of working memory in some detail since we wish to argue that it is sufficiently successful in handling a broad range of results to make it worth exploring as a potential model for auditory imagery. However, as mentioned earlier, phenomenological reports of imagery have never been included as part of the experimental paradigm, and consequently the evidence for the plausibility of such a hypothesis has at this stage to be indirect. Furthermore, for the most part it consists of evidence indicating that some of the assumptions mentioned in our definition of imagery can plausibly be made for the phonological store. While few studies directly investigate the phenomenology of phonological storage, there has been a good deal of interest in the topic of phonological awareness, mainly in connection with hypotheses about its role in normal reading, and we therefore consider the evidence from this source.

Further, we argue that the phonological store does offer a stage which is accessible both to auditory stimuli and to internally-generated stimuli, and that these two interact. Much of the memory literature has been concerned with speech, and for that reason we need to consider whether the phonological store is limited to speech-like material or can be used more broadly, because it seems obvious to us that auditory imagery is not limited to spoken material. While there is some research on processing environmental sounds, the main evidence for nonverbal short-term storage comes from studies of the effects of music. Finally, we discuss the case for and against the phonological store as the seat of auditory imagery.

Phonological Awareness and Judgments of Rhyme

While there appear to be few direct studies of auditory imagery, there are a number of techniques that have attempted to study phonological judgments indirectly, for example by requiring judgments of homophony and rhyme. Let us assume that in order to perform these tasks the subject sets up and compares phonological images. This being the case, one might expect that anything that disrupts phonological storage would impair the capacity to make judgments of homophony and rhyme.

There has in fact been a good deal of controversy over the question of whether articulatory suppression influences either or both of these tasks. A series of studies carried out by Baddeley and Lewis (1981), replicating some unpublished data by Folkard, reported that articulatory suppression had no effect on rhyme judgments. However, as Besner (1987) has subsequently pointed out, although the instructions Baddeley and Lewis gave their subjects concerned judgments of rhyme, the tasks in fact all involved judgments of homophony since all the rhyming words presented were homophones such as *QUAY* and *KEY*, or involved homophonous word–nonword judgments such as *PHYTE, FIGHT*, or involved deciding whether a nonword was homophonous with a real word (e.g., *HOAM*). While this and a number of other studies find relatively little disruption from articulatory suppression, Besner showed that those studies which have required a true rhyme judgment in which the words were not homophonous (e.g., *TEA, KEY*) do typically show impairment. Johnston and McDermott (1986) also have shown that whenever a delay is inserted between the two comparison stimuli, then articulatory suppression impairs performance.

How then should we interpret the data in this area? Certainly, one cannot regard the area as offering particularly strong support to the idea that the phonological store is the seat of auditory imagery, because even when judgments of rhyme rather than homophony are used, the effects of articulatory suppression are far from dramatic. However, even if there proved to be no effect of articulatory suppression, the data would not be totally damaging to the hypothesis inasmuch as articulatory suppression is assumed to influence the articulatory control process rather than the phonological store itself. As such, a strong effect of suppression would indicate that creating a phonological representation demands the subvocal articulatory process. The absence of a strong effect implies that such a representation can be set up in other ways, possibly via the direct visual-to-semantic route, which in turn is set up via a link from the semantic system to phonological input. Either way, articulatory suppression does not speak strongly to the nature of the representation of the image, as opposed to its mode of access.

In as far as we are assuming that the image depends on the short-term phonological store, a more direct way of testing the hypothesis than articulatory suppression, might be to use the irrelevant speech effect. This is assumed to have its effect directly on the phonological store. As noted below, irrelevant speech produces a clear impairment in the short-term storage of both verbal and musical sequences. However, Baddeley and Salamé (1986) found no evidence for a disruptive effect of irrelevant speech on either rhyme or homophony judgments, suggesting that neither of these depends crucially on the phonological store.

The various measures of phonological awareness might seem to offer a much more direct way of exploring auditory imagery. Tests of phonological awareness typically require subjects to perform tasks such as consonant deletion, i.e., what word is left if you delete the first consonant from *CLIP?* Another test of phonological awareness is to ask the subject to take the initial consonant of a person's first and second name and reverse them, so-called spoonerisms (e.g., *Margaret Thatcher* becomes *Thargaret Matcher*). Unfortunately, although these are assumed to measure phonological awareness, the validity of this assumption is by no means clear. Furthermore the relationship between tests of phonological awareness and the short-term phonological store remains obscure.[2]

The Phonological Store
as an Auditory-Articulatory Interface

Before discussing the phonological store in this regard, it is perhaps worth mentioning briefly that there is an alternative candidate for the seat of auditory imagery, namely echoic memory. The term echoic memory was given by Neisser (1967) to the brief temporary storage of auditory information. When a list of items is presented auditorily, the last few items are very well recalled, in contrast to the same items presented visually. However, if the sequence of items is followed by a spoken suffix such as the instruction "recall," then this marked recency effect is wiped out, a phenomenon that Crowder and Morton (1969) attributed to the over-writing of a precategorical acoustic store (PAS). Should this brief store be regarded as the prime candidate for the seat of auditory imagery?

We suggest not, for two reasons. The first is that the simple hypothesis of an auditory store has proved far too simple for the complex pattern of data that has emerged from subsequent studies (see, e.g., Penney, in press, for a recent review). However, even if one were to accept the simple PAS model, it would not appear to offer a good interpretation of imagery since its operation is tied to modality of input, whereas one of the main criteria of imagery as we define it is its capacity to be evoked in the absence of auditory stimulation. When memory for a sequence of visually presented letters is tested, the marked recency effect that characterizes studies of the PAS system is absent. Nonetheless, clear evidence of phonological coding is found in the form of a marked effect of phonological similarity (Conrad & Hull, 1964).

The fact that visually presented letters are encoded phonologically is *prima-facie* evidence for optional access to the phonological store in the absence of

---

[2]Evidence has recently appeared to suggest that phonological memory and phonological awareness are dissociable. This comes from the study of a patient, T. B., originally reported by Baddeley and Wilson (1988) as a patient with impaired memory span and comprehension. A follow-up study (Wilson & Baddeley, in prep.) found that his memory span and comprehension performance had totally recovered (digit span = 9), while he still showed very poor performance on tests of phonological awareness including consonant addition and spoonerisms.

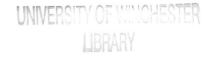

auditory input. Further evidence for the interaction between self-generated phonological codes and auditory input is, of course, offered by the irrelevant speech
effect. Performance is impaired by unwanted spoken material, with the crucial
feature of the material being its phonological rather than its semantic characteristics, again suggesting that the interaction is occurring at a common phonological level (Salamé & Baddeley, 1982). It should be pointed out at this stage,
however, that the nature of the irrelevant sound is crucial. While speech in a
foreign language is quite disruptive to performance, white noise is not, even
when the intensity of the noise is pulsed so as to resemble the intensity envelope
of the speech signal that has been shown to disrupt memory (Salamé & Baddeley,
1989).

Does this mean then that the system is capable only of handling speech? This
is clearly not the case, since Salamé and Baddeley found that memory for
visually presented digits was disrupted by vocal music to the same extent as by
irrelevant spoken material and was significantly, though somewhat less disrupted
by instrumental music.

The fact that memory is more disrupted by vocal than by nonvocal music
might seem to suggest that the system is essentially speech based. It is possible,
however, that the greater disruption by speech reflects the nature of the primary
task, namely remembering digits, a task that is likely to operate principally in
terms of the spoken names of the digits. It is entirely conceivable that a different
primary task would lead to a different degree of disruption. One possibility then
might be to look at studies investigating memory for environmental sounds.
Unfortunately, the evidence in this area seems to be relatively sparse. Shallice
and Warrington (1974) showed that their patient was better at remembering
environmental sounds than spoken digits, but, unfortunately, it is possible that
the task was done by first identifying the sounds and then remembering them
semantically.

A more recent, as yet unpublished study by Jack (1990) has explored the
effects of irrelevant environmental sounds on recall of visually presented sequences of nine digits. Jack replicated the disruptive effects of instrumental
music reported by Salamé and Baddeley (1989). In addition he found that continuous environmental sounds (running water, a vacuum cleaner or continuous
typing) also disrupted recall of visually presented digit sequences. Moreover, the
degree of disruption for environmental sounds was very similar to that found in
his study for instrumental music. This further generalizes the Salamé and Baddeley findings to suggest that the phonological storage of digits also appears to be
automatically accessed by environmental sounds, possibly in the same way as it
is accessed by instrumental music. However, there is as yet little evidence for the
characteristics of a system that would temporarily store such environmental
sounds (Bartlett, 1977; Bower & Holyoak, 1973; Ferrara, Puff, Gioia, & Richards, 1978; Rowe, Philipchalk, & Cake, 1974). For these reasons, we next
explore memory for music, which might offer some useful clues.

The Phonological Loop and Memory for Tones

We have described some of the work that has examined the processing and temporary storage of verbal material. It is apparent that the phonology of the words has a major role to play in such retention of verbal material. It might seem reasonable to suggest that a system responsible for retention of word sounds might well have developed from a more primitive system responsible for temporary storage of environmental sounds. For example, an animal may hear leaves rustling followed by the crack of a twig. The sounds have to be retained in memory long enough to make a decision as to whether they indicated the effects of a light breeze or the approach of a predator.

In contemporary human cognition, we apparently have the ability to remember a sequence which may be recognized as a familiar tune, and many people can, given conducive conditions, echo back a novel sequence of notes. Moreover, people can make judgments as to whether or not two notes, presented one after the other, are identical in pitch (e.g., Deutsch, 1969). All of these tasks require some form of temporary storage of the acoustic information, for periods of perhaps several seconds. This is well in excess of the period necessary for initial perceptual processing of material (Moore & Rosen, 1979).

There is an extensive literature on the processing and storage of nonverbal, auditory information, particularly music, including studies at both the psychoacoustic level (e.g., Moore & Rosen, 1979; Patterson, Peters, & Milroy, 1983), and at a cognitive level. These latter studies demonstrate that the average listener is equipped with highly structured templates and schemas that allow him or her to impose structure on sequences of tones and chords. For example, Krumhansl (1983) has argued that cognitive structures for tonal music mirror musical structure.

However, it remains unclear as to how we retain such material over short periods of time. It seems reasonable to suggest that there might be some overlap between the functional mechanisms involved in retention of tone sequences and the provision of similar functions for the auditory components of verbal material. The results reported by Salamé and Baddeley (1989), that irrelevant music disrupts the retention of visually presented digit sequences, certainly bears on this issue. However, it would be useful to consider whether the Phonological Loop might also be involved in the temporary storage of musical sequences. For example, do subjects retain arbitrary sequences of tones by means of a form of "subvocal singing"? If so, we might expect that retention of such sequences would be disrupted by articulatory suppression.

A second issue concerns whether retention of musical sequences requires cognitive functions which overlap with the ability to make judgments of phonology. Baddeley and Lewis (1981) have found that homophone judgments do not appear to be disrupted by concurrent articulatory suppression. Subjects reported being able to "hear inside their heads" the sounds of the words that they were reading under suppression. To what extent would subjects be able to use this same system for retention of nonverbal auditory material?

These issues were explored in a series of experiments by Logie and Edworthy (1986). In the first experiment, subjects were presented with a pair of tone sequences played one after the other. The first sequence of each pair was constructed by selecting tones at random from the tonal scale. For half of the trials, the sequences in each pair were identical, while on the remaining trials, the sequences differed by one note; the difference could occur anywhere in the sequence. Thus the task involved a recognition procedure with subjects deciding whether or not the sequences in each pair were identical.

The task was performed on its own, or concurrently with each of three secondary tasks. The first task involved articulatory suppression. The second task involved word–nonword homophone judgments (e.g., *Colonel-Kurnel*) as used by Baddeley and Lewis (1981). It is possible that the tone sequence recognition task might be disrupted simply by the requirement to carry out any secondary task, regardless of the nature of that task. Therefore a third secondary task involved matching of strings of nonalphabetic characters, (e.g., @#*&. . . . @!*&). This was intended to be formally equivalent to the homophone matching task, but required a visual comparison rather than a phonological one.

Table 8.1 shows the percentage of incorrect responses in each condition. There was a significant deterioration in performance with the presence of a secondary task. However, this disruption was shown only by articulatory suppression and by concurrent homophone matching. There was no disruption by the visual matching task.

These results cannot easily be explained in terms of differential difficulty of the secondary tasks. One might argue that making homophone judgments is more difficult than making visual string comparisons. However, it is much more difficult to argue that repeating an irrelevant word requires more cognitive resources than comparing novel strings of characters.

The finding that articulatory suppression and homophone judgments both showed about the same amount of interference is particularly interesting. One interpretation might be that both homophone judgments and articulatory suppression rely equally on the use of the Phonological Loop. However we know from Baddeley and Lewis (1981) that these two tasks do not interfere with one another, suggesting that they reflect two separate mechanisms. One distinction made by Besner (1987) is between tasks that involve phonological *processing,* and those that require the *storage* of phonological material. For example, if we assume that the tone sequence comparison task involved both storage and processing, this might imply that the homophone judgments disrupted the processing component of the task, that is comparison of the sequences while articulatory suppression disrupted the storage of the sequences.

Therefore, in a second experiment, Logie and Edworthy (1986) used a pitch comparison task. This required the storage of just one tone for later comparison with a second tone that was identical or slightly different in pitch. Results are shown in Table 8.1. In this experiment, homophone judgment was the only

TABLE 8.1
Percent Incorrect Responses in Recognition of Tonal and Atonal Sequences and in Pitch
Discrimination, with Articulatory Suppression, Homophone Judgments, and Visual Comparison

	Tonal Sequence	Pitch	Atonal Sequence
Control	32%	28%	33%
Suppression	40%	28%	40%
Homophones	40%	35%	43%
Visual Comparison	35%	30%	37%

secondary task to disrupt pitch comparison. Neither articulatory suppression nor visual string comparisons had any effect on performance.

In a third, unpublished experiment, Logie and Edworthy repeated the procedure for their Experiment 1, but with atonal sequences. The use of atonal sequences was intended to minimize the use of prior knowledge of tonal melodies or tonal melodic structure in retention of the sequences. The results are shown in Table 8.1 and essentially replicate those for Experiment 1.

These data seemed to support the view that articulatory suppression and homophone judgments involve separate mechanisms, and that memory for tone sequences involves both of these mechanisms. It is interesting that temporary storage of verbal material also appears to involve two mechanisms, namely subvocal rehearsal and a phonological store. One very neat characterization of the Logie and Edworthy data would be to suggest that these same mechanisms appear to be involved in tone sequence memory. The data are certainly consistent with the view that subvocal rehearsal or subvocal "singing" of tone sequences acts as an aid to accurate retention of tones in a prescribed sequence. Pitch comparison clearly does not reflect the operation of the articulatory control process, however it leaves open the question as to whether judgments of pitch might involve the phonological store.

THE PHONOLOGICAL LOOP
AND AUDITORY IMAGERY?

To what extent do these data clarify the case for or against the Phonological Loop as the seat of auditory imagery? Let us examine this by considering in turn the two components of the articulatory loop. Much of the evidence that we have considered appears to provide only modest support for an involvement of subvocal rehearsal in auditory imagery. We have presented some evidence which suggests a role for this form of rehearsal in retaining tone sequences. However, the amount of the disruption, although statistically significant, was quite small in absolute terms.

Crowder (1989) reported a series of studies involving memory for pitch and musical timbre (see also chapter 2 by Crowder and Pitt in this volume). Subjects were required to remember the pitch of a tone played on a guitar, a flute or a trumpet and compare this with a pitch played 500 msec later on either the same or a different musical instrument. Subjects were much faster in responding correctly when the same instrument was used for both the target and the comparison tone. In a follow-up experiment subjects were presented with a pure sine-wave tone, and they were required to image that tone as it would sound when played on one of the musical instruments. The comparison tone was then played on one or other of the instruments. Subjects were faster if the timbre of the comparison tone matched that of the imaged tone.

Crowder argued that this task cannot involve "a strictly motoric representational model," inasmuch as subjects can have an auditory image of sounds that they could not reproduce overtly with their vocal system. This might rule out "subvocal singing" as being involved in auditory imagery in Crowder's tasks because we do not have the vocal apparatus to mimic the timbre of different musical instruments. The argument seems even more compelling if we consider that we can retain and experience auditory images of environmental sounds such as rushing water or animal noises, although just how we do this remains to be explored.

There are two reasons why we are not wholly convinced by this argument. First, we should consider that Crowder used a pitch comparison task and, as Logie and Edworthy (1986) demonstrated, the processing and storage requirements of pitch comparison are different from the requirements of a task involving memory for the order of tones in a sequence. Thus, Crowder's view of no "motoric" involvement may apply only to a narrow range of tasks such as pitch comparison, with less to offer auditory imagery tasks in general.

Second, Crowder's argument that auditory imagery is not dependent on subvocalization rests on the assumption that sounds which cannot be reproduced overtly also cannot be rehearsed subvocally. It is true that we may not have the vocal apparatus to reproduce timbre, environmental sounds, or the several simultaneous voices of choral singing. We can nevertheless "hear" such sounds inside our heads. Moreover, we have argued that patients without overt speech can nevertheless demonstrate phenomena such as the word length effect (Baddeley & Wilson, 1985; Logie et al., 1989). That is, subvocal rehearsal does not necessarily require overt speech, but rather seems to require some deeper form of processing. Informal discussion with one of these anarthric patients (Patient 'LB,' Logie et al., 1989) revealed that she could indeed "hear inside her head" the names of pictures and words with which she had been presented. This being the case, we could extend the argument to suggest that the system responsible for subvocal rehearsal need not be limited by the constraints of the physical vocal apparatus, and that it is probably more closely associated with preparation for speech output (e.g., Ellis, 1980; Logie et al., 1989). On this view, the operation of subvocal rehearsal places constraints on overt vocalization, rather than the other way around, and these constraints are reflected, at least in part, in the speed of overt articulation.

Thus we would suggest that Crowder's subjects were indeed subvocalizing, in the sense that they were "rehearsing inside their heads," but in a fashion that was not constrained in the same way as is overt vocalization.

Other recent evidence on "auditory mental scanning" also bears on this issue. Halpern (1988; see also chapter 1, this volume) investigated "mental scanning" of familiar songs. In her experiments, subjects were required to compare two different selections from the lyrics of songs such as the American "National Anthem," or "Hark the Herald Angels Sing," and decide whether or not the lyrics were selected from a particular song. Lyrics chosen from the later parts of a song resulted in longer response times than lyrics chosen from a section near the beginning of the song. A similar result was obtained when subjects were asked to compare the pitches of notes corresponding to lyrics in the songs. Halpern suggested that subjects scanned a temporal auditory image of the songs in order to perform the task. These data are certainly consistent with the use of some form of subvocal singing.

What about the phonological storage component of the Phonological Loop? The results from Salamé and Baddeley (1989) and from Logie and Edworthy (1986) seem to point to some processing of musical material by the phonological store, which is also responsible for storing verbal material in a phonological form. We would suggest that when a single pitch is to be stored along with its timbre, this involves the phonological store. Such a store would not necessarily be restricted to storage of material that the subject was able to overtly reproduce. Subvocal rehearsal may be of benefit where a sequence of sounds is to be retained in a particular order, but it remains a moot point regarding how this latter function might be constrained by the vocal apparatus. For example, it would of interest to combine paradigms with Crowder's approach to examine the effects of suppression on the retention of sequences of tones each with a different timbre. In chapter 5, this volume, Smith, Reisberg, and Wilson report an experiment along these lines. Their finding is that blocking subvocalization removes the effects reported by Crowder (1989), a result that lends considerable support to the importance of subvocalization in auditory imagery tasks. This in turn makes the Phonological Loop a more plausible candidate for the seat of auditory imagery.

CONCLUSIONS

In this chapter we have attempted to apply the phonological loop component of working memory to the analysis of auditory imagery. The phonological loop assumes two relatively simple functional mechanisms, a phonological store and an articulatory control process. To what extent can these hypothesized mechanisms account for the phenomenon of auditory imagery?

In defining auditory imagery at the start of this chapter we specified four criteria, each of which can be evaluated in terms of the evidence from studies of phonological storage and phonological judgment. The first of these concerns the assumption that auditory imagery involves conscious experience. As noted earlier, we know of virtually no research concerned with the phenomenological aspects of working memory in general or the Phonological Loop in particular. It remains to be seen whether auditory imagery depends crucially on the Phonological Loop, the central executive, or indeed neither of these. Any adequate test of the hypothesis must explore directly the phenomenology of imagery.

The second assumption was that auditory imagery resembles the experience of hearing a sound directly. The evidence here is equivocal, because studies of irrelevant speech and music indicate that sound is capable of interfering with the storage of phonological sequences but does not appear to impair phonological judgments. This is consistent with the distinction between processing and storage, suggesting that the retention of auditory imagery possibly does involve the Phonological Loop, but that the system may not be necessary for imagery based judgments.

The third assumption is that the image can be evoked in the absence of any auditory stimulus. The fact that visual presentation is entirely adequate for producing both a phonological similarity effect in immediate serial recall, and for judgments of rhyme and homophony, strongly support this assumption. The same phenomena also support the fourth assumption, namely that an auditory image can be evoked intentionally by the subject.

To summarize, the evidence seems reasonably strong for the role of the Phonological Loop in the temporary storage of auditory images, but it is much less strong for the processes involved in evoking and experiencing images of this kind. The most urgent need in this area, therefore, is for studies that address directly the role in auditory imagery of phenomenological awareness.

ACKNOWLEDGMENTS

A. D. Baddeley is grateful to the ESPRIT BRA (ACTS 3207) contract on Auditory Connectionist Techniques for Speech. Some of the work described in the chapter was carried out when R. H. Logie was at the Medical Research Council Applied Psychology Unit, Cambridge, U.K.

REFERENCES

Atkinson, R. C., & Shiffrin, R. M. (1968). Human memory: A proposed system and its control processes. In K. W. Spence (Ed.), *The psychology of learning and motivation: Advances in research and theory* (Vol. 2, pp. 89–195). New York: Academic Press.
Baddeley, A. D. (1966). Short-term memory for word sequences as a function of acoustic, semantic and formal similarity. *Quarterly Journal of Experimental Psychology, 18,* 362–365.

Baddeley, A. D. (1986). *Working Memory*. Oxford, England: Oxford University Press.

Baddeley, A. D. (1990). *Human memory: Theory and practice*. London, England: Lawrence Erlbaum Associates.

Baddeley, A. D., & Hitch, G. J. (1974). Working memory. In G. Bower (Ed.), *The psychology of learning and motivation (Vol. VIII*, 47–90). New York: Academic Press.

Baddeley, A. D., & Lewis, V. J. (1981). Inner active processes in reading: The inner voice, the inner ear and the inner eye. In A. M. Lesgold & C. A. Perfetti (Eds.), *Interactive processes in reading* (p. 107–129). Hillsdale, NJ: Lawrence Erlbaum Associates.

Baddeley, A. D., Lewis, V. J., & Vallar, G. (1984). Exploring the articulatory loop. *Quarterly Journal of Experimental Psychology, 36*, 233–252.

Baddeley, A. D., Papagno, C., & Vallar, G. (1988). When long-term learning depends on short-term storage. *Journal of Memory and Language, 27*, 586–595.

Baddeley, A. D., & Salamé, P. (1986). The unattended speech effect: Perception or memory? *Journal of Experimental Psychology: Learning, Memory, and Cognition, 12*, 525–529.

Baddeley, A. D., Thomson, N., & Buchanan, M. (1975). Word length and the structure of short-term memory. *Journal of Verbal Learning and Verbal Behavior, 14*, 575–589.

Baddeley, A. D., & Wilson, B. (1985). Phonological coding and short-term memory in patients without speech. *Journal of Memory and Language, 24*, 490–502.

Baddeley, A. D., & Wilson, B. (1988). Comprehension and working memory: A single case neuropsychological study. *Journal of Memory and Language, 27*, 479–498.

Bartlett, J. C. (1977). Remembering environmental sounds: The role of verbalization at input. *Memory and Cognition, 5*, 404–414.

Besner, D. (1987). Phonology, lexical access in reading, and articulatory suppression: A critical review. *Quarterly Journal of Experimental Psychology, 39A*, 467–478.

Bishop, D. V. M., & Robson, J. (1989). Unimpaired short-term memory and rhyme judgement in congenitally speechless individuals: Implications for the notion of "articulatory coding." *Quarterly Journal of Experimental Psychology, 41A*, 123–140.

Bower, G. H., & Holyoak, K. (1973). Encoding and recognition memory for naturalistic sounds. *Journal of Experimental Psychology, 101*, 360–366.

Campbell, R., & Wright, H. (1989). Immediate memory in the orally trained deaf: Effects of "lipreadability" in the recall of written syllables. *British Journal of Psychology, 80*, 299–312.

Case, R. D., Kurland, D. M., & Goldberg, J. (1982). Operational efficiency and the growth of short-term memory span. *Journal of Experimental Child Psychology, 33*, 386–404.

Colle, H. A. (1980). Auditory encoding in visual short-term recall: Effects of noise intensity and spatial location. *Journal of Verbal Learning and Verbal Behavior, 19*, 722–735.

Colle, H. A., & Welsh, A. (1976). Acoustic masking in primary memory. *Journal of Verbal Learning and Verbal Behavior, 15*, 17–32.

Conrad, R., & Hull, A. (1964). Information, acoustic confusion and memory span. *British Journal of Psychology, 55*, 429–432.

Crowder, R. G. (1989). Imagery for musical timbre. *Journal of Experimental Psychology: Human Perception and Performance, 15*, 472–478.

Crowder, R. G., & Morton, J. (1969). Precategorical acoustic storage (PAS). *Perception and Psychophysics, 5*, 365–373.

Davis, R., Moray, N., & Treisman, A. (1961). Imitative responses and rate of gain of information. *Quarterly Journal of Experimental Psychology, 13*, 78–90.

Deutsch, D. (1969). Music recognition. *Psychological Review, 76*, 300–307.

Ellis, A. W. (1980). Errors in speech and short-term memory: The effect of phonemic similarity and syllable position. *Journal of Verbal Learning and Verbal Behavior, 19*, 624–634.

Ferrara, R. A., Puff, C. R., Gioia, G. A., & Richards, J. M. (1978). Effects of incidental and intentional learning instructions on the free recall of naturalistic sounds. *Bulletin of the Psychonomic Society, 11*, 353–355.

Gathercole, S., & Baddeley, A. D. (1989). Evaluation of the role of phonological STM in the development of vocabulary in children: A longitudinal study. *Journal of Memory and Language, 28,* 200–213.

Gathercole, S., & Baddeley, A. D. (1990). Phonological memory deficits in language disordered children: Is there a causal connection? *Journal of Memory and Language, 29,* 336–360.

Halpern, A. R. (1988). Mental scanning in auditory imagery for songs. *Journal of Experimental Psychology: Learning, Memory, and Cognition, 14,* 434–443.

Hitch, G. J., Halliday, M. S., Dodd, A., & Littler, J. E. (1989). Development of rehearsal in short-term memory: Differences between pictorial and spoken stimuli. *British Journal of Developmental Psychology, 7,* 347–362.

Hitch, G. J., Halliday, M. S., & Littler, J. (1989). Item identification time and rehearsal rate as predictors of memory span in children. *Quarterly Journal of Experimental Psychology, 41A,* 321–337.

Hitch, G. J., Halliday, M. S., Schaafstal, A. M., & Schraagen, J. M. C. (1988). Visual working memory in young children. *Memory and Cognition, 16,* 120–132.

Hulme, C., Thomson, N., Muir, C., & Lawrence, A. (1984). *Journal of Experimental Child Psychology, 38,* 241–253.

Jack, A. (1990). *Effects of instrumental music and environmental sounds on phonological short-term memory.* Unpublished BSc thesis, Aberdeen, Scotland: University of Aberdeen.

Johnston, R. S. & McDermott, E. A. (1986). Suppression effects in rhyme judgement tasks. *Quarterly Journal of Experimental Psychology, 38A,* 111–124.

Kosslyn, S., Brunn, J., Cave, K., & Wallach, R. (1985). Individual differences in mental imagery ability: A computational analysis. *Cognition, 18,* 195–243.

Krumhansl, C. L. (1983). Perceptual structures for tonal music. *Music Perception, 1,* 28–62.

Logie, R. H. (1989). Characteristics of visual short-term memory. *European Journal of Cognitive Psychology, 1,* 275–284.

Logie, R. H. (1991). Visuo-spatial short-term memory: Visual working memory or visual buffer? In C. Cornoldi & M. McDaniel (Eds.), *Imagery and cognition* (pp. 77–102). New York: Springer-Verlag.

Logie, R. H., Cubelli, R., Della Sala, S., Nichelli, P., & Alberoni, M. (1989). Anarthria and verbal short-term memory. In J. R. Crawford & D. M. Parker (Eds.), *Developments in clinical and experimental neuropsychology* (pp. 203–211). New York: Plenum.

Logie, R. H., & Edworthy, J. (1986). Shared mechanisms in the processing of verbal and musical material. In D. G. Russell, D. Marks, & J. Richardson (Eds.), *Imagery 2,* pp. 33–37. Dunedin, New Zealand: Human Performance Associates.

McKellar, P. (1965). *The investigation of mental images.* In S. A. Barnett & A. McClaren (Eds.) *Penguin Science Survey.* Harmondsworth, England: Penguin Books.

McLeod, P., & Posner, M. (1984). Privileged loops from percept to act. In H. Bouma & D. G. Bouwhuis (Eds.), *Attention and performance X,* pp. 55–66. Hore, England: Lawrence Erlbaum Associates.

Moore, B. C. J., & Rosen, S. M. (1979). Tune recognition with reduced pitch and interval information. *Quarterly Journal of Experimental Psychology, 31,* 229–240.

Morris, N., & Jones, D. M. (1990). Habituation to irrelevant speech: Effects on a visual short-term memory task. *Perception and Psychophysics, 47,* 291–297.

Murray, D. J. (1965). Vocalization-at-presentation with varying presentation rates. *Quarterly Journal of Experimental Psychology, 17,* 47–56.

Murray, D. J. (1968). Articulation and acoustic confusability in short-term memory. *Journal of Experimental Psychology, 78,* 679–684.

Neisser, U. (1967). *Cognitive Psychology.* New York: Appleton Century-Crofts.

Nicholson, R. (1981). The relationship between memory span and processing speed. In M. P. Friedman, J. P. Das & N. O'Connor (Eds.), *Intelligence and learning* (pp. 179–183). New York: Plenum Press.

Pascual-Leone, J. A. (1970). A mathematical model for the transition rule in Piaget's developmental stages. *Acta Psychologica, 32,* 301–345.

Patterson, R. D., Peters, R. W., & Milroy, R. (1983). Threshold duration for melodic pitch. In R. Klinke & R. Hartmann (Eds.), *Hearing-Physiological Basis and Psychophysics* (pp. 321–326). Berlin: Springer-Verlag.

Penney, C. G. (1989). Modality effects and the structure of short-term verbal memory. *Memory and cognition, 17,* 398–422.

Richardson, J. (1980). *Mental Imagery and Human Memory.* New York: St. Martins.

Rowe, E. J., Philipchalk, R. P., & Cake, L. J. (1974). Short-term memory for sounds and words. *Journal of Experimental Psychology, 102,* 1140–1142.

Salamé, P., & Baddeley, A. D. (1982). Disruption of short-term memory by unattended speech: Implications for the structure of working memory. *Journal of Verbal Learning and Verbal Behavior, 21,* 150–164.

Salamé, P., & Baddeley, A. D. (1989). Effects of background music on phonological short-term memory. *Quarterly Journal of Experimental Psychology, 41A,* 107–122.

Shallice, T., & Warrington, E. K. (1970). Independent functioning of verbal memory stores: A neuropsychological study. *Quarterly Journal of Experimental Psychology, 22,* 261–273.

Shallice, T., & Warrington, E. K. (1974). The dissociation between long-term retention of meaningful sounds and verbal material. *Neuropsychologia, 12,* 553–555.

Vallar, G., & Baddeley, A. D. (1984). Fractionation of working memory: Neuropsychological evidence for a phonological short-term store. *Journal of Verbal Learning and Verbal Behavior, 23,* 151–161.

Vallar, G., & Cappa, S. (1987). Articulation and verbal short-term memory: Evidence from anarthria. *Cognitive Neuropsychology, 4,* 55–78.

Wilson, B., & Baddeley, A. D. (in preparation). Spontaneous recovery of impaired memory span: Does comprehension recover?

9 The Representation of Pitch in Musical Images

Timothy L. Hubbard
Eastern Oregon State College

Keiko Stoeckig
Glassboro State College

Imagine that you are in a darkened concert hall. The conductor approaches the podium and raises the baton, and the orchestra plays the first pounding chords of Beethoven's *Fifth Symphony*. Can you imagine what the music sounds like— "hear" it in your "mind's ear"—as you would if you were actually in the concert hall? Or, imagine a snowy Christmas Eve. Carollers arrive outside your home and begin to sing "Silent Night." Can you hear the voices lifting in unison, the snow crunching lightly beneath their feet, the lyrics and melody wafting gently through your living room? What do these two examples have in common? They are examples of musical imagery, examples of the recreation of a musical experience in the absence of the musical stimulus and direct perceptual experience.

One of the most common aspects of musical images, indeed of all types of images, is their experiential aspect, that is, the creation of an image seems to be a re-creation of the sensory experience, the qualia, in a way that mere abstract knowledge of what that something sounds like is not. For example, I can know that the opening strains in Strauss' *Thus Spake Zarathustra* are built upon the I, V, and I' tones of a major scale or that the NBC chimes include a major sixth, but knowledge of this type is different from "hearing" what those notes sound like. Musical images, re-creations of musical experience, all possess a qualia, a sensory quality or "raw feel" that makes the experience of imaging similar to the experience of perceiving in a way that abstract representation is not. Additionally, musical images can vary greatly in their length or degree of detail, as one can "hear" a single note in isolation, well known melodies such as "Twinkle Twinkle Little Star" or "White Christmas," or entire symphonies.

Musicians often rely on musical imagery and its richness of qualia to compose music, guide their performances and memorize new music. This richness of qualia in musical imagery is illustrated in this passage from Seashore (1938/1967):

> The musician lives in a world of images, realistic sometimes even to the point of a normal illusion. . . . he is able to "hear over" a musical program which he has heard in the past as if it were rendered in the present. He creates music by "hearing it out," not by picking it out on the piano or by mere seeing of the score or by abstract theories, but by hearing it out in his creative imagination through his "mind's ear." That is, his memory and imagination are rich and strong in power of concrete, faithful, and vivid tonal imagery. . . . This capacity, I should say, is the outstanding mark of a musical mind at the representation level—the capacity of living in a representative tonal world. This capacity brings the tonal material into the present; it colors and greatly enriches the actual hearing of musical sounds; it largely determines the character and realism of the emotional experience; it is familiarity with these images which makes the cognitive memory for music realistic. Thus, tonal imagery is a condition for learning, for retention, for recall, for recognition, and for the anticipation of musical facts. Take out the image from the musical mind and you take out its very essence. (pp. 5–6)

For the majority of people, especially nonmusicians, music is primarily experienced through the auditory modality; music is foremost something that is heard. Although music may perhaps be experienced in other modalities (e.g., visually from reading musical scores), such experiences will not be addressed here. We will consider musical imagery to be a special case of auditory imagery. Auditory imagery includes re-creations of auditory sensory-experiences in general, including, for example, the slamming of a car door, the crack of the bat at a baseball game, or the crashing of waves upon the beach, whereas musical imagery includes re-creations of the auditory experiences of explicitly musical stimuli.[1] In this chapter we focus on the mental representation of musical pitch in images (for reviews of related properties, such as timbre, loudness, and duration, see chapters 1, 2, and 3, this volume). The vast majority of research examining imagery has focused on visual imagery (e.g., Block, 1981; Kosslyn, 1980; Shepard & Cooper, 1982); where appropriate, we note these findings and consider the implications they might have on theories of musical imagery. One purpose of this is to consider work in visual imagery as a fruitful source of hypotheses or explanations for findings in musical imagery research. We also take occasional forays into the literatures of both visual perception and music perception for the same purpose.

---

[1]A discussion of the necessary and sufficient properties distinguishing expressly musical stimuli from generic auditory stimuli is beyond the scope of this chapter; for a comprehensive discussion, see Dowling and Harwood (1986) and Davies (1978). For our purposes, musical stimuli will refer to auditory stimuli possessing melodic and/or harmonic properties (primarily of Western music).

We begin by examining how recent models of music perception and memory have addressed the representation of pitch in memory. Inasmuch as images can be generated based on information in memory, understanding the form of that information is vital to understanding imagery. In addition, the data from which theories of musical representation are derived will ultimately constrain theories of musical imagery. Theories concerning the mental representation of music may, in turn, be constrained by data derived from studies of musical imagery, although the experience of "having an image" need not necessarily tell us anything about the form of the underlying long-term representation (Marschark, Richman, Yuille, & Hunt, 1987)—any cognitive phenomenon can be explained by a variety of models, albeit more or less parsimoniously (Anderson, 1978). Moreover, it is important to consider whether any of these types of models can account for the qualia, the subjective experience, of musical imagery, because any model that cannot account for these properties will be in need of revision or rejection.

MODELS OF THE MENTAL REPRESENTATION OF MUSICAL PITCH

There are a myriad of theories and models purporting to describe the way that music, especially musical pitch, is cognitively represented. Although the cognitive representation of music and pitch has been the source of speculation at least as early as the days of classical Greece, our focus will be on the more recent empirically derived models of pitch representation. The majority of these modern models fall primarily into one of three classes of models, which we refer to as the (a) psychoacoustical, (b) rule-based, and (c) schematic/connectionist approaches.

Psychoacoustical Models

Psychoacoustic models tend to emphasize the purely acoustical aspects of the musical signal and concentrate on low-level (neural) explanations of pitch representation. For example, early psychophysical and acoustical models hypothesized that pitch could be represented by a single dimension (e.g., Stevens & Volkmann, 1940; Stevens, Volkmann, & Newman, 1937), roughly equivalent to frequency. The "representations," as such, were believed to be located along the length of the basilar membrane; tones with relatively short wavelengths (high frequency) were located near one end of the basilar membrane and tones with relatively long wavelengths (low frequency) were located near the other end of the basilar membrane. The similarity of any two tones was thus a function of the distance of their representations along the basilar membrane, that is, the difference in their absolute pitches. Although parsimonious, this type of explanation was often unable to account for findings in which pairs of pitches that were further apart (in absolute frequency) were rated as more similar than pairs of pitches that were closer. For example, a pitch of 1046 Hz (C_6) is perceived to be more similar to a pitch of 523 Hz (C_5) than to a pitch of 783 Hz (G_5), even though the frequency difference is greater for the first pair than for the second pair (Krumhansl & Shepard, 1979). However, when the frequency ratios are compared, the first ratio ($2 : 1$) is simpler than the second ratio ($3 : 2$). Although the relationship between the ratios of the frequencies of pitches and their consonance or dissonance has been known since the time of classical Greece, the way in which pitch was represented in memory in psychoacoustical models rarely seemed to incorporate these rather complex relationships.

Rule-Based Models

Rule-based models tacitly exploit some of the outward similarities between music and language. In language, there are a limited number of letters that can be combined to form valid words and words that can be combined to form grammatical sentences. In music, there are a limited number of tones (12 tones in Western music, cycling through approximately six octaves) that can be combined to form melodies and accompanying harmonies. Just as not every combination of letters forms a valid word, not every combination of tones forms an acceptable melody or harmony. The rules that govern the combination of letters in language are specified by the rules of grammar; the rules that govern the combination of tones in music are specified by the rules of music theory. Although there are a number of rule-based models, this class is perhaps best exemplified by the models of Deutsch and Feroe (1981) and Lerdahl and Jackendoff (1983). Deutsch and Feroe presented a model in which music can be represented by a language consisting of pitch sequences that are represented by a pitch alphabet, which can then be acted upon by a set of formal rules that can then organize these pitches into higher level (hierarchical) structures. These higher level structures are themselves represented by higher order alphabets with their own organizational rules. Using these sets of rules, in conjunction with the appropriate alphabets, a hierarchical code, or language, is developed that recreates the harmonic structure of the musical sequences quite well.

Lerdahl and Jackendoff have developed an extensive generative grammar of music founded on a rule-based approach. The elements constituting a musical piece, which they referred to as the *surface structure* (thus further extending the analogy between music and linguistics), are grouped together using various sets of rules to obtain an underlying hierarchical organization. Lerdahl and Jackendoff specify four sets of rules: (a) a set that specifies intuitions about how to group elements into musical motives, phrases and sections (grouping structure), (b) a set that specifies intuitions that events within the piece are organized into alternating weak and strong beats that are organized in a hierarchical way (metrical structure), (c) a set that assigns structural importance to hierarchically organized pitches according to their positions within the grouping and metrical structures (time-span reduction), and (d) a set that assigns hierarchical importance of harmonic and melodic elements (prolongation reduction). Each of the four sets of rules is further divided into two major types: well-formedness rules and general preference rules. Well-formedness rules are applied to the surface structure and specify possible structural outcomes. Once possible outcomes have been generated, preference rules are applied to designate which outcome corresponds to the listener's experience at any one time.

Much as rule-based grammars may offer an excellent accounting of the syntax of any production of language, ruled-based models of pitch representation may offer an excellent accounting of the syntax of any production of music. As pointed out by Chomsky (1972), the rules of grammar of language allow for an infinity of grammatical combinations. If the history of music is any indication, the rules of music theory also allow an infinity of grammatical combinations. However, especially in the realm of music, these rule-based models are often better at generating *post hoc* descriptions of musical compositions than at explaining how music is actually represented in memory. Moreover, much like its linguistic counterpart, musical syntax does not satisfactorily explain the semantics, the "meaning," of a production. The issue of meaning in music is a highly controversial one (e.g., Bernstein, 1976; Meyer, 1956), and it is not addressed here. We raise the issue as an example of at least one aspect of the experience of music that is not explained by a purely rule-based approach. We would suggest that qualia may be similarly nonexplainable by appeal to rule-based approaches. While a rule-based approach may adequately describe how to manipulate some aspects of qualia, it does not shed light on the nature of qualia per se.

Schematic/Connectionist Models

Schematic models, the most recent approach to pitch representation, are also the most popular approach within psychology. In these models, pitch is represented through some sort of music schema that often consists of at least three, and often more, dimensions. Although there are a great many schematic models, we present only two representative models—one by Longuet-Higgins (1978) and one by Shepard (1982). Longuet-Higgins proposed a three-dimensional framework in which intervals along one dimension increase by major fifths, intervals along a second dimension increase by major thirds, and intervals along the third dimension increase by octaves. A schematic of the first two dimensions of Longuet-Higgins' model may be seen in Fig. 9.1. One property of Longuet-Higgins' model is that all of the notes belonging to a particular key are located near to each other in the "tonal space." This is illustrated in Fig. 9.1 where all of the notes belonging to the key of C major have been enclosed by the solid line. There are many other properties of this model—for example, major triads are obtained by taking a note and its immediately higher neighbors along the x- and y-axes—but

	B	F#	C#	G#	D#	A#	E#	B#
Major 3rds	G	D	A	E	B	F#	C#	G#
	Eb	Bb	F	C	G	D	A	E
	Cb	Gb	Db	Ab	Eb	Bb	F	C

Perfect 5ths

FIG. 9.1. The first two dimensions of Longuet-Higgins' model. From Longuet-Higgins (1978).

the point of note for our purposes is that the model does not specify the nature of the representation within the tonal space. That is, what exactly is it that is labeled as C, E, G, etc.? As we discuss further, it is not clear whether these points represent images or abstractions of images, nor whether qualia are or can be represented in this way; however, we shall return to this issue later.

A more complex four-dimensional schema has been proposed by Shepard (1982). One dimension is circular in form and reflects the tone chroma (the letter name) of a pitch; one way to think of this dimension is as a piano keyboard collapsed across octaves. The second dimension is roughly analogous to "pitch height" and reflects the overall frequency level of the stimulus. Consideration of these two dimensions yields a helical (screw-like) structure in which the notes an octave apart (and thus sharing the same chroma or name) are aligned vertically along the outside of the resulting cylinder; the perimeter of the cylinder thus forms the chroma circle. An additional helix, which further wraps around the first, consists of triangles constructed of three successive tones, representing the harmonic closeness shared by the tonic and fifth of a scale. This produces a "double helix" arrangement whereby relationships between both fifths and octaves are preserved. As a final step, Shepard wound the double helix around a torus, producing a four-dimensional representation (see Fig. 9.2). Although there

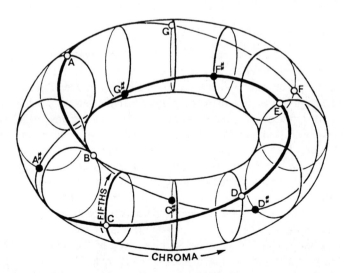

FIG. 9.2. Shepard's double helix model of the structure of pitch. From Shepard (1982).

are many ramifications to this type of model (see Shepard, 1982, for details), for our purposes one critical aspect of pitch representation remains unclear—the nature of the tonal "points" on the torus: specifically, if these points can account for the "raw feel," or qualia, of subjective experience. Although the relative positions and overall structure of the representations of specific pitches are clearly specified, the nature of the representations in themselves is not addressed.

Although schematic models preserve both tonal and harmonic relationships quite well, they have traditionally been static in form, showing possible links but offering no specified way of accessing those links and no way to account for learning or other changes in the representation. Newer schematic models have borrowed from the computational approaches to learning found in recently developed parallel distributed processing, or connectionist, models (e.g., McClelland & Rumelhart, 1986; Rumelhart & McClelland, 1986). An early version of a connectionist model of the representation of harmonic relationships was introduced by Bharucha and Stoeckig (1986, 1987). In this model musical chords are represented by nodes in a network (see Fig. 9.3). These chord nodes are connected via links to their parent key nodes (presumably there are also separate tone nodes that are linked to their parent chord nodes; the appearance of tone nodes are specified in later versions of this model). Chord nodes are activated through auditory experience, and activation spreads via the links to key nodes. The activation of key nodes causes activation to reverberate to the daughter chord nodes of the activated parent key, thus generating harmonic expectancies of what is to come. Newer versions of such a connectionist model (e.g., Bharucha, 1987; see Fig. 9.4) appear able to acquire the same pattern of responses to harmonic stimuli as are found with human subjects. These models share with traditional schematic models a representation of both tonal and harmonic structure but also have the advantage of a dynamic and elastic structure. Such elasticity is essential if we are to account for any changes over time (e.g., learning) in the schema.

All of the schematic and connectionist models of pitch perception preserve the

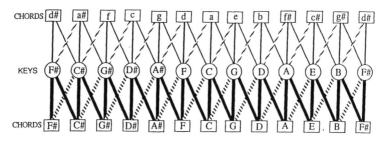

FIG. 9.3. An early connectionist model of Bharucha and Stoeckig. Major and minor chords are indicated by upper and lower case letters, respectively; link strength is indicated by thickness of the connecting lines. From Bharucha and Stoeckig (1986). Copyright (1986) by the American Psychological Association. Reprinted by permission.

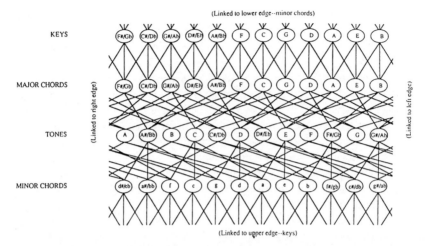

FIG. 9.4. A recent connectionist model of Bharucha. Major and minor chords are indicated by upper and lower case letters, respectively; links between units reflect the membership of tones in chords and the membership of chords in keys. From Bharucha (1987). © 1987 by the Regents of the University of California. Reprinted from Music Perception. Vol. 5. No. 1 (Fall, 1987), pp. 1–30, by permission.

types of relationships defined and required by rules of harmony. They specify the relative distance between two given pitches and the strength of any relationship between those pitches within a hypothetical pitch space of some minimum number of dimensions. Many of the schematic models of pitch perception, and especially the connectionist models, adopt the view that activation of the network begins with the activation of pitch nodes, nodes in memory that represent musical pitches and are usually thought to be frequency specific (or tuned to specific frequency channels, as proposed by Deutsch, 1969). Activation of such a pitch node might, then, correspond to having a memory of that pitch. But whether activation of the node also corresponds to having an image of the pitch, with all the qualia inherent in a musical image, has rarely, if ever, been addressed.

Even though a rule-based or schematic/connectionist model might offer us a complete description of how musical representation might be accomplished, it is not clear that such an understanding or such a representation would necessarily include the subjective elements of imagery so commonly reported. Pylyshyn (1984, p. 45) points out that information-processing types of theories have "set aside questions about what constitutes qualia, or 'raw feels'—dealing only with some of their more reliable functional and semantic correlates (for example, the *belief* that one is in pain, as opposed to the *experience* of the pain)." Nagel (1974), in his provocative essay, "What is it like to be a bat?," suggested that even though humans may possess a complete understanding (i.e., belief) of how bat sonar works, we still are unable to imagine the experience (i.e., qualia) of being a bat (we can, however, imagine the experience of what it would be like for a *human* to pretend to be a bat, even though we cannot imagine what it is like for a *bat* to be a bat). Again, we see an emphasis on belief about an experience rather than experience itself. In the present case, even though we understand or believe (via schematic/connectionist models) how music representation works, is this belief structure equivalent to the experience?

To make the case a bit clearer, we may adapt the logic of Jackson (1982) and postulate the existence of Mary, a sophisticated, dedicated, highly educated cognitive neuroscientist. Mary, alas, has been deprived of the experience of hearing music for all of her life, yet she has courageously studied her cognitive psychology, cognitive science, neuroscience, and music theory and has learned everything there is to know about the representation and processing of music. Although Mary may indeed have all the appropriate *beliefs* about music representation, does the possession of these beliefs equate with the *experience* of music? It would not seem so (but see Churchland & Churchland, 1981; Dennett, 1978 for contrasting views). Interestingly, Mary would be no better off if she were interested in the qualia of perception than if she were interested in the qualia of imagery—in both cases the "raw feel" of the experience would not be available. This similarity of qualia of perception and imagery is considered in more detail in the section on *Functional Equivalence of Musical Images and Percepts*.

A related philosophical notion involves the idea of an inverted spectrum (Block & Fodor, 1980). The inverted spectrum argument postulates the possible existence of a person whose apparent functioning would be identical to a normal person's, but who would nonetheless see the colors of the spectrum in reverse order. The intriguing aspect of the inverted spectrum problem is that there is no clear difference in functioning (e.g., both say "blue" when presented with the same object), although the sensation of appearing-as-blue to a person with an inverted spectrum would be the same as the sensation of appearing-as-yellow to a person with a noninverted spectrum. The appearing-as-blue and appearing-as-yellow qualia would be different, but functional accounts could not account for this difference. A more extreme version of the inverted spectrum argument postulates an absent qualia (perhaps in an intelligent-appearing machine, e.g., Block, 1980b). Thus, even though the neural or behavioral responses of a normal person and a person with an inverted spectrum might be identical, the internal experiences upon which those responses would be based would be totally different. It would not be difficult to construct an analog of the inverted qualia problem involving musical imagery—an "inverted scale" problem. In such a case, there would be no clear difference in functioning (e.g., both say "low" when presented with the same pitch), although the sensation of sounding-as-low to a person with an inverted scale would be the same as the sensation of sounding-as-high to a person with a noninverted scale. Again, even though their responses might be similar, the internal experiences upon which those responses would be based would be totally different. If models are unable to distinguish among inverted spectrum cases, it is unclear how they will be able to account for cases of inverted scale.

The inverted or absent qualia arguments are often raised as objections against functionalism, an approach underlying much of the computer simulation and modeling upon which most of the previously discussed schematic and connectionist models are based (e.g., discussion in Bechtel, 1988; readings in Block, 1980a), and to the extent that the inverted and absent qualia arguments are successful, then a portion of the response, the qualia, would remain unaccounted for. Within the philosophical community there have been various responses to the inverted and absent qualia problems. Some philosophers suggest that qualia may be characterized only so far as they cause beliefs (Shoemaker, 1980), while others have argued that only functional criteria are important and that cases of inverted qualia could not arise (Churchland & Churchland, 1981). Nonetheless, the issue of qualia remains a troubling one to many philosophers, as there subjectively seems to be some aspect of experience beyond that which can be captured in purely mechanistic models of the mind (Bechtel, 1988; however, see Dennett, 1978).

The critical question, then, is whether each of the models discussed to this point preserves the qualia that we have come to associate with imagery. Can these models account for that experience of actively hearing the sound as though it were perceived? It is logically possible that activation of a node or group of nodes interconnected by a network corresponds to an experience of qualia, although by the very nature of the abstraction inherent in such models, the schematic and connectionist models would not seem able to account for the concrete qualia quality of imagistic recreations of sensory experience. The qualia seem to be missing from network representations—but where can they be? We begin our search by looking at studies of absolute pitch and functional equivalence.

MEMORY FOR ISOLATED TONES

The models for the representation of pitch examined in the previous section were developed primarily from data collected in tasks in which subjects made some type of comparison or judgment of one or two stimuli that had been presented in a relatively minimal context. Judgments were made while subjects were actively attending to and perceiving the stimuli. In this section we examine data from studies in which subjects made some type of judgment about a musical stimulus while remembering or imaging that stimulus.

Absolute Pitch

Absolute or perfect pitch is the ability to identify the specific frequency or name of a given tone (Ward & Burns, 1982; Miyazaki, 1988; Van Krevelen, 1951) or the ability to produce a specific tone or frequency without using any objective reference tone as a standard of comparison (Seigel, 1972). This should be distinguished from the more common characteristic of relative pitch, in which individuals can identify particular relations among a group of pitches. In the simplest case, a subject could identify an interval between two pitches (as a octave, minor third, etc); in a more complex case, a subject could identify a melody based on relationships between subsequently presented notes.

Absolute pitch can be conceived of as an ability to retrieve an image of a particular pitch (say, A 440), and compare it with a stimulus pitch. Siegel (1974) reports that when subjects possessing absolute pitch compared two pitches differing by ¹⁄₁₀ semitone, those subjects reported using a sensory coding (imagistic) type of strategy, but if the standard and comparison differed by a larger amount, ¾ semitone, subjects possessing absolute pitch shifted to a verbal coding strategy (G, G#, A, etc.), while subjects not possessing absolute pitch continued to use a sensory trace strategy. The use of a verbal coding strategy by absolute pitch possessors is in keeping with what we know about strategies to overcome constraints of short-term memory. To keep these pitches in memory it is more efficacious to assimilate the stimulus into an existing pitch schema. Once the appropriate schema has been selected, that is, once the appropriate verbal label has been selected, that schema guides retrieval and hence assumedly organizes the memory. Dependence upon qualia may indeed then reflect a lower, less organized, form of pitch memory. The idea of assimilation of a pitch to a schematic organization is in the same spirit as many of the schematic models discussed earlier. A subject not possessing absolute pitch, that is, a subject continuing to use a sensory trace strategy, would be prolonging the "raw feel" of the stimulus in the image. What is it about an image that allows it to have this "raw feel" of perception?

The Notion of Functional Equivalence

The similarity of the "raw feels" of imagery and perception might result from imagery sharing or otherwise utilizing at least some of the processes or structures that are normally used in perception. The idea that images may use some of the same cognitive processes or structures that are used by perceptual processes has been referred to as *functional equivalence,* and it suggests that observed performances in perception tasks and imagery tasks are mediated by similar or overlapping internal structures or processes (Finke & Shepard, 1986). Mediation by similar processes is assumed to result in patterns of responses that will be similar. Furthermore, if the internal processing is similar, then similar experimental methods ought to be capable of quantifying that processing. Shepard and Podgorny (1978) pointed out that many cognitive processes seem to resemble, to some extent, the corresponding perceptual processes, and they suggested that some of the techniques developed for the study of perceptual processes might be fruitfully adapted to the study of cognitive processes. To a surprising extent, this has been true for use of multidimensional scaling (e.g., Shepard & Chipman, 1970; Shepard, Kilpatric, & Cunningham, 1975), chronometric analysis (e.g., Kosslyn, 1980), and psychophysical scaling (e.g., Algom, in press).

To apply the notion of functional equivalence to music perception and musical imagery, we examine studies in which methods originally developed for the study of the perception of music have been adapted to the study of musical imagery. In addition to examining equivalences between music perception and music imagery, we will also look for equivalences in processing between visual imagery and musical imagery. It may be that some commonalities, by virtue of a generic imagery resource or capacity, arise. Although many researchers have proposed that images are processed by mechanisms similar to or even identical with those used in the processing of percepts (e.g., Farah, 1985, 1988; Finke, 1985; Finke & Shepard, 1986; Kosslyn, 1980, 1987), such a position is not universally accepted (e.g., Pylyshyn, 1984; Chambers & Reisberg, 1985). After an extensive review of the literature, Finke and Shepard (1986) concluded that, while different alternative hypothesis to each functional equivalent result can be given, the hypothesis of a functional equivalence between imagery and perception is the single best overall explanation for results across a wide domain of tasks.

In one of the early experiments dealing with functional equivalence between perception and imagery, Brooks (1968) reported that visual imagery seemed to interfere with a visual task. In one of Brooks' experiments, subjects would visualize a block letter, such as an F, and then scan around the perimeter of the letter. As subjects scanned the letter, they indicated whether each corner they encountered was at the extreme top or bottom of the figure. When subjects responded vocally or by tapping, their response times were approximately twice as fast as when they responded by pointing to Ys and Ns that were arranged in a complex pattern. Brooks reasoned that visual activity would be necessary in order for subjects to point to the correct location; such visual activity would not be necessary for the other response methods. Therefore, to the extent that a person's image is visual, that is, invokes visual processing resources, subjects found it difficult to respond using methods that also require visual resources. Even though weaknesses in Brooks' design have since been discussed (e.g., level of difficulty of the three response methods may not have been equal, interference notwithstanding), it did serve to motivate research on interferences between imagery and perception.

Another early seminal work was conducted by Segal and Fusella (1970), who requested subjects to form either a visual image or an auditory image. After subjects indicated that they had successfully formed and were maintaining an image, either a faint visual stimulus, a faint auditory stimulus, or no stimulus was presented. Segal and Fusella found that visual images interfered with visual perception and that auditory images interfered with auditory perception. Interestingly, visual images did not appear to interfere with auditory perception nor did auditory images interfere with visual perception. The data were interpreted as suggesting that same-modality imagery interferes with perception more than does cross-modality imagery. A key to these results was that the objects to be detected in the same-modality task were different from the objects being imaged. Peterson and Graham (1974) modified Segal and Fusella's method so that subjects imaged either a visual stimulus identical to the one to be detected or different from the one to be detected. Subjects who imaged a compatible object performed better on the detection task than subjects who imaged an incompatible object, thus leading Peterson and Graham to suggest that the image "tailors" attention for the coming percept. Another way to conceive of this is that an image "primes" the appropriate mental representation; this idea is expanded below.

Functional Equivalence of Musical Images and Percepts

The findings of Segal and Fusella (1970) and Peterson and Graham (1974) initially seem contradictory—on the one hand, same-modality images seemed to interfere with perception, but on the other hand, at least some same-modality images seemed to facilitate perception. However, in Segal and Fusella's work, the image was concurrent with the percept, whereas in Peterson and Graham's work the image preceded the percept. Farah and Smith (1983) combined both of these conditions into one experimental procedure in which subjects had to detect whether or not an auditory signal had been presented. The signal was one of two different frequencies (715 Hz or 1000 Hz), and subjects were instructed as to which of the two frequencies to image. In one session they imaged one of the frequencies during the detection interval on each trial; in the other session they imaged the frequency immediately prior to the detection interval. The dependent measure was the threshold intensity measure necessary to detect the perceptual auditory signal.

Farah and Smith found that the signal strength necessary for detection was lower when subjects imaged the specific frequency that was to be detected. This is consistent with the Peterson and Graham results and suggests that same-frequency images are able to prime detection of a same-frequency target; however, this selective facilitation was no greater in the image-before than in the image-during condition. Farah and Smith interpreted this as showing that frequency information is represented in images. Inclusion of frequency information in auditory images is, of course, perfectly consonant with ideas of functional equivalence, as percepts inarguably include a representation of a frequency component. If musical images preserve pitch, as Farah and Smith's data suggest, then we should expect to see the same effects of harmonic relatedness (e.g., harmonic priming) for imaged pitches that we do for perceived pitches. Thus, we would expect response patterns and accuracy rates for imaged stimuli to match those obtained for perceived stimuli.

Hubbard and Stoeckig (1988) looked at this prediction. In their studies, subjects were presented with a cue stimulus that was either a single tone or chord and then formed an image of what that tone or chord would sound like if it were raised in pitch one whole step. (Subjects imaged a higher pitch, rather than the presented pitch, in order to eliminate contributions of echoic memory to performance.) When subjects indicated that they had formed the proper image, a tone or chord probe stimulus was played to them and they judged whether the pitch(es) of the probe was *same* or *different* from the pitch(es) that they were imaging. If the cue had been a tone, then the probe was a tone; if the cue had been a chord, then the probe was a chord. The relationship between the pitch(es) of the probe and the pitch(es) of the image varied along the continuum of harmonic relatedness. The probe either matched the pitch(es) of the image, was different but closely harmonically related, or was different and distantly harmonically related. Response times and accuracy rates were measured.

The accuracy rates mirrored patterns that had been found when people make tonal discriminations given a harmonic context (e.g., Cuddy, Cohen, & Miller, 1979); subjects were most accurate in the same condition, followed by the different-unrelated condition, and least accurate in the different-related condition. Response times were consistent with patterns found in previous music perception experiments (e.g., Bharucha & Stoeckig, 1986, 1987); subjects were fastest in the same condition, followed by the different-unrelated condition, and slowest in the different-related condition. In a control experiment, subjects instructed not to use imagery predicted how other subjects using imagery would perform. The control subjects correctly predicted that *same* responses would be faster than *different* responses, but incorrectly predicted different-related tones would be faster than different-unrelated tones and there would be no difference between different-related chords and different-unrelated chords. The similarity of patterns obtained from imagery subjects with patterns previously obtained from perception subjects, in conjunction with the failure of control subjects to accurately predict these patterns, is consistent with the notion that images were processed in the same way that percepts were, thereby lending support to the notion of an equivalence in the representations underlying imagery and perception.

Another type of equivalence was examined in the Hubbard and Stoeckig (1988) experiments, a level of equivalence not between musical imagery and musical perception, but between musical imagery and visual imagery. Work in visual imagery has shown that more complex images take longer to form than less complex images. Kosslyn, Reiser, Farah, and Fliegel (1983) presented subjects with line drawings of different animals; three versions of each drawing were used. In the first version, all of the animal was drawn on a single page. In the second version, the drawing was split up over two pages so that one page contained the torso and the other page contained the appendages. In the third version, the drawing was split up over five pages. When subjects were instructed to form an image of the entire animal, Kosslyn et al. found a linear relationship between the number of pages upon which the drawing had been presented and the time required to form the image.

Single tones might be considered analogous to the one-page drawings used in Kosslyn et al., and the major chords (constructed from three tones) might be considered analogous to the multi-page drawings. Thus chords, the more complex stimuli, should require more time to image than tones, the less complex stimuli. This was precisely what was found, as chord images took longer to form than tone images. Additionally, in the two experiments in which the time to image tones and chords was measured, the ratio of tone image formation time to chord image formation time was nearly constant (approximately 1.15). Were subjects forming the chords a tone at a time and then "mentally gluing" the single tones together to form one chord, we would have expected that chords would have taken approximately three times longer to form than did tones, but in fact, although the chord image formation time was longer than that for tones, it did not approach being three times longer. There are two possible interpretations of the longer image formation time for the chords. The first is that the chord images were activated as single units. The additional time required may have been due to the more complex nature of the representation. In an analogous case of forming an image of a three letter word, the word itself can be directly imaged without first needing to image the individual letters sequentially (Weber, Kelley, & Little, 1972). The second possibility is that the single tones composing the chord were activated singly but in parallel. The additional time required was then used to merge the separate elements into a single entity. The data to this point cannot distinguish between these possibilities, but it remains an enticing idea for further research.

In summing up the research on the representation of imaged pitch of isolated tones and chords, it certainly appears as though there are at least some functional equivalences between perception and imagery in the processing of musical pitch. Pitches imaged with a specific frequency can prime or inhibit subsequently presented stimuli in a manner similar to that of perceived pitches. More convincingly, imaged pitches exhibit the same kinds of harmonic relationships to perceived pitches as other perceived pitches would. Although it is possible that imaged pitches and perceived pitches obtain this similarity by using separate but equal representational systems, it is more parsimonious to posit a common representational system that is utilized by both imagery and perception.

MEMORY FOR FAMILIAR SONGS

Our discussion in the preceding section focused on imagery for isolated musical elements—single tones and chords. Even in these relatively isolated contexts, though, we were able to see effects of harmonic relatedness on imaged tones and chords, and these patterns paralleled those found in studies of music perception.

Now we move beyond isolated tones and chords and cast our net wider so that we can look at memories and images of entire melodies (sequences of tones and chords). It seems intuitively obvious that we possess memories for familiar songs. With little effort, you can imagine the way a song goes (even if you cannot produce it, you can at least imagine how it would sound if you or someone else sang or played it). When images of familiar songs are accessed, are there any properties that we might be able to document? One possible property that might be included is the temporal course of the melody. Melodies are extended across time, and much as we can scan across a visual image that is extended in space, we should be able to scan across a melodic image that is extended in time.

Scanning of Imaged Melodies

Before we examine studies of the scanning of imaged melodies in musical imagery, we review studies of the scanning of imaged objects in visual imagery that may serve as partial inspiration. One of the best-known studies in imagery, indeed in perhaps all of cognitive psychology, is the original study of mental rotation reported by Shepard and Metzler (1971; also see Shepard & Cooper, 1982). Subjects in these experiments typically saw line drawings of two different three-dimensional objects which were either identical or mirror images of each other. The subjects' task was to decide whether the two objects were the same object differing only in orientation or if they were different objects. Shepard and Metzler found that the time required to make this decision was a linear function of the degree of angular disparity between the two objects. The larger the angular disparity, the more time subjects took to respond.

Shepard used these results to argue the subjects mentally rotated a mental analog of one object, and this "mental rotation" continued until the orientation of the mentally rotated object matched the orientation of the other object. A key point in Shepard's conceptualization is that the mental representation was an analog one; this notion of analog representation entails a number of important features. The important feature for our purposes is that the mental representation passed through intermediate points. For example, in rotating an object from a 45° to a 90° orientation, the representation of the object had to pass through an intermediate orientation of 60° (see also Cooper, 1976). This was an important claim, because it seemed to suggest some basic properties of the human cognitive system. Other models of cognitive processing (e.g., propositional networks) could not easily accommodate the mental rotation results, and over the next decade a fierce debate ensued concerning which properties (such as taking longer to rotate greater distances) were truly basic ones in cognition and which properties were not basic, that is, could be influenced by other cognitive factors (see Kosslyn, Pinker, Smith, & Schwartz, 1979; Kosslyn & Pomerantz, 1977; Pylyshyn, 1981, 1984).

Another of the oft-cited studies in the visual imagery literature that also has a bearing on our consideration of image scanning was conducted by Kosslyn, Ball, and Reiser (1978). They examined the relationship between distance in a visual image and the amount of time required to mentally scan that distance. In one experiment, subjects memorized a map of a fictitious island that contained several landmarks (hut, well, rock, etc.). After subjects had memorized the map, the experimenter would name a landmark and subjects would visualize the map and focus their attention on that landmark. The experimenter would then name a second landmark, and if that landmark was located on the map, subjects imagined a small black speck flying from the landmark where they were focused to the second landmark. The dependent variable was the time required to scan from the first to the second landmark. Kosslyn et al. reported a linear relationship between distance and scanning time. The larger the distance to be scanned, the more time subjects took to respond.

Extrapolation from the results of Shepard and Metzler (1971) and Kosslyn et al. (1978) leads to some very specific predictions about the scanning of musical images. Just as a physical object unfolds across space, so a melody unfolds across time. Instead of using a metric of inches across a map or degrees of angular disparity, however, scanning through a melody involves a metric of the number of beats in the melody increases. Using this analogy, we would predict a monotonic (possibly linear, if subjects maintained a constant tempo) relationship tion in which the musical image should pass through intermediate points of the melody on its journey from one point in the lyric to another, much as Shepard and Metzler's subjects imaged the rotation of an object through intermediate orientations and Kosslyn et al.'s subjects imaged the black speck at intermediate locations. Given a constant tempo, more time is required to play a melody as the number of beats in the song increases. Using this analogy, we would predict a monotonic (possibly linear, if subjects maintained a constant tempo) relationship between the number of beats to be scanned in the imaged melody and the time required to do so.

This prediction was recently examined by Andrea Halpern (1988; see also Halpern, chapter 1, this volume). There were two conditions: imagery and nonimagery instructions. On each trial, both groups of subjects were presented with the title of a well known melody and then with two lyrics and had to judge whether those two lyrics were from that song. If they knew immediately that the second lyric was not contained within the song, they responded *false* as rapidly as possible, but if the second lyric was indeed contained within the song, imagery subjects were to imagine singing from the first lyric to the second lyric and, when they arrived at the second lyric, compare the pitches of the two lyrics. Nonimagery subjects were merely told to respond as quickly and as accurately as possible. Both imagery and nonimagery groups increased in reaction time as number of beats between the first and second lyrics increased, suggesting that subjects were operating on an analog mental representation of the song, that is, mentally "playing" the song. Additionally, lyrics close together seemed to be scanned proportionally faster than those farther apart, and there was a tendency for imagery subjects to be slower for trials in which the starting point was further into the song, suggesting that imagery subjects were starting their images at the beginning of the songs, even though this was not explicitly required of them. The larger the pitch separation between Lyric 1 and Lyric 2, the smaller the error rates. A follow-up study explicitly designed to control for pitch separation found significantly fewer errors with greater pitch separations and a nonsignificant trend for larger separations to result in faster response times.

Hubbard and Stoeckig (in preparation) have replicated the trends in melody scanning times reported by Halpern, and have also adapted the methods used by Deutsch (1972) in her studies of tonal memory. Deustch (1972) had subjects judge whether two tones (called the standard and the comparison, respectively) separated by a short time interval were the *same* or *different*. When the interval between the presentation of the standard and the presentation of the comparison was filled with silence, subjects were very accurate in their discriminations. When the interval was filled with distractor pitches, the subjects' accuracy varied with the composition of the tone pair and the nature of the distractors. More specifically, Deustch found that if the standard and comparison were the same, then if a tone of the same pitch was included within the distractors, accuracy increased. However, if the standard and comparison were different, accuracy increased if the distractors included a tone at the pitch of the standard, but decreased if the distractors included a tone at the pitch of the comparison. If images are functionally equivalent to perceptions, and subjects are "going through the intervening notes" in a melody scanning tasks, then the same pattern of responses ought to be found when subjects merely image the intervening melodic material as when they perceive it.

To test these hypotheses, Hubbard and Stoeckig (in preparation) presented subjects with a starting pitch, a song title, and a target lyric. When subjects had formed an image of the first word of the melody on the starting pitch, and were ready to begin imaging the melody, they pressed a designed key and a tone (i.e., the standard) was played. After the standard finished playing, subjects imaged singing the song to themselves; they began the melody on the starting pitch and scanned the image until they reached the target lyric. When they reached the target lyric, they pressed another key and a second tone (i.e., the comparison) was played. Subjects compared the pitch of the standard and the pitch of the comparison and judged whether they were the *same* or *different*. For example, subjects saw "Old MacDonald—farm." When they had formed an image of "Old," and were ready to begin scanning the image, they pressed a key and heard the standard. They then scanned through the melody until they reached the word "farm," and when they reached this target lyric, they pushed another key, heard the comparison pitch, and judged whether the it was the *same* as or *different* from the standard.

The parts of songs imaged between the presentation of the standard and comparison tones took one of three forms: a tone at the pitch of either the standard or comparison was not included, a tone at the pitch of the standard was included, or a tone at the pitch of the comparison was included in the interpolated imaged song. Thus, the structure of the task exactly mirrored that used by Deutsch (1972) in her studies of memory for tones, except that the distractors in her study were perceived, whereas the distractors in this study were imaged.

Although this study is not yet completed, preliminary analysis has revealed some marginally significant trends. When the standard and comparison were the same pitch, accuracy increased if a tone of the same pitch was included in the interpolated imaged melody. However, when the standard and comparison were different, accuracy increased if a tone at the pitch of the standard was included in the imaged melody, but decreased if a tone at the pitch of the comparison was included. This pattern of accuracies matches the accuracy pattern found by Deutsch (1972, 1982) in her perceptual studies. Should this pattern hold, these results would be consistent with the notion that imaged pitches result in the same kind of facilitation/inhibition of pitch memory as obtained from perceived pitches, providing yet more evidence of a functional equivalence between perception and imagery processes.

To this point we have been looking at melody and ignoring lyric aspects. To the extent that lyrics have been involved at all, they have functioned merely as landmarks for particular locations within a melody. However, even casual inspection of musical material suggests a substantial role of lyrics in music, so now we turn our attention more explicitly to the role of lyrical text in musical imagery.

Melody–Text Integration

Serafine and her colleagues (Serafine, Crowder, & Repp, 1984; Serafine, Davidson, Crowder, & Repp, 1986) have examined the way that melody and lyric (text) are integrated in the memory for songs. One possibility is that the memory representations for melody and lyric form an integrated unit; if such an integration occurred, it would be difficult to produce or recognize either melody or lyric without activating the mental representation of the other (at least subvocally). As Serafine et al. (1986) have pointed out, this often does appear to be the case, for it is often difficult to recognize even a very familiar melody if the words have been changed. For example, many people do not recognize the melody line of "Baa Baa Black Sheep" when they hear "Twinkle Twinkle Little Star," even though the two songs have the same melody line. Likewise, many people do not realize that "Merrily We Roll Along" has the same melody as "Mary Had a Little Lamb."

Serafine, Crowder, and Repp (1984) looked at the independence of memory for melody and memory for lyrics. Subjects heard excerpts from folksongs and then were given a recognition test. There were four types of items in the recognition test: new melody with new lyric, old melody with new lyric, new melody with old lyric, old melody with old lyric that had been sung to a different tune in the original presentation. Serafine et al. reasoned that if subjects integrate melody and lyric in memory, then they should recognize previously heard melodies or lyrics more accurately when those melodies or lyrics were paired with their original lyric or melody than when paired with a different lyric or melody. If melody and lyric are independent, then subjects should recognize melodies and lyrics equally well regardless of the lyric or melody with which they are paired. It was found that melodies and lyrics are better recognized when the lyric or melody with which they are heard is the same as the lyric or melody with which they had been originally learned, and Serafine et al. referred to this idea as an *integration effect.*

Serafine, Davidson, Crowder, and Repp (1986) looked at several alternatives to the integration idea. One alternative is the *semantic hypothesis,* which suggests that the integration effect is driven by semantic connotations that the words impose on a melody. The semantic hypothesis suggests that the melody becomes imbued with qualities implied by the text's meaning; for example, a lyric referring to a cobbler may make short repetitive notes resembling hammering or a lyric referring to a bluebird may include a series of ascending notes which suggest taking flight. A second alternative is the *decrement hypothesis,* which suggests that the integration effect is an artifact of the distracting influence that a "wrong" element has on an already familiar component. The melody representation may be quite independent of its lyric, and under normal circumstances may be just as easily recognized in one context as in another. However, a mismatch of melody and lyric may distract or confuse subjects and thus depress recognition. Subjects were presented with excerpts from 24 folksongs and then were given a recognition test which varied whether a lyric was presented at learning or testing and the level of semanticity of the lyric; neither the semantic hypothesis nor the decrement hypothesis were supported (although the decrement hypothesis narrowly missed significance). Serafine et al. cast their interpretation in line with Tulving's (1983) ideas of encoding specificity, that is, recreating the context (e.g., producing the original melody or lyric that accompanied the lyric or melody to be recognized) greatly facilitates retrieval.

What do these studies of the memory of familiar songs tell us? In the Halpern (1988) and Hubbard and Stoeckig (in preparation) experiments subjects were scanning across time, and it was seen that the musical image seems to preserve temporal aspects of melodic space in the same way the visual image preserves spatial aspects of visual space. Of course, this parallel is not complete, as evidence suggests that scanning is more difficult in some directions (backwards) in auditory images than in others, and this sort of asymmetry has not typically been found in scanning visual images. Nonetheless, the results are suggestive. In the experiments of Serafine et al. (1984; 1986), musical images were shown, in some conditions, to include both text (lyric) and melody (pitch) elements integrated tightly together. The representation of pitch is thus associated, in some instances at least, with nonpitch representations of a possibly extra-musical source. We will now consider all of the data we have reviewed and attempt to cull a parsimonious model from them.

THE FORM
OF THE UNDERLYING REPRESENTATION

Do all of these studies tell us anything about the form of the underlying representation? There is no single, well developed model of musical imagery, so again, let us first consider the analogous visual imagery results. The most fully developed theory of visual imagery is surely that put forward by Kosslyn (1980, 1981); we now examine aspects of that theory and see if selected portions of it may be useful as a first approximation toward a model of musical imagery. To understand Kosslyn's model, we need to distinguish between two components of imagining: (a) the medium underlying imagery, and (b) the data structures that occur within that medium. To use an analogy, consider Plato's conception of memory as a wax tablet. In this view, specific memories are likened to specific impressions in different locations on the tablet. The clearness of the impression (memory) depends upon the sharpness of the instrument that produced it, and the impression, or memory, would tend to fade with time. In this example, the wax is the medium that supports the impression, and the relationships between the elements in the impression are the data structures.

In Kosslyn's theory the medium is quasi-pictorial; that is, it performs many of the same functions as a picture, the most important of which is the preservation of metric space. That is, if in a real object points A and B are farther apart than points C and D, then this spatial relationship will be preserved in the image of that object. This does *not* mean that images are pictures in the head, as such a position is clearly untenable (for example, an image of a green elephant would then itself have to be green and shaped like an elephant). Rather, the theory holds that the medium in which images occur preserves those (spatial) relationships that would be found in the object, although the nature of this preservation need not be physically isomorphic with the object. Shepard and Chipman (1970) have referred to this functional preservation as *second-order isomorphism*.

Kosslyn posits two major components to visual images: (a) the surface representation, and (b) the deep representation. The surface representation is analogous to the impression on the wax tablet—it is the subjective sense of image, or what we "see" when we see an image. More specifically, the surface representation depicts an object. The idea that images depict (rather than describe) an object has several implications about the nature of images, the most important of which is that color, size, shape, orientation, and location information are not independent within an image, and specification of value on one dimension requires simultaneous specification of value along other dimensions. To see that this is true, try to image a square that doesn't have a specific size or location or is not oriented in any direction. Try to imagine the color red without extending that color over any space. It is quite difficult—probably impossible—to form these images. In contrast, it is quite easy to achieve a nonimaginal format (such as a propositional network) in which values for qualities such as these could be listed without specifying values on other qualities. The other component of visual imagery, the deep representation, contains the information held in long-term memory that gives rise to or is used in creation of the surface representation.

Once the surface representation is created, there are a number of processes that operate on it. Among these, Kosslyn (1980) has elaborated on procedures that generate, inspect, and transform a visual image. Image generation occurs when a surface representation is formed and involves such processes as those that create, inspect, find and add new parts to an image. Inspection occurs when that surface representation is examined and involves processes that look for separate parts on a depicted object, zoom in on particular areas, or pan back for a wider view. Transformation occurs when an existing image is changed and involves processes such as rotation and scanning of the image. There are two classes of transformation: field general refers to transformations involving the entire surface of the image and region bounded refers to transformations involving only a limited, bounded region of the surface representation. Additionally, there are two ways in which each type of transformation may be carried out: shift transformations involve gradual changes in the image by which the image approaches its goal state by closer and closer approximations (e.g., mental rotation), and blink transformations involve wiping clean the entire surface representation and then creating an entirely new image.

Is it possible to adapt parts of Kosslyn's model of visual imagery in order to specify a model of musical imagery? If the surface representation of a visual image depicts a visual object, then the surface representation of the musical image should depict a musical event in the same way. Just as the depiction of a visual object by a visual image specifies basic information about the color, size, shape, orientation, and location of that object, so then must the depiction of a musical event by a musical image specify basic information about a particular musical event. The basic information for a musical event, however, will probably differ from that of a visual event and could include such characteristics as pitch, loudness, duration, timbre, and temporal sequence. The medium in which musical images occur should preserve those relationships that would be found in the musical event, and, as with visual imagery, the nature of that preservation need not have a simple or first-order isomorphism with the object, but would demonstrate a higher-order isomorphism. Moreover, this sort of information must be specified in a non-independent way, similar to the non-independence of shape, size and color in the visual image. Does that seem possible with musical stimuli? Probably yes. Intuitively, it seems quite difficult to image a specific pitch without extending it in time, without some degree of loudness, or without some particular timbre.[2] Again, it seems that such isolation of attributes is not possible within an image, whereas it would be possible in a nonimaginal format in which values on some qualities could be listed without specifying values on other qualities.

Once we have generated a musical image, we ought to be able to apply processes similar to the inspection and transformation procedures specified by Kosslyn for visual imagery. If so, then we could examine the data for any functional equivalence between music perception and music imagery. In fact, the melody scanning studies of Halpern (1988) and Hubbard and Stoeckig (in preparation) and the studies of image priming by Hubbard and Stoeckig (1988) show just that: images preserve the functional relationships of the original stimuli. We have seen that it takes less time to scan to words that occur relatively early in the course of a lyric than to scan to the words that occur later in a lyric. Moreover, this time difference (roughly) corresponds to the number of musical beats between the words in the melody. As with mental rotation and image scanning, the distances and relationships (in these cases, temporal and harmonic) between parts of the stimulus seem to be maintained, offering implicit evidence for the notion that such musical image scanning involves an analog medium—in scanning through the lyric of a melody, subjects are thought to proceed through the song and pass through the intermediate beats precisely as the images in mental rotation studies are thought to pass through intermediate orientations. Further, the harmonic relationships of those parts are also maintained (as are the spatial relationships in a visual image), as can be seen in the ability of an image to prime a judgment about a perceived stimulus (Hubbard & Stoeckig, 1988) and an imaged interpolated melody to affect judgment of a standard and a comparison tone (Hubbard & Stoeckig, in preparation).

Such a model of musical imagery would lead to a number of predictions. For example, is there a musical analog of the region bounded and field general

---

[2]Intons-Peterson (1980) has suggested that loudness information is only an optional component of auditory imagery. This assertion is based on the findings that while differences between loudness ratings affect the times to match and to make comparative judgments of described sounds, loudness ratings are not related to the time required to generate auditory images. However, there are at least two reasons why failure to find a relationship between loudness ratings and image generation time does not mean that loudness is not present in the image: (a) It is not necessary that it should take longer to image a louder sound. Instead of having loudness generated by beginning with a soft sound and then rapidly incrementing the loudness level of the imaged sound until the desired level of loudness is obtained, it is possible that loudness can be imaged initially at the desired volume, without the necessity of incrementing further. (b) Perhaps the total range of loudness portrayed in an image is reduced or scaled from that of perception. Such a reduction or scaling is not without precedent, for example, maximum size of the visual field in perception is approximately 180 degrees, but the maximum size of the visual field in visual imagery is much smaller (e.g., Hubbard & Baird, 1988; Kosslyn, 1978), and imaged magnitude is often smaller than perceived magnitude when the psychophysical exponent is less than 1 (for review, see Hubbard, 1990). Such a scaling or reduction of imaged magnitude would reduce any effects of differences in loudness level.

distinction? Intuitively this seems possible; for example, a region bounded transformation might involve imaging the sound of an orchestra and then focusing (and amplifying) a particular part, such as the oboe line, and a field general transformation might involve changing the subjective volume level of the entire orchestra. Another possibility concerns the time it takes to transpose from one key into another. Mental transposition may be analogous to mental rotation in that both types of transformations preserve the relationships between the constituent parts while changing the absolute relationship of those parts to the observer (as also suggested by Shepard, 1982). Since larger degrees of mental rotation require larger increments of time, would transposing a musical piece into more distant keys similarly require larger increments of time? This is, of course, an empirical question, and it is unclear whether the analogy should be carried so far. However, if we do so, two results may be predicted. If the piece to be transposed is fairly complex, or if harmonic information is necessary for the transposition, we might expect transposition time to increase as key distance increased. If, however, the piece is relatively simple, with a starting pitch given (as commonly found while singing), we might expect no difference in transposition time as key distance increased. Why? In this case, once the starting pitch is given, all the performer has to do is recreate the proper intervals (a task for which the precise starting note should be irrelevant), and no additional harmonic information is necessary. The issue of whether a subject transposes through intervening keys or creates an entirely new image is reminiscent, of course, of the distinction between shift and blink transformations in Kosslyn's model.

Our theorizing to this point has dealt with relatively "surface-type" representations of this model. The surface representation may correspond somewhat to the notion of qualia with which we began our discussion. However, in his model Kosslyn explicitly disavows any concern or attention to the qualia or the "raw feel" so characteristic of the phenomenal aspect of imagery and focuses instead on a functional level of analysis, that is, on what information is contained within an image and how that information influences cognitive processes. In fact, Kosslyn's model has been instantiated in a computer program (Kosslyn & Schwartz, 1977), and the computer assumedly would not (or need not) experience the same qualia as a human being (or could this even be determined?—see pp. 207–208). Given Kosslyn's disavowal of qualia, where does that leave a model that appears to draw heavily on analogies to his? The model as stated, like Kosslyn's, may rest on nonimagistic deep representations, and some of these deep representations may correspond or be similar in form to some of the models of pitch representation reviewed earlier. The deep representation (which need not be analog or imagistic) may be a convenient place for the interfacing of musical representations with nonmusical representations and, as such, is a convenient level for the representation of text or lyric of a musical passage. If lyric is associated with the pitch representation, then activation of the pitch would in turn activate the representation of the lyric, accounting for the integration of lyric and melody reported by Serafine and her colleagues. The appropriateness of a comparison between the surface representation and the qualia remains to be determined, however.

If we borrow heavily from Kosslyn's model, we almost by definition buy into the idea of an analog medium, at least at one level of representation. A different conception of visual imagery, which does not utilize an analog medium, has been proposed by Neisser (1976). Specifically, Neisser suggests that images may be conceptualized as schemata that have been decoupled from a perceptual cycle. In his book, *Cognition and Reality,* Neisser sketched out what he referred to as a "perceptual cycle." This cycle consists of three activities, which in turn influence each other (see Fig. 9.5). The schemata direct exploration of the world. This exploration samples objects in the world, and this sampling in turn modifies the schemata of the world. These modified schemata direct sampling of the world, and so on. When the schemata become detached from this schema-exploration-object cycle, those schemata in isolation are experienced as images. Since schemata by practice (if not by definition) are generally considered to be implemented in nonanalog forms, images that result from decoupled schemata are nonanalog.

Neisser's model, like many of the models of pitch representation reviewed earlier, is considered to be a schematic model. As in most schematic models, it is assumed that music schemata have been built up over a lifetime of experience. In this case, a lifetime of experience with the music of Western culture would have led to the build up of strong musical expectancies; when these expectancies were detached from the perceptual cycle (as would occur when a subject imaged a musical stimulus), the effects of those schematic harmonic expectancies on purely imaged stimuli could be observed. Given that the schemata were developed during the perception of and interaction with the world, it would not be surprising, and indeed would be expected, that imaged stimuli would produce response patterns similar to the response patterns produced by perceived stimuli.

However, schematic conceptions cannot easily account for the depictive ele-

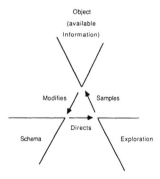

FIG. 9.5. Neisser's view of the perceptual cycle in which images correspond to detached schemata. From Neisser (1976).

ment of images. Why could we not image a color without an extent, or a pitch without a timbre, as we could easily do if we were merely describing rather than depicting the stimulus? One possibility is that schemata can include these depictive elements as covarying terms, but that seems unjustifiably *post hoc*. Additionally, evidence from other areas of cognitive psychology indicates that the memory representation is far richer and more detailed than schema models can generally account for (for review, see Alba & Hasher, 1983). Perhaps a part of the richness that schematic models have difficulty accounting for includes qualia, as qualia are by definition concrete and specific and not abstract and general. A person may be capable of experiencing the richness of qualia during perception (or even in memory) and yet not possess a schema of sufficient detail to allow precise specification and abstraction of that stimulus. Such a richness could be experienced by a person with no musical training or who does not possess absolute pitch; although such a person could experience the qualia, he or she would not be able to then assimilate that stimulus to a specific schema (e.g., give the pitch a verbal label). Given the schematic nature of Neisser's conceptualization and the difficuties of schemata in accounting for qualia discussed earlier, it is not clear how an approach based solely on Neisser's ideas of decoupled schemata might account for qualia.

An alternative approach that may indirectly touch on the issue of the qualia inherent in images is the episodic/semantic distinction proposed by Tulving (1972, 1983, 1985). In this model, the long-term memory store consists of two classes of memory: semantic memory, consisting of general world knowledge, and episodic memory, consisting of memory for the specific events (or episodes) experienced by a particular person. Tulving has suggested a number of distinctions between episodic and semantic memory (see Tulving, 1983); for example, the primary source of information for semantic memory is comprehension, the basic units of information are concepts or ideas, and the organization is conceptual and posseses little attached emotional content. On the other hand, the primary source of information for episodic memory is sensory, the basic units of information are episodes and events, and the organization is temporal (time related) and possesses greater attached emotional content. Other classes of memory, such as autobiographical memory (memory for episodes or events specifically from one's own life; e.g., Groninger & Groninger, 1984) and flashbulb memory (vivid memory of a surprising and emotionally arousing event; e.g., Brown & Kulik, 1977), appear to be highly related to Tulving's conception of episodic memory in that these types of memory are generally embedded in other personal contexts, are associated with temporal qualities, possess emotional qualities, and often involve vivid visual images.

Some of the qualities ascribed to episodic memories appear very similar to the qualities ascribed to musical images. Flashbulb memories, for example, appear to share the substantial experiential sensory qualia manifested in musical images. Although the representation of qualia in theories of episodic memory, autobiographical memory, and flashbulb memory has not yet been explicitly addressed, perhaps models of musical imagery might be able to adapt ideas from such theories of memory as a first approximation toward a theory of qualia. Similarly, perhaps ideas from imagery could be adapted to account for sensory aspects of episodic memory. Considerations of episodic memory, however, have rarely addressed the nature of imagery, and so it is not yet clear to what extent models of episodic memory could account for qualia. It is possible, for example, that the cognitive structures or processes involved with imagery and with flashbulb memory are interconnected in some way or are two manifestations of the same underlying representational system.

In sum, we have examined a number of approaches to account for the representation of pitch in musical imagery, and we have found that none of the approaches (as currently specified) seem to provide an adequate accounting of qualia in imagery. Perhaps the most promising possibility for future research would involve a combination of several of the previous approaches. For example, one possibility would involve a modular system consisting of a "surface" representation module whose outputs might correspond to the experienced qualia of pitch and other musical characteristics. The surface representation for musical images would, of course, exhibit a temporal rather than spatial medium, and could partially account for the depictive (rather than descriptive) nature of images (why, for example, it is difficult to image a color without extending it over a space or a tone without extending it over time). The output of a module, while possibly based on schematic input, a more analog form of long-term memory, or some combination of sources, would not have the independent and isolable abstraction typical of schemata.

In the case of perception, the input to such a module would come through the sense organs, but in the case of imagery, the input could come from a memory store, possibly from an abstract or decoupled schema. By utilizing the same structural or processing modules, similar outputs for imagery and perception would be obtained, thus accounting for the similarity in perceptual and imagery qualia. Such an approach allows us to account for both the qualia and the more abstract representations (such as rule-based or schematic/connectionist models thought by many to underlie pitch representation) and also allows us to combine the more sensory images of the melody or harmony with the more verbal representations of lyric. Even though this approach capitalizes heavily on the notion of functional equivalence, we must be careful not to generalize wholesale from perception processes to imagery processes (e.g., witness the failure of psychoacoustical models to account for basic phenomena like musical consonance and dissonance). Music and musical imagery possess unique characteristics, and part of the challenge and fun of research in this area is delineating those characteristics.

In our discussion of the representation of pitch to this point, we have repeatedly stressed the idea that qualia are an inherent and an important part of musical images. The study of qualia are, however, notoriusly difficult because qualia are not directly observable by an experimenter and can be studied only indirectly. One early method involved the use of self-report, but the difficulties with self-report and introspective data have been extensively documented (e.g., Nisbett & Wilson, 1977). Other methods, namely chronometric measures, have been developed and used extensively (e.g., Kosslyn, 1980). Given that qualia are best exemplified in imagery, it is appropriate for us to examine the ways that properties and characteristics of imagery are typically studied.

EVALUATION OF THE IMAGERY APPROACH
TO MUSIC COGNITION

In this section we evaluate some of the difficulties in investigating imagery and also consider if studies using musical stimuli reveal anything about imagery in general that studies using visual stimuli cannot. There are a number of criticisms of the methodology used in conducting research on imagery, but these criticisms are hardly specific to strictly musical types of imagery. Some of the difficulties that have been cataloged include the use of tacit knowledge, cognitive penetrability, demand characteristics, and experimenter bias (for review, see Finke, 1985; Pylyshyn, 1981, 1984). Most of these objections were developed in the arena of research on visual imagery; we will consider each of these in turn and evaluate its impact on music imagery research.

Tacit Knowledge and Cognitive Penetrability

The first criticism of imagery paradigms we consider involves the use of tacit knowledge on the part of the subjects (see Pylyshyn, 1981). The *tacit knowledge* explanation claims that the responses of subjects reflect their beliefs about the way the world works (however, these beliefs are not always valid, see Gentner & Stevens, 1983). Subjects' performance would thus not reflect properties of an imagery medium of representation, but rather their knowledge about physical or perceptual processes. For example, consider the case of mental rotation. Subjects may be aware that an actual physical object undergoing rotation must pass through intermediate orientations, so they then use this knowledge to simulate rotation by having their mental representation also pass through intermediate points. The important point is that, under the tacit knowledge objection, such a simulation is not necessary and does not reflect a basic-level property of the cognitive system. Pylyshyn (1981) noted that it is critical to distinguish between two interpretations of instructions to "use imagery": (a) solve a particular problem by using a particular form of representation (i.e., imagery), and (b) attempt to recreate as accurately as possible the sequence of perceptual events that would occur if you were actually observing a certain real event happening. Different criteria of success should be used depending on which interpretation is used. While many experimenters might hope subjects interpreted "use imagery" as in *a,* Pylyshyn suggested that subjects may often interpret "use imagery" as in *b.* Rather than revealing properties of the "mind's eye," what we instead see is how well other nonimaginal processes can simulate perceptual events.

Closely related to tacit knowledge is the idea of cognitive penetrability. *Cognitive penetrability* refers to the ability of a subject's knowledge, beliefs, or desires to influence his or her performance on a task. If a subject's performance can be so altered, the task is said to be cognitively penetrable; if the performance cannot be so altered, the task is said to be cognitively impenetrable. A process that is sensitive to the contents of subjects' beliefs, that is, cognitively penetrable, may contain at least some symbolic and inferential aspects. If this be granted, we cannot then infer from subjects' performance on a given task any attributes basic to that level of representation since the performance on that task would be controlled by cognitive structures residing at a different level of cognitive representation. Structural theories of imagery (such as Kosslyn's) use the performance on imagery tasks to infer characteristics of the representation that underlies imagery. However, if that task is cognitively penetrable, inferences can only be made about the nature of subjects' knowledge (tacit or conscious) which controls the performance of their "imagery" and not about the nature of the underlying representation.

Before considering the impact of the tacit knowledge idea on music imagery, we should make a distinction between the phrase "tacit knowledge" as used in critiques of the literature on visual imagery and the phrase "tacit knowledge" as used in the literature on the psychology of music. The former has been explained at length above as the beliefs, knowledge, or desires that may affect performance. Tacit knowledge in this case may differ from other knowledge in that, unlike normal knowledge, tacit knowledge is not introspectable or otherwise verbally articulable. Tacit knowledge in the second sense, the sense used in psychology of music, refers to knowledge of a culture's musical norms. Such knowledge, especially in the case of a nonmusician, is also normally not verbally available. Like a nonlinguist's knowledge of grammar, it has been picked up primarily through exposure to a culture and not necessarily through explicit instruction. In the first (Pylyshyn's) sense, an immediate change in belief would lead to an immediate change in performance, and so the task would be considered cognitively penetrable. In the second (music-theoretic) sense, an *immediate* change in representational structures is not possible, and so the task would be relatively cognitively impenetrable by Pylyshyn's standards. Even though knowledge of harmonic structure is often thus "tacitly" acquired, this type of tacit knowledge is not the type referred to by Pylyshyn.

While not yet extensively investigated, there is some evidence that the type of tacit knowledge and cognitive penetrability contamination feared by Pylyshyn need not be a critical obstacle for studies of musical imagery. For example, consider the image priming study by Hubbard and Stoeckig (1988). In that study, subjects imaged a particular tone or chord and then had another tone or chord played to them. Subjects then compared the pitch(es) of their imaged tone or chord with the pitch(es) of the perceived probe tone or chord and judged whether they were the *same* or *different*. Pylyshyn's account would suggest that upon hearing the probe that subjects accessed knowledge of the appropriate harmonic structure, identified the harmonic relationship between the image and the percept, determined what response latency and accuracy rate they should produce for that particular relationship, consciously modified their response on each trial to produce that response, and then implemented that response, all within the span of under a second. Such a position is extremely untenable, especially in light of the fact that most subjects have difficulty even correctly identifying the intervals between two perceived stimuli when given unlimited time. To expect subjects to do all that Pylyshyn's objection would require, in the brief time allowed, is simply unreasonable.

In fact, what image priming studies such as Hubbard and Stoeckig's, as well as more general studies of the representation of music such as Bharucha (1987) and Shepard (1982), are tapping is precisely the tacit knowledge that has been built up in the subject over a lifetime of enculturation. Within that experience, there would be no reason to expect a subject to be able to rapidly change his or her patterns of belief and response (although, that is, of course, an empirical question). Hence, while a change in a subject's belief, knowledge, and desires might change performance in a visual image scanning task (where subjects had relatively more time available on each trial), it would not change performance in a speeded decision such as that used in the image priming music imagery task.

Demand Characteristics and Experimenter Bias

The previous objections, tacit knowledge and cognitive penetrability, arise from consideration of knowledge the subject brings to the experimental situation. The next objection we will consider, demand characteristics, arises out of knowledge the subject is able to glean from the experimental setting itself. The *demand characteristics* objection points out that goals or hypotheses in imagery experiments may often be transparent, and that subjects may often be able to determine what form of response the experimenter expects or wants to receive. Being the good subjects that they are, they then modify their natural response so that they produce the response that they think the experimenter wants. There is no absolute way to rule out demand characteristics in any experiment (not just those involving an imagery manipulation), but current approaches to minimize the impact of demand characteristics involve questioning experimental (imagery) subjects thoroughly upon debriefing (which is, of course, also subject to further demand characteristics) and asking a control group of subjects to predict the responses of the experimental group. If some experimental group subjects are able to guess the purposes or hypotheses of the experiment, then their data are examined separately from that of other experimental group subjects who were not able to guess the hypotheses, because if they knew the hypotheses they might have been able to modify their responses either toward or away from the predicted pattern. If the control group can predict the pattern produced by the experimental group, the responses of the experimental group *may* have been due to demand characteristics. We stress *may* because this outcome suggests that subjects may have been able to figure out the responses desired and tailored their behavior to fit, but it does not show that they necessarily did so. If the pattern the control group predicts does not match that produced by the experimental group, this is usually taken as evidence that responses of the experimental group are not due to demand characteristics (see also Denis & Carfantan, 1985).

Another objection, experimenter bias, arises from knowledge that the experimenter brings to the experimental setting. The *experimenter bias* objection suggests that the behavior of the experimenter may inadvertently bias the responses of the subject. The frequently ambiguous nature of many imagery experiments may make them vulnerable to this problem, as subjects search for confirmation from the experimenter that they "are doing the right thing." The effect of experimenter expectation has been examined in the visual image scanning literature, and Intons-Peterson (Intons-Peterson, 1983; Intons-Peterson & White, 1981) has presented evidence that experimenter's expectation can affect subjects' performance across a range of visual imagery tasks. Goldston, Hinrichs, and Richman (1985) also presented data suggesting that subjects' performance on a visual image-scanning task could be affected somewhat by instructional set. However, Jolicoeur and Kosslyn (1985), using naive experimenters, failed to find a difference in visual image-scanning performance as a function of instructional set. Musical imagery studies, especially those studies based on speeded responses, would seem to be relatively immune to these problems because for any given trial type, the subject would still have to determine what type of response the experimenter expects and modify his or her response accordingly within a very limited amount of time. Given the length of response time typically obtained in these types of studies, this simply may not be possible.

All of these objections to imagery methodology—tacit knowledge, cognitive penetrability, demand characteristics, experimenter bias—are of course highly related to each other. The common denominator concerns whether subjects are able to determine the hypotheses of the experimenter and modify their responses according to whatever knowledge they can bring to bear. We have argued that with speeded decision methods (like the image priming method used in Hubbard & Stoeckig, 1988), subjects do not have time to engage in the type of cognitive processes postulated by these criticisms, but what about the application of these criticisms to methods in which subjects possess more time? One example might be imaged melody scanning, in which a subject has essentially as much time as he or she would like (scan times in Halpern, 1988, ranged as high as 9 seconds, and scan times in Hubbard & Stoeckig, in preparation, ranged as high as 14 seconds). In this case it is possible that subjects may figure out the relationship under investigation and modify their responses accordingly. A useful control here would parallel methods in Intons-Peterson (1983) and Jolicoeur and Kosslyn (1985), that is, a group of naive experimenters, each of whom is led to expect different results, runs a group of subjects. If the same patterns are found in all conditions, we are justified in having more confidence in the results. Such a control assumes, of course, that if the naive experimenters do not know the true hypothesis, neither can the subjects. This may or may not be a reasonable assumption. Of course, the instructional set of the naive experimenters may still be inadvertently biased.

Benefits of Using of Musical Stimuli to Study Imagery

Now that we have considered possible difficulties with experiments involving imagery in general, are there any benefits to using explicitly musical materials in the study of imagery? One benefit to using musical materials as stimuli for the study of imagery is that because very few people possess absolute pitch, very few people can assign verbal labels to the stimuli. One cost to using visual materials as stimuli for the study of imagery is that people can often assign names to the objects to be imaged. The verbal label, rather than the qualia, may then be utilized in answering questions or making comparisons. If subjects are unable to assign a verbal label to a musical stimulus, they may have to depend on sensory qualities (the qualia) of the stimulus in order to be able to answer questions about the stimulus or use it in any form of comparison. Thus, use of musical materials minimizes the chance of subjects using a nonimagistic (e.g., verbal) coding scheme. Therefore, music may potentially be an arena in which contributions of pure imagery as relatively unconfounded by verbal labels may be studied.

Another benefit to the use of explicitly musical materials in the study of imagery is that there is a wide range of musical expertise in the general population, so the study of imagery in the musical realm allows study of how one form of representation may change with the development of expertise in that area. Such a wide range is not necessarily available with visual stimuli, as visual inspection is a highly overlearned skill in much of the population. In the image priming experiments, similar patterns of results are found with highly trained as well as untrained subjects (although the pattern is often stronger or more accentuated in subjects who have had extensive musical training; see Hubbard & Stoeckig, 1988), raising the question of how much of the representational structure is explicitly learned. Some theories of the development of expertise propose that stimuli within the area of expertise are abstracted as learning and expertise are acquired (and hence more easily associated to relevant schemata, e.g., Chase & Simon, 1973; Lesgold, 1984), suggesting that the representation of pitch in highly trained musicians may be more abstract and less imagistic than the representation of pitch in untrained subjects. Although no firm data are available, some theorists have speculated that the representation of pitch by musicians differs qualitatively as well as quantitatively from that of nonmusicians (e.g., Halpern & Bower, 1982); the role of imagery in those representations is an interesting theoretical question with many implications for theories of human cognition.

CONCLUSIONS AND FUTURE DIRECTIONS

Throughout this chapter we have emphasized the critical role of qualia in musical imagery. Psychoacoustic, rule-based, and schematic/connectionist models did not seem easily able to account for qualia. We then discussed three general types of approaches that might eventually be able to account for qualia. The first alternative, adapted from Kosslyn's model of visual imagery, was based on an imagistic surface representation and a more abstract deep representation. The second alternative, based on Neisser's conceptualization of images as decoupled perceptual schemata, suggested that images may result from the use of schemata that normally guide perception. This approach, however, does not shed light on how qualia are incorporated or represented within a perceptual schema. The third alternative, based on parallels between elements of episodic memory and imagery, namely the vivid sensory qualities of flashbulb memories and qualia qualities of images, suggested that research on episodic types of memory could shed light on aspects of imagery (and vice versa). None of these alternative approaches, however, was able to offer an adequate or compelling accounting of qualia.

We then suggested that a more thorough accounting of qualia might result from a combination of these approaches. We sketched out a rather preliminary model of musical imagery in which musical images are generated in a temporal analog medium by a modular system based upon input from either sense organs (perception) or memory (imagery). Inputs from memory could be in the form of abstract schematic/connectionist networks, other analog representations, or some combination of these. The merging of analog and schematic elements allows us to represent successfully much of the complex hierarchical structure inherent in music and also account for the interfacing of musical and nonmusical (lyric text) representations. Mere activation of a schema itself, without further processing of that information by the module, might result in the availability of the abstract knowledge contained within the schema but without the accompanying qualia (this might be akin to the experience of musically untrained listeners who have general expectancies about upcoming events [e.g., in Bharucha & Stoeckig, 1986] but who are not able to image a specific tone or chord). In passing, we would also note that people who did not possess the appropriate schema, upon hearing a stimulus, would have to rely on a sensory-trace strategy in order to remember it. As noted above, this is precisely what happens in

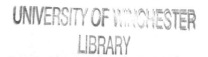

subjects who do not possess absolute pitch. By postulating such an analog module utilized by both perceptual and imagistic processes, it is possible to account for the qualia that our musical images often seem to have and for the many functional equalivalences that seem to exist between imagery and perception.

Where to go next? With burgeoning amounts of research being done in both music perception and visual imagery, there seems to be a fresh store of ready hypotheses for the testing. One of the most useful hypotheses has been that of a functional equivalence between cognitive structures or processes used in music perception and the structures or processes used in music imagery. A wealth of data supports the equivalence hypothesis, as musical images seem to facilitate and inhibit processing of perceived musical stimuli in the same way that other perceived musical stimuli would. Another hypothesis that has been quite useful has been that of a similarity between processes and structures involved in visual or auditory imagery and those involved in music imagery. Both of these ideas have been very useful in early investigations, but they have certainly not yet been tapped to their fullest.

REFERENCES

Alba, J. W., & Hasher, L. (1983). Is memory schematic? *Psychological Bulletin, 93,* 203–211.

Algom, D. (Ed.). (in press). *Psychophysical approaches to cognition.* New York: Elsevier.

Anderson, J. R. (1978). Arguments concerning representations for mental imagery. *Psychological Review, 85,* 249–277.

Bechtel, W. (1988). *Philosophy of mind: An overview for cognitive science.* Hillsdale, NJ: Lawrence Erlbaum Associates.

Bernstein, L. (1976). *The unanswered question.* Cambridge, MA: Harvard University Press.

Bharucha, J. J. (1987). Music cognition and perceptual facilitation: A connectionist framework. *Music Perception, 5,* 1–30.

Bharucha, J. J., & Stoeckig, K. (1986). Reaction time and musical expectancy: Priming of chords. *Journal of Experimental Psychology: Human Perception and Performance, 12,* 403–410.

Bharucha, J. J., & Stoeckig, K. (1987). Priming of chords: Spreading activation or overlapping frequency spectra? *Perception and Psychophysics, 41,* 519–524.

Block, N. (1980a). *Readings in the philosophy of psychology* (Vol. 1). Cambridge, MA: Harvard University Press.

Block, N. (1980b). Troubles with functionalism. In N. Block (Ed.), *Readings in the philosophy of psychology* (Vol. 1). Cambridge, MA: Harvard University Press.

Block, N. (Ed.). (1981). *Readings in philosophy of psychology* (Vol. 2) Cambridge, MA: MIT Press.

Block, N., & Fodor, J. A. (1980). What psychological states are not. In N. Block (Ed.), *Readings in the philosophy of psychology* (Vol. 1). Cambridge, MA: Harvard University Press.

Brooks, L. R. (1968). Spatial and verbal components of the act of recall. *Canadian Journal of Psychology, 22,* 349–368.

Brown, R., & Kulik, J. (1977). Flashbulb memories. *Cognition, 5,* 73–99.

Chambers, D., & Reisberg, D. (1985). Can mental images be ambiguous? *Journal of Experimental Psychology: Human Perception and Performance, 11,* 317–328.

Chase, W. G., & Simon, H. A. (1973). The mind's eye in chess. In W. G. Chase (Ed.), *Visual information processing*. New York: Academic Press.

Chomsky, N. (1972). *Language and mind*. New York: Harcourt, Brace Jovanovich.

Churchland, P. M., & Churchland, P. S. (1981). Functionalism, qualia, and intentionality. *Philosophical Topics, 12*, 121–145.

Cooper, L. A. (1976). Demonstration of a mental analog of an external rotation. *Perception and Psychophysics, 19*, 296–302.

Cuddy, L. L., Cohen, A. J., & Miller, J. (1979). Melody recognition: The experimental application of musical rules. *Canadian Journal of Psychology, 33*, 148–157.

Davies, J. B. (1978). *The psychology of music*. Stanford, CA: Stanford University Press.

Denis, M., & Carfantan, M. (1985). People's knowledge about images. *Cognition, 20*, 49–60.

Dennett, D. C. (1978). Toward a cognitive theory of consciousness. In C. W. Savage (Ed.), *Minnesota studies in the philosophy of science* (Vol. 9). Minneapolis: University of Minnesota Press.

Deutsch, D. (1969). Music recognition. *Psychological Review, 76*, 300–307.

Deutsch, D. (1972). Effect of repetition of standard and comparison tones on recognition memory for pitch. *Journal of Experimental Psychology, 93*, 156–162.

Deutsch, D. (1982). The processing of pitch combinations. In D. Deutsch (Ed.), *The psychology of music* (pp. 271–316). New York: Academic Press.

Deutsch, D., & Feroe, J. (1981). The internal representation of pitch sequences in tonal music. *Psychological Review, 86*, 503–522.

Dowling, W. J., & Harwood, D. L. (1986). *Music cognition*. New York: Academic Press.

Farah, M. J. (1985). Psychophysical evidence for a shared representational medium for mental images and percepts. *Journal of Experimental Psychology: General, 114*, 91–103.

Farah, M. J. (1988). Is visual imagery really visual? Overlooked evidence from neurophychology. *Psychological Review, 95*, 307–317.

Farah, M. J., & Smith, A. F. (1983). Perceptual interference and facilitation with auditory imagery. *Perception and Psychophysics, 33*, 475–478.

Finke, R. A. (1985). Theories relating mental imagery to perception. *Psychological Bulletin, 98*, 236–259.

Finke, R. A., & Shepard, R. N. (1986). Visual functions of mental imagery. In K. R. Boff, L. Kaufman, & J. P. Thomas (Eds.), *Handbook of perception and human performance. Vol. 2: Cognitive processes and performance* (pp. 37.1–37.55). New York: Wiley.

Genter, D., & Stevens, A. L. (1983). *Mental models*. Hillsdale, NJ: Lawrence Erlbaum Associates.

Goldston, D. B., Hinrichs, J. V., & Richman, C. L. (1985). Subjects' expectations, individual variability, and the scanning of mental images. *Memory and Cognition, 13*, 365–370.

Groninger, L. D., & Groninger, L. K. (1984). Autobiographical memories: Their relationship to images, definitions, and word recognition. *Journal of Experimental Psychology: Learning, Memory and Cognition, 10*, 745–755.

Halpern, A. R. (1988). Mental scanning in auditory imagery for songs. *Journal of Experimental Psychology: Learning, Memory, and Cognition, 14*, 434–443.

Halpern, A. R., & Bower, G. H. (1982). Musical expertise and melody structure in memory for musical notation. *American Journal of Psychology, 95*, 31–50.

Hubbard, T. L. (1990). Mental psychophysics. *Manuscript submitted for publication*.

Hubbard, T. L., & Baird, J. C. (1988). Overflow, first-sight, and vanishing point distances in visual imagery. *Journal of Experimental Psychology: Learning, Memory, and Cognition, 14*, 641–649.

Hubbard, T. L., & Stoeckig, K. (1988). Musical imagery: Generation of tones and chords. *Journal of Experimental Psychology: Learning, Memory, and Cognition, 14*, 656–667.

Hubbard, T. L., & Stoeckig, K. (in preparation). *Scanning of melodic images*.

Intons-Peterson, M. J. (1980). The role of loudness in auditory imagery. *Memory and Cognition, 8*, 385–393.

Intons-Peterson, M. J. (1983). Imagery paradigms: How vulnerable are they to experimenters' expectations? *Journal of Experimental Psychology: Human Perception and Performance, 9,* 394–412.

Intons-Peterson, M. J., & White, A. R. (1981). Experimenter naiveté and imaginal judgments. *Journal of Experimental Psychology: Human Perception and Performance, 7,* 833–843.

Jackson, F. (1982). Epiphenomenal qualia. *Philosophical Quarterly, 32,* 127–136.

Jolicoeur, P., & Kosslyn, S. M. (1985). Is time to scan visual images due to demand characteristics? *Memory and Cognition, 13,* 320–332.

Kosslyn, S. M. (1978). Measuring the visual angle of the mind's eye. *Cognitive Psychology, 10,* 356–389.

Kosslyn, S. M. (1980). *Image and mind.* Cambridge, MA: Harvard University Press.

Kosslyn, S. M. (1981). The medium and the message in mental imagery: A theory. *Psychological Review, 88,* 46–66.

Kosslyn, S. M. (1987). Seeing and imaging in the cerebral hemispheres: A computational approach. *Psychological Review, 94,* 148–175.

Kosslyn, S. M., Ball, T. M., & Reiser, B. J. (1978). Visual images preserve metric spatial information: Evidence from studies of image scanning. *Journal of Experimental Psychology: Human Perception and Performance, 4,* 47–60.

Kosslyn, S. M., Pinker, S., Smith, G., & Schwartz, S. P. (1979). On the demystification of mental imagery. *The Behavioral and Brain Sciences, 2,* 535–581.

Kosslyn, S. M., & Pomerantz, J. R. (1977). Imagery, propositions, and the form of the internal representation. *Cognitive Psychology, 9,* 52–76.

Kosslyn, S. M., Reiser, B. J., Farah, M. J., & Fliegel, S. L. (1983). Generating visual images: Units and relations. *Journal of Experimental Psychology: General, 112,* 278–303.

Kosslyn, S. M., & Schwartz, S. P. (1977). A simulation of visual imagery. *Cognitive Science, 1,* 265–295.

Krumhansl, C. L., & Shepard, R. N. (1979). Quantification of the hierarchy of tonal functions within a diatonic context. *Journal of Experimental Psychology: Human Perception and Performance, 5,* 579–594.

Lerdahl, F., & Jackendoff, R. (1983). *A generative theory of tonal music.* Cambridge, MA: MIT Press.

Lesgold, A. M. (1984). Acquiring expertise. In J. R. Anderson & S. M. Kosslyn (Eds.), *Tutorials in learning and memory.* New York: W. H. Freeman.

Longuet-Higgins, H. C. (1978). The perception of music. *Interdisciplinary Science Review, 3,* 148–156.

Marschark, M., Richman, C. L., Yuille, J. C., & Hunt, R. R. (1987). The role of imagery in memory: On shared and distinctive information. *Psychological Bulletin, 102,* 28–41.

McClelland, J. L., & Rumelhart, D. E. (1986). *Parallel distributing processing: Explorations in the microstructure of cognition, Vol. II.* Cambridge, MA: MIT Press.

Meyer, L. B. (1956). *Emotion and meaning in music.* Chicago: University of Chicago Press.

Miyazaki, K. (1988). Musical pitch identification by absolute pitch possessors. *Perception and Psychophysics, 44,* 501–512.

Nagel, T. (1974). What is it like to be a bat? *The Philosophical Review, 83,* 435–450.

Neisser, U. (1976). *Cognition and reality.* New York: W. H. Freeman.

Nisbett, R. E., & Wilson, T. D. (1977). Telling more than we know: Verbal reports of mental processes. *Psychological Review, 84,* 231–259.

Peterson, M. J., & Graham, S. E. (1974). Visual detection and visual imagery. *Journal of Experimental Psychology, 103,* 509–514.

Pylyshyn, Z. W. (1981). The imagery debate: Analogue media versus tacit knowledge. *Psychological Review, 88,* 16–45.

Pylyshyn, Z. W. (1984). *Computation and cognition.* Cambridge, MA: MIT Press.

Rumelhart, D. E., & McClelland, J. L. (1986). *Parallel distributing processing: Explorations in the microstructure of cognition* (Vol. I) Cambridge, MA: MIT Press.

Seashore, C. E. (1967). *Psychology of music*. New York: Dover. (Original work published in 1938)

Segal, S. J., & Fusella, V. (1970). Influence of imaged pictures and sounds on the detection of visual and auditory signals. *Journal of Experimental Psychology, 83,* 458–464.

Serafine, M. L., Crowder, R. G., & Repp, B. H. (1984). Integration of melody and text in memory for songs. *Cognition, 16,* 285–303.

Serafine, M. L., Davidson, J., Crowder, R. G., & Repp, B. H. (1986). On the nature of melody-text integration in memory for songs. *Journal of Memory and Language, 25,* 123–135.

Shepard, R. N. (1982). Structural representations of musical pitch. In D. Deutsch (Ed.), *The psychology of music* (pp. 343–390). New York: Academic Press.

Shepard, R. N., & Chipman, S. (1970). Second-order isomorphism of internal representations: Shapes of states. *Cognitive Psychology, 1,* 1–17.

Shepard, R. N., & Cooper, L. A. (1982). *Mental images and their transformations*. Cambridge, MA: MIT Press.

Shepard, R. N., Kilpatric, D. W., & Cunningham, J. P. (1975). The internal representation of numbers. *Cognitive Psychology, 7,* 82–138.

Shepard, R. N., & Metzler, J. (1971). Mental rotation of three-dimensional objects. *Science, 171,* 701–703.

Shepard, R. N., & Podgorny, P. (1978). Cognitive processes that resemble perceptual processes. In W. K. Estes (Ed.), *Handbook of learning and cognitive processes* (Vol. 5, pp. 189–237). Hillsdale, NJ: Lawrence Erlbaum Associates.

Shoemaker, S. (1980). Functionalism and qualia. In N. Block (Ed.), *Readings in the philosophy of psychology* (Vol. 1, pp. 251–267). Cambridge, MA: Harvard University Press.

Siegel, J. A. (1972). The nature of absolute pitch. In I. E. Gordon (Ed.), *Studies in the psychology of music* (Vol. 8, pp. 65–89). Iowa City: University of Iowa Press.

Siegel, J. A. (1974). Sensory and verbal coding strategies in subjects with absolute pitch. *Journal of Experimental Psychology, 103,* 37–44.

Stevens, S. S., & Volkmann, J. (1940). The relation of pitch to frequency: Revised scale. *American Journal of Psychology, 53,* 329–353.

Stevens, S. S., Volkmann, J., & Newman, E. B. (1937). A scale for the measurement of the psychological magnitude of pitch. *Journal of the Acoustical Society of America, 8,* 185–190.

Tulving, E. (1972). Episodic and semantic memory. In E. Tulving & W. Donaldson (Eds.), *Organization of memory* (pp. 381–403). New York: Academic Press.

Tulving, E. (1983). *Elements of episodic memory*. London: Oxford University Press.

Tulving, E. (1985). How many memory systems are there? *American Psychologist, 40,* 385–398.

Van Krevelen, A. (1951). The ability to make absolute judgments of pitch. *Journal of Experimental Psychology, 42,* 207–215.

Ward, W. D., & Burns, E. M. (1982). Absolute pitch. In D. Deutsch (Ed.), *The psychology of music* (pp. 431–45). New York: Academic Press.

Weber, R. J., Kelley, J., & Little, S. (1972). Is visual imagery sequencing under verbal control? *Journal of Experimental Psychology, 96,* 354–362.

10 The Climate of Auditory Imagery and Music*

Diana Deutsch
University of California, San Diego

John R. Pierce
Stanford University

THE TRADITION OF IMAGERY

> From where do I take my ideas? That I cannot say with certainty. They come uncalled, directly and indirectly. I could grasp them by my hands in the freedom of nature, on walks in the silence of the night or in the early morning through moods which turn into tones which sound, blow, storm, until the notes are standing before me. (Cited in Dorian, 1947, p. 8)

These words were written by Beethoven in 1824, three years before his death. The astonishing creations of this great composer which were written decades following the onset of his deafness are perhaps the most striking examples of imagery, in any modality.

Indeed, the procedures generally employed by the masters of composition indicate that feedback, whether auditory, or in the form of symbolic description, is not a necessary part of the compositional process, and might even interfere with it. Composers have frequently asserted that they work over an entire piece mentally, elaborate and polish it in considerable detail, before they set anything down in writing. Again from Beethoven:

> I carry my thoughts a long time, often very long before I write them down. Therein my memory remains loyal to me, since I am sure not to forget a theme even after years, once I have conceived it. Some things I change, reject, try all over again until I am satisfied. (pp. 251–252)

*This chapter is based on numerous discussions between the authors when one of us (DD) was a Visiting Scholar at the Center for Computer Research in Music and Acoustics (CCRMA) at Stanford, in the Spring of 1989. The authorship is listed alphabetically, but should be considered as equal.

Other composers have given similar accounts. As Gluck wrote:

Once I am clear about the composition of the whole and about the characterization of the main parts, I consider the opera finished, although I have not yet written one single note. (p. 254)

And again:

First I go through each individual act, later through the whole work. The plan of the composition I sketch in my mind while sitting in the parterre (of the theatre). Such a preparation usually takes one entire year. (p. 254)

And from Weber:

Before I approach the execution of the detail, I figure out the great plan of the tonal picture through determining its main colors and its individual parts; namely, I outline for myself the exact sequence of the keys . . . and I strictly weigh the use of the instruments. (p. 255)

This process occurred with such precision that, as his son Max wrote:

Without any intermediary stage, the whole score would flow out of his pen from the flute to the double bass like an etching. (p. 255)

Mozart also adopted this procedure as his favorite mode of composing, regarding the final writing of the score as an irksome process. As he wrote in 1780 "Composed is everything, written not yet a single note" (Dorian, 1947, p. 256).

Indeed, many composers were not only able to write scores without preliminary sketches, but they also wrote their music directly for the different instrument parts without reference to a full score. For this reason, much music has come down to us in the form of individual parts alone. Composers frequently intended to conduct their pieces themselves, and full scores would for them have been redundant. It was therefore frequently left to others to assemble together the different parts of an orchestral piece (Dorian, 1947).

The process of musical composition not only furnishes us with examples of highly specific and elaborate long term auditory memory, but also gives us insight into how such imagery might be formed. Musical ideas were frequently described as sudden inspirations, often occuring dramatically, for example in dreams. Thus Wagner in his autobiography describes how the Prelude for his *Rheingold* was conceived:

I fell into a kind of somnolent state, in which I suddenly felt as though I were sinking in swiftly flowing water. The rushing sound formed itself in my brain into a musical sound, the chord of E-flat major, which continually reechoed in broken forms; these broken chords seemed to be melodic passages of increasing motion, yet the pure triad of E-flat major never changed, but seemed by its continuance to impart infinite significance to the element in which I was sinking, I awoke in sudden terror from my doze, feeling as though the waves were rushing high above my head. I at once recognized that the orchestral overture to *Das Rheingold,* which must have long lain latent within me, though it had been unable to find definite form, had at last been revealed to me. (p. 55)

Other composers, such as Berlioz, Chopin, Bruckner, and Cesar Franck, have also described the emergence of musical images in their dreams, and as sudden inspirations.

So far we have been considering musical composition, which constitutes an exceptional example of imagery. However, we should note that the successful performance of a piece also requires a high degree of imagery, and even naive listeners must use this faculty to a considerable extent.

EARLIER CONFLICTS

Given such considerations, it is remarkable that for the last few decades, auditory imagery has been neglected in most of the literature on psychoacoustics, and its existence has essentially been denied by many experimental psychologists. This situation is historically anomalous: in previous times the approach to hearing in terms of low-level or peripheral factors has coexisted with considerations of higher-level processing.

Aristoxenus, perhaps the leading music theorist in ancient Greece, argued strongly for a high-level approach. As he wrote in his Harmonics:

And we must bear in mind that musical cognition implies the simultaneous cognition of a permanent and of a changeable element, and that this applies without limitation or qualification to every branch of music. (Cited in Macran, 1974, pp. 189–190)

And later:

It is plain that the apprehension of a melody consists in noting with both ear and intellect every distinction as it arises in successive sounds—successive, for melody, like all branches of music, consists in a successive production. For the apprehension of music depends on these two faculties, sense-perception and memory; for we must perceive the sound that is present and remember that which is past. In no other way can we follow the phenomena of music. (p. 193)

The epoch of the scientific revolution was a very fertile one for the study of hearing; most of those responsible for the striking advances in mathematics, astronomy and mechanics of this period also made important contributions to music. Amongst these were Mersenne, Galileo, Kepler, Huygens, and Descartes. It was at this time that the relationships between pitch and rate of vibration in strings, pipes and bells were determined; the phenomenon of beats was discovered; as was the overtone series; and in addition issues such as tuning and temperament, and consonance and dissonance hotly debated.

On this last issue, both low-level and high-level factors were proposed. For example, Galileo espoused a low-level approach, a sort of rhythmic theory of consonance. Consonance resulted from a distinct pattern of two tones beating on the eardrum, and dissonance from irregular beats.

> The Offence [the Dissonances] give, proceeds, I believe, from the discordant and jarring Pulsations of two different Tones, which, without any Proportion, strike the Drum of the Ear: And the Dissonances will be extreme harsh, in case the Times of the Vibrations are incommensurable [. . .] Those Pairs of Sounds shall be Consonances and will be heard with Pleasure, which strike the *Timpanum* in some Order, which Order requires, in the first Place, that the Percussions made in the same Time be commensurable in Number, that the Cartilage of the *Timpanum* or Drum may not be subject to a perpetual Torment of bending itself two different Ways, in submission to the ever disagreeing Percussion. (Cited in Cohen, 1984, p. 90)

Mersenne also adopted a low-level approach, but placed the locus of the interactions a little further along the auditory pathway:

> . . . the external air excites the air inside the ear, and it impresses a state of motion upon the auditory nerve that resembles the one it received; and the mind that is present in each part of the body, and consequently in the said nerve, perceives at once the movement of the organs of the ear, and thereby judges the qualities of the motion of the sound, and of the external objects that produce it. Now one could imagine that the mind is like an indivisible and intellectual point, to which all sense impressions taper, like all lines of a circle towards their center, or like all the threads of the web of the spider that spins and weaves them . . . (p. 110)

Kepler, in contrast, argued that low-level factors were inadequate to explain the phenomena:

> If the velocity of one string has the ability to move another, proportionate string that to the eye appears not to be moved, then would not the equal velocities of two strings have the ability pleasantly to titillate the ear, since in a certain sense it is excited uniformly by both strings, and since the two strokes of both tones or vibrations coincide every moment? No, I say, this is too simple a way to settle the matter [. . .] For please, what relationship could there be between the titillation of the sense of hearing, which is a corporal thing, and the incredible delight that we perceive deep within our soul through the harmonic consonances? If the delight comes from the titillation, would not then the main part of this delight be played by

the organ that sustains the titillation? In my *Dioptrics* it seemed best to me to define any sense organ in such a way that the sense perception that brings forth pleasure or grief is not completed until the species of the organ that is destined for the perception in question, as it is affected from outside, has reached inwards, through the guidance of the spirits, the tribunal of the general sense. Hence I now ask, what part in this delight in hearing consonant voices and notes the ear has? Do we not sometimes feel pain in our ears when we listen to music and, because of the horrible blare, shut them with our hands, although we continue to perceive the consonances and our heart jumps? Add to this that the explanation taken from motion is applied in the first place to the unison; but sweetness does not primarily lie in the unison; but in the other consonances and the combination thereof. Much [more] might be adduced in order to destroy this alleged explanation of the sweetness that comes from the consonances; but for the moment I prefer to desist from a more detailed disquisition. (p. 31)

Descartes also had misgivings about invoking a low-level explanation of consonance alone, and proposed what today is described as the difference between sensory consonance and musical consonance:

For it should be observed that all these calculations [on coinciding strokes] serve only for showing which consonances are the simplest, or, if you prefer, the sweetest and the most perfect ones, but not on that account the most agreeable [. . .] . But in order to determine what is most agreeable, one should consider the capacity of the listener, that changes like taste, according to the person in question; thus some will prefer to hear one single melody, others part-music, etc; just as the one prefers what is sweet, and the other what is somewhat bitter or acid, etc. Concerning the sweetness of the consonances, two things should be distinguished: namely, what renders them simpler and more accordant, and what renders them more agreeable to the ear. Now, as to what renders them more agreeable, that depends on the places where they are employed: and there are places where even dimished fifths and other dissonances are more agreeable than consonances, so that one could not determine absolutely that one consonance is more agreeable than another. One could, indeed say, however, that, normally speaking, the thirds and sixths are more agreeable than the fourth; that in cheerful songs major thirds and sixths are more agreeable than minor ones, and the opposite in sad [songs], etc., in that there are more occasions where they can be employed agreeably. But one can say absolutely which consonances are the most simple and the most accordant ones; for that depends only on how often their sounds unite, and how closely they approach the nature of the unison; so that one can say absolutely that the fourth is more accordant than the major third, while ordinarily it is not so agreeable, just as cassia is definitely sweeter than olives, but not so agreeable to our taste.[1] (p. 169)

One can indeed sympathize with the desire to invoke partially understood peripheral structures as explanatory devices, and to avoid resorting to more

---

[1]We may note that Descartes wrote after thirds had been admitted to music.

abstract types of explanation; however this approach is not without its pitfalls. Such pitfalls are illustrated in a report by Everard Home, in his 1799 Croonian lecture to the Royal Society of London on the "Structure and Uses of the Membrana Tympani of the Ear." Having described his researches on the tympanic membrane in elephants (reasoning, as Bekesy did in our time, that the animal's size makes it easier to observe its anatomical features) he compared the ear drum to a monochord "of which the membrana tympani is the string; the tensor muscle the screw, giving the necessary tension to make the string perform its proper scale of vibrations; and the radiated muscle acting upon the membrane like the moveable bridge." He then proceeded to assert that accuracy of music perception is determined by the degree of perfection in the activity of these muscles:

> The difference between a musical ear and one which is too imperfect to distinguish the different notes in music, will appear to arise entirely from the greater or less nicety with which the muscle of the malleus renders the membrane capable of being truly adjusted. If the tension be perfect, all the variations produced by the action of the radiated muscle will be equally correct, and the ear truly musical; but, if the first adjustment is imperfect, although the actions of the radiated muscle may still produce infinite variations, none of them will be correct: the effect . . . will be similar to that produced by playing upon a musical instrument which is not in tune. (Cited in Miller & Cohen, 1987, p. 30)

THE TURN OF THE CENTURY

Let us consider next the approach to hearing taken by those in the latter part of the last century and the beginning of this one. Here again we find that representation of complex structures was not neglected, and imagery was considered alongside phenomena that allowed for peripheral explanations.

The work that was perhaps the most influential for twentieth century psychoacoustics was Helmholtz's *On the Sensations of Tone* (1885/1954). Helmholtz not only dealt with issues that were consistent with peripheral explanations, such as the pitch of complex tones, beats, and combination tones, but he also gave detailed consideration to higher-level musical phenomena such as scales, modes, root progressions of chords, systems of key relationships, and the concept of tonality. Our ability to learn, remember, recall and call up played a considerable part in his thought. Amongst his several discussions of imagery he wrote:

> The effort felt in singing the leading note does not lie in the larynx, but in the difficulty we feel in fixing the voice upon it by mere volition while another tone is already in our mind, to which we desire to pass . . . (pp. 286–287)

and later:

Supposing that I have been used to hearing Fifths taken at all possible pitches, and have recognized them by aural sensation as having a very close melodic relationship, I should know the magnitude of this interval by experience for every tone in the scale, and should retain the knowledge thus acquired by the actions of a man's memory of sensations, even of those for which he has no verbal expression . . .

And just in the same way I shall be able to recognise, as previously known, other melodic passages or whole melodies which are executed in simple tones, and even if I hear a melody for the first time in this way, whistled with the mouth or chimed by a clock, or struck on a glass harmonicon, I should be able to complete it by imagining how it would sound if executed on a real musical instrument, as the voice or a violin.

A practiced musician is able to form a conception of a melody by merely reading the notes. If we give the prime tones of these notes on a glass harmonicon, we give a firmer basis to the conception by really exciting a large portion of the impression on the senses which the melody would have produced if sung. (pp. 289–290)

The Gestalt psychologists, who were primarily concerned with issues of high-level representation, made frequent reference to music in their discussions. At that time, Mach (1898/1943) raised the question of "Whether there is anything similar to the symmetry of figures in the province of sounds".

Now, although in all the preceding examples I have transposed steps upward into equal and similar steps downward, that is, as we may justly say, have played for every movement the movement which is symmetrical to it, yet the ear notices little or nothing of symmetry. The transposition from a major to a minor key is the sole indication of symmetry remaining. The symmetry is there for the mind but is wanting for sensation. No symmetry exists for the ear, because a reversal of musical sounds conditions no repetition of sensations. If we had an ear for height and an ear for depth, just as we have an eye for the right and an eye for the left, we should also find that symmetrical sound-structures existed for our auditory organs. (p. 103)

Mach was canny in differentiating what is pattern to the eye and what is pattern to the ear.

DOCTRINES IN MUSIC AND SCIENCE

Figure 10.1 illustrates the potential symmetry of which Mach writes. It is interesting to compare Mach's conclusion with the following statement by Schoenberg (1975) who, although not a psychologist, propounded what he thought

FIG. 10.1. Musical example given by Mach, presented in both original and inverted form. This was used to illustrate Mach's conclusion that passages related by inversion are not perceptually equivalent. Adapted from Mach (1898/1943), Fig. 26, p. 102.

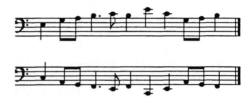

should be or must be true of musical images as a justification for his method of twelve-tone composition:

THE TWO-OR-MORE DIMENSIONAL SPACE IN WHICH MUSICAL IDEAS ARE PRESENTED IS A UNIT . . . The elements of a musical idea are partly incorporated in the horizontal plane as successive sounds, and partly in the vertical plane as simultaneous sounds . . . *The unity of musical space demands an absolute and unitary perception.* In this space . . . there is no absolute down, no right or left, forward or backward . . . To the imaginative and creative faculty, relations in the material sphere are as independent from directions or planes as material objects are, in their sphere, to our perceptive faculties. Just as our mind always recognizes, for instance, a knife, a bottle or a watch, regardless of its position, and can reproduce it in the imagination in every possible position, even so a musical creator's mind can operate subconsciously with a row of tones, regardless of their direction, regardless of the way in which a mirror might show the mutual relations, which remain a given quantity. (pp. 220–223)

His theory of abstract representation of tones series is illustrated in Fig. 10.2. In referring to the illustration he writes "The employment of these mirror forms corresponds to the principle of the absolute and unitary perception of musical space" (p. 225). For Schoenberg, musical space must be just like the space of vision.

In sharp contrast to the concerns of composers, the general approach of 20th-century psychoacoustics has been to disregard issues of higher-level representation, and to focus instead on highly circumscribed phenomena which could, it is assumed, be explained in terms of simple neural activity, preferably in terms of the actions of the peripheral hearing apparatus. A huge amount of data has amassed concerning, for example, absolute thresholds, difference thresholds for frequency and loudness, the masking of one tone by another, the lateralization of sinusoids and noise bands, adaptation and fatigue. Similarly, auditory physiologists have focused on the response of the auditory system to narrowly defined stimuli, and have addressed a few circumscribed problems; for example they have examined the response of the basilar membrane to clicks and to sinusoids, plotted tuning curves for neural units in various parts of the auditory system, described relationships between stimulus amplitude and firing rate, mapped out tonotopic organization in central auditory structures; and so on.

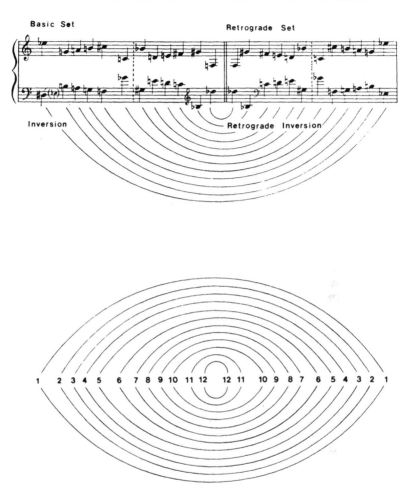

FIG. 10.2. Musical example given by Schoenberg. This was used to
illustrate Schoenberg' assumption that passages related by inversion
and retrogression are perceptually equivalent. Adapted from Schoenberg (1975), Example 4, pp. 224–225.

This reductionistic approach has gathered much particular information, some
of which has value. Unfortunately, it has been coupled with the doctrine that
higher-level issues should be excluded from consideration until low-level functioning is entirely understood. The problem here is that one cannot, logically,
come to any satisfactory conclusion by following this approach. More specifically, one cannot exclude central or complex factors by focusing only on low-level
stimuli or on explanations in terms of peripheral mechanisms; the perceptual

characteristics at issue could in principle be taking place anywhere in the processing chain. On the contrary, it is *peripheral* or *simple* explanations which can logically be excluded, by demonstrating that effects occur as a result of central interactions, or as a result of some complex process. Thus, even assuming that one's sole aim is to understand the action of peripheral mechanisms, it is necessary to generate stimulus patterns which enable the determination that observed effects are indeed peripheral rather than central in origin, or that they are based on simple rather than on complex operations. Thus issues involving central structures and complex operations cannot, logically, be avoided.

We attribute the reluctance to consider high-level processing in hearing to a number of factors. The first has been the difficulty involved in generating complex stimuli with sufficient stimulus control; this severely inhibited researchers from embarking on experiments using such stimuli. Fortunately, over the last few decades this problem has been overcome. With new advances in sound generation and analysis by computer, stemming primarily from work begun around 1960 by Max Mathews (see Mathews, 1969), researchers now have available the tools with which to address any issues concerning sound perception, however complex, and they can do so with both versatility and precision.

A second factor that led researchers to focusing on low-level parameters was the enthusiasm resulting from new understandings of the workings of the inner ear. It is understandable that researchers would attempt to attribute as much as possible to the characteristics of newly discovered mechanisms. We are reminded here of Galileo's enthusiasm for the tympanic membrane as the organ responsible for the perception of consonance and dissonance, ignoring the rather obvious points made by Kepler and by Descartes. On the other hand, we see clearly in Home's Croonian lecture on the muscles controlling this membrane the pitfalls inherent in being overly enthusiastic about some known peripheral structure as an explanatory device.

A third factor (and this is perhaps the most important one) is a lack of awareness of musical issues in our culture. In the case of vision, specialized knowledge is not required in order to pinpoint some of the analyses that the nervous system would need to perform in order for useful perception to occur. Obvious operations include, for example, the recognition of objects when these are presented in different orientations, or at different distances from the observer. However, in the case of hearing, analogous operations do not readily present themselves, except to the musically initiated. As we have seen, in previous times scientists were musically knowledgeable, and this enabled them to consider, as Helmholtz and Mach did, high-level along with low-level factors in their explanations of the hearing process.

In this context we can also consider the approach taken by experimental psychologists to auditory memory. The framework that has generally been adopted for work on human memory is a three-stage model consisting of a sensory register, a short term store, and a long term store. The first detailed version of this model was proposed by Broadbent (1958), who hypothesized that information presented to the observer is first retained in a large capacity sensory system, where it decays very rapidly. The material is saved from obliteration only through a process of verbal encoding, which enables it to enter short term memory. Information is there saved from obliteration by verbal rehearsal, until it is transferred to long term memory. Several later versions of the three-stage model have been proposed (see, for example, Neisser, 1967).

Despite the general implausibility of the notion of an extremely short term store for auditory memory, certain experimental results have been cited in its favor (for example, Pollack, 1972; Treisman & Rostron, 1972). However, the results of these experiments are also consistent with alternative explanations in terms of interference effects that occur under highly specialized stimulus conditions (see Deutsch, 1975a, for an extended discussion). The incontrovertible fact remains that most people can remember quite complex music over entire lifetimes. This cannot be reconciled with the view that auditory memory decays within a second or two unless it is recoded into verbal form. Again, we attribute the widespread acceptance of this view, which must surely be incorrect, to the lack of consideration of musical phenomena.

A fourth factor has arisen through the advanced computer technology that, through the work of Max Mathews, has so expanded the complexity and variety of sounds that can be generated and used in experiments on music and musical imagery. With the computer has come work on artificial intelligence and work on neural networks and other varieties of computational neural science.

Artificial intelligence, or AI, purports to gain insight into human function by programming computers to perform a variety of "human" tasks. Computational neural science, or CNS, purports to gain insight into human behavior by proposing computer models of the functioning of the nervous system. Both deal with high-level as well as low-level behavior.

What have AI and CNS told us about human capabilities and human behavior? Both deal with the behavior of complicated computer programs rather than with the behavior of actual organisms. It is not clear that, in general, workers in AI and CNS are aware of what is actually known about human behavior and its neurophysiological substrate—or particularly care.

SEARCH FOR SYNTHESIS

We have discussed some of the conflicts and hazards in the current relation among science and technology on the one hand and music and its imagery on the other. The interrelations involve conflicting doctrines various in source and scope. Yet, our time is a time of unprecedented resources for exploration and enlightenment.

Computer technology has supplied us with resources for generating complex musical sounds, and for generating quasi-musical sounds in which various aspects of quality and perception have been intensified or eliminated. Computer technology has also made it far easier to devise and conduct experiments and to gather data.

Audio technology, including the computer generation of sounds and their recording and distribution on audio cassettes, and lately, on compact disks, have opened new potentialities of illustration and demonstration in the study of musical perception and imagery.

In the field of vision, illustrations in books and the projection of patterns fixed or in motion have played an essential role in discovering, confirming, and demonstrating various visual phenomena. Today the illustration of auditory and musical phenomena through recordings, or through direct digital sound generation, can have a similar value in auditory perception.

Our argument from here forward is that science and technology have provided us with new and varied opportunities for studying music and musical imagery. In exploiting these profitably, we must choose wisely among fields of endeavor that are widely different in procedures, standards, modes of presentation, and relevance to musical imagery.

Among other things, we must keep in mind that it is clear from current psychological studies that the human being is no *tabula rasa*. Some of our capabilities are built in. Some capabilities must be learned. But, we can learn only skills that are within our scope. Some distinctions, ready reactions to some sort of formal order, are beyond our inherent capabilities.

Along with the nature and variety of the physical phenomena essential to musical instruments, human capabilities of perceiving and distinguishing must be the stuff of which music is made. Fortunately, some realization of this is becoming apparent among psychoacousticians and cognitive psychologists, if not in the fields of AI and CNS.

It is easy to say that we should be cautious of wrongheaded simplification in psychoacoustic demonstrations and experimentation. It is also easy to say that we should get at the root of important matters, rather than carefully gathering huge amounts of narrow data that give us no deep insight. Our hope and belief is that various different and competing *aspects* of perception can be sorted out and studied in a meaningful, insightful way.

In any simplification important things are bound to be left out. We can only recommend caution in interpreting and applying to music and its perception the results of experiments and demonstrations made with simplified, quasi-musical sounds in a non-musical or barely musical environment.

THE ROLE OF NEUROPHYSIOLOGICAL STUDIES

We have advocated a holistic approach and inveighed against a specialization that loses meaning in detail. Nonetheless, detail can be important. Between the instrument and the ear, music travels as sound waves. Within the ear vibrations of air excite vibrations of little bones, and these excite vibrations in the fluid of the cochlea and the basilar membrane. The basilar membrane performs a rough frequency analysis, and different regions, corresponding to different small ranges of frequency, excite different nerve endings of the auditory nerve. The nerve impulses on the auditory pathways up to the auditory cortex are processed in various interconnecting and bypassed way stations. When we speculate about mechanisms of perception and imagery, we should try to keep our ideas consistent with what is known about the auditory system.

In the past 20 or so years a great deal has been learned about the structure and functions of auditory pathways. A volume such as *Auditory function: Neurobiological bases of hearing* (Edelman, Gall, & Cowan, 1988) will convince any reader that it is not easy to understand the current status of auditory neurophysiology. It is clear, however, that important advances have been made over the background given in recent books on hearing. Rhode (1970, 1971) found that in live animals the frequency analysis performed by the basilar membrane is much finer grained than deduced by von Bekesy (1960) through studying cadaver material; nevertheless, fairly current textbooks on hearing still show von Bekesy's drawings. It is found from animal studies (Schreiner & Langer, 1988) that in general only low time rates of excitation are preserved up to the auditory cortex—at most a few tens of changes a second will be followed. Time response is faster lower down in the neural pathways of the auditory system, but it is only as far as the first interaction of the two ears that response is followed to a small fraction of a millisecond, and that time differences of around 10 microseconds can be distinguished.

Some aspects of animal hearing have been worked out inconsiderable detail. This is particularly true of the auditory system of barn owls (Konishi, Takahashi, Sullivan, Wagner, & Carr, 1988; Knudsen, 1988). The details of binaural time and loudness comparisons for various frequency ranges, and the neural pathways that, through inhibition, overcome ambiguities in source location have been explicated. The bringing together in one part of the brain of visual and auditory clues to object location has been demonstrated.

Where does the relevance of such knowledge to musical imagery lie? It lies chiefly in restricting our range of sensible speculation. It does not tell us what to believe about human perception, but it can indicate things that we should not believe.

It is very difficult to use what little we know about auditory pathways in the study of music perception. Certainly, however, we should not hypothesize functions or processes that seem grossly at odds with what we know of the anatomy and physiology of hearing.

THE THREAT OF MODELS

As we have noted, the capabilities of human hearing are astonishing. Complicated anatomical structures and physiological processes must lie behind these capabilities. We are certain concerning some of these, as the rough frequency analysis performed in the cochlea, and the importance of both relative intensity and relative time of arrival of sounds in the two ears in judgment of the location of a source of sound. Many details of the processes of perception are not known, even when we sense important aspects.

The psychoacoustic literature is full of models, including models of pitch perception. Some models have been worked out in analytical detail beyond present sure neurophysiological or psychophysical verification. Autocorrelation models of pitch perception (Licklider, 1951) call for functions that have not been found in the auditory system, and involve amounts of delay of waveform or its features that seem neurophysiologically dubious.

One model for the perception of virtual pitch (Terhardt, 1974) calls for the internal creation of a subharmonic frequency that early work (Fletcher, 1924) indicates to be perceptually unimportant when present. In the work cited, Fletcher himself felt impelled to hypothesize the generation of such a fundamental frequency internally through nonlinearities, presumably because Helmholtz had erroneously concluded that pitch is perceived only through the fundamental frequency.

As we have noted, psychoacoustic speculators have turned to electronic or computer simulated "neural networks," or have made various computational models in seeking explanation of auditory perception. Such work is commonly pursued without any adequate demonstration that the networks or functions hypothesized actually correspond to processes found in behavioral and neurophysiological explorations of animal hearing.

An engineer may wish to make a machine that will do something previously done by people or animals. Often there will be several possible avenues open, as in the case of flying. We should not argue from the success of the airplane that birds fly by spinning a propeller. Some psychoacousticians write as if the making-up of an unverified and sometimes unverifiable model lends creditability to a proposed explanation, even when there is no evidence for that the processes hypothesized have been found in animals, or are plausible on the basis of what is known. In our view, most models are a distraction from thought and an inspiration to certitude for the uncertain.

CAUTIONS ON THE USE
OF TRAINED LISTENERS

We have all heard of Pavlov's dogs which, through training, salivated at the sound of a bell. This does not mean that the sound of a bell and the smell or sight of food are similar sensations. It means that through training the same "objective" behavioral response can be evoked by different stimuli.

Is it fanciful that the evocation of the same responses through different sensations could lead to erroneous conclusions in psychoacoustic experiments? We don't think so. Let us note that a tune can be recognized through listening to it, or through a musician examining a score. And, that a tune can be recalled either as a sequence or sounds that just "come to" the person who sings or whistles the tune. Or, as a sequence of note names and durations.

There seems to be no danger here. But suppose that we are studying the perception of pitch. A tune with a very characteristic rhythmic pattern may be recognized by the rhythmic pattern alone. So, in experiments aimed at the study of pitch we should avoid tunes with rhythmic patterns. But a familiar tune can be recognized by its melodic contour, even when it is played with stretched or otherwise distorted intervals. Here we are on shaky ground, but the ground can be shakier.

The rate of periodic bursts of high-frequency tones can be distinguished as faster or slower. But, up to a few hundred tonebursts a second, the match of different patterns of tonebursts is on tonebursts per second, not on fundamental frequency or harmonic spacing, as it is at higher rates. And, when the match is on rate rather than fundamental frequency, changing the rate in a ratio of $5:4$ does not result in the perception of a musical interval of a major third (Pierce, 1990).

Subsequent informal experiments have shown that for a subject with absolute pitch tonebursts with rates up to a few hundred a second periodic tonebursts sound like a buzz with no pitch. No identification occurs with a note of the scale or position on the keyboard. Yet, faster or slower can be distinguished.

Because faster or slower can be distinguished, it seems plausible that with sufficient training a subject could be taught to respond to higher rates with the term "higher pitch," and to lower rates with the terms "lower pitch," and perhaps even to respond with position on a keyboard, just as in the presentation of a note on a staff. Here is a chance for a real confusion.

In psychoacoustic experiments, much is made of well-trained subjects. Yet, objective responses to stimuli may depend on training. Thus, the similarity that musicians find in isolated chords and their inversions is not found in data on subjects without musical training (Mathews, Reeves, Pierce, & Roberts, 1988).

In the study of musical perception, experimental outcomes will in some cases depend on musical talent and training. In part, the responses of subjects without formal musical training will depend on exposure to and degree of care in listening to music. This makes it difficult to distinguish inherent abilities from those resulting from exposure to music.

In particular studies, prolonged training of subjects could lead to responses more characteristic of the training than of anything else. And, to "the right," "the expected," or "the requested" response as to sensation or image.

EXPERIMENTS VERSUS DEMONSTRATIONS

In connection with visual perception, we have seen wonderful demonstrations that leave the participant utterly convinced. These include apparent motion of flashing lights, errors of relative size of figures in perspective drawings, depth perception of random-dot stereograms—and a host of others. Such demonstrations establish a general fact concerning human response beyond all question, though details and quantitative laws may have to be worked out through time-consuming experiments.

Convincing demonstrations work when the salient fact to be demonstrated can be disentangled from other effects that would make it less clear and obvious. Alas, the psychoacoustic literature is full of wonderfully detailed experiments in which any clear point is hidden by obscuring processes, and any conclusion must be teased out by detailed analysis.

We hold that good demonstrations are more convincing than experiments. A good demonstration need not be preceded by special training which just *might* influence what we hear, or how we respond to it. In a good demonstration, that which is demonstrated is right out front; we can't approach a demonstration with a kit of statistical tools. But, a good demonstration is less easily arrived at than a "careful" experiment.

The good auditory demonstrations we know of involve ingeniously simplified stimuli whose perception casts light on other stimuli, such as musical sounds or our reactions to them. However there is some danger here. A powerful demonstration may not be applicable to what we really want to understand.

AMATEURS AT WORK

Computers and synthesizers have put tools of unprecedented power into the hands of talented musicians and, indeed, of talented tinkerers who are unused, as was Galileo, to the laborious protocols of experiment and analysis that have become standard in psychoacoustic literature.

Such "amateurs" are interested chiefly in powerful and demonstrable results. Some have contributed very important synthesis techniques and insights as, Chowning (1973) in fm synthesis, in his vividly convincing evocation of moving sound sources (1971) and in fm voice synthesis (1980, 1989); Risset in various paradoxical sounds and brass and bell sounds (Risset & Wessel, 1982), and Rodet, Potard, & Barriere (1984) in synthesis of the singing voice. Much of such work is to be found in print, other such work has been presented at computer music conferences, and some becomes scuttlebutt among the like minded. Much real insight is not to be found in the standard literature. One of us (JRP) was surprised to find that improvement of consonance by adequate frequency separation of higher harmonics is to be found in U.S. patent 4,117,413 filed by Robert A. Moog in 1977.

A wealth of important or potentially important insights, observations, and techniques may be escaping the scientific literature. It is not escaping those who wish to use it. Much of it is unlikely to be available as standard papers in standard journals. It is available through word of mouth and through publication in new journals with new standards. And, often it is available through a very convincing demonstration on a tape or even compact disc.

ANALYSIS BY SYNTHESIS

Analysis by synthesis is a very powerful tool. In essence, the investigator seeks a (usually simple) algorithm for producing a perceptual effect. In this search he may as legitimately be guided by hunches or black magic or chance observations as by keen experimental or analytical insight. It doesn't matter *how* he arrives at the algorithm. But, he succeeds only if the algorithm works, and works well.

Risset (Risset & Wessel, 1982) sought an algorithm for producing brasslike sounds. He waded through much analytical detail, relevant and irrelevant. What he finally found was that for a sound to be brasslike the components of higher frequency must rise later than those of lower frequency. Guided by this result, Mathews processed bowed tones in such a way that they sounded brassy.

Analysis by synthesis can be subject to abuse. The algorithm arrived at must be patently successful. It must not be "just sort of." It must find what is clearly a chief and sufficient, or almost sufficient ingredient. The origin of some consonants in frequency motions toward a following vowel (Cooper et al., 1952) is convincing, we guess, but we'd be more convinced and happier with examples that sounded more like human speech.

SOME STRONG EFFECTS
AND THE DEMONSTRATIONS THEREOF

In this section we call attention to some powerful aspects of music perception, and illustrations of the decisive impact that ingenious demonstrations can have.

The Ratios of Small Integers and Harmonic Effects

The sense of consonance, of harmony, and of progression to a resolution are central to Western music. Since the day of the Greeks, the sense of consonance has been associated with the ratios of small integers: the octave $2:1$, fifth $3:2$, fourth $4:3$, major third $5:4$, and minor third $6:5$.

The traditional explanation of Helmholtz, as elaborated by Plomp (1966), is that for these intervals, harmonic partials of the two tones will not beat disagreeably, because many either coincide in frequency (or for tempered intervals very nearly coincide), or are well separated in frequency. But, musicians recognize musical intervals and chords when the individual tones are sine waves, for which there is no such beating. Could it be that the ratios of small integers somehow gave us the diatonic scale and its intervals, and that the considerations that

Helmoltz and Plomp put forward are sufficient but not necessary in the appreciation of Western music? How could we possibly find out?

That beats, or the interactions of partials lying within a critical bandwidth, are absolutely essential in music of several voices is conclusively demonstrated by demonstration 31, tracks 58–61 of the IPO NIU ASA compact disc of Houtsma, Rossing, and Wagenaars (1987). The musical material is a four-part Bach chorale. The tones used have 9 partials. There are two versions of the scale: normal and logarithmically stretched to replace the octave by a ratio 2.1 : 1. There are two versions of the frequencies of the partials: harmonic (which goes with the normal, 2 : 1 octave) and stretched logarithmically to conform to the stretched scale.

When the stretched partials are used with the stretched scale the partials of two notes that coincide before stretching will coincide after stretching, and partials that lie well apart in frequency before stretching will lie well apart after stretching. Thus, if relative positions of the partials of the several simultaneous tones are the harmonically important criterion, the unstretched scale and tones will sound all right together, and the stretched scale and stretched tones will sound all right together, while the stretched tones will sound bad with the unstretched scale, and the unstretched tones with the stretched scale. This is what one hears in the demonstration, very strongly. It is clear that even small departures in scale *or* partials undermines the harmonic basis of Western music, while the same departure from scale *and* partials can be acceptable.

Percussive sounds may play a larger part in African and Indonesian music than in western music. In many percussive instruments, overtones are not harmonic in frequency. Do the intervals of the scales in such cultures depart somewhat from diatonic intervals, perhaps to produce intervals with less beating?

Perceptual Fusion

Chowning (1973) showed how complex spectra can be produced efficiently through fm (frequency modulation) of a sinusoidal carrier frequency. When he used this approach in synthesizing the singing voice (1980, 1989) he found that the harmonic frequency components depicting the formant structure of a sung vowel simply did not fuse with the fundamental frequency to produce the sound of a vowel. Rather, the percept was that of a nondescript collection of tones, a collection of tones that could lead to no sensible musical percept, to no image of a singer.

When all frequency components were given a common vibrato, they fused into a sung vowel sound. Chowning found that he could use this technique to attain the effect of three voices singing a major triad together, and, beyond that, of several voices singing together a note of the same pitch. Without the use of vibrato, there was no sensible musical image. With appropriate vibrato, the image of a chorus could be invoked.

The value of a common vibrato in making a complex sound evoke a musical image had been appreciated before Chowning's work. Chowning's contribution is that there can be an absolute necessity for common small erratic deviations in pitch and/or amplitude if a complicated assortment of component frequencies are to be heard as a fused sound coming from one source. Such common erratic variations are of course characteristic of the human voice and of traditional musical instruments.

Octave Equivalence

It is traditional to take into account two aspects of pitch: the note within the octave (called the *pitch class* or *chroma*) as, C, E, G, and the octave within which the note lies (sometimes called *pitch height*), which can be designated C4 (middle C), C5, C6, and so on.

Shepard (1964) produced well-known tones in which one goes around the pitch class circle, seemingly without changing pitch height.[2] These tones consist of octave-related partials whose amplitudes are given by a rising, then falling curve fixed with respect to frequency. As these octave-related partials are moved up together in small steps along the log frequency continuum (and so clockwise along the pitch class circle) new partials enter at the low-frequency end at levels below the threshold of perception, and exit at the high-frequency end, again at levels below the threshold of perception. An impression of an ever-increasing pitch can thus be attained. For this particular pattern, then, pitch height appears virtually constant. Physically, the C at the beginning of an octave's span of such movement results in the identical tone as the C at the end of the octave's span of such movement.

These quasi-musical tones exhibit stepwise changes of pitch class from note to note. But the final note at the beginning of what would be expected to be the next higher octave is instead identical to the initial note. This is octave equivalence with a vengeance.

What about octave equivalence for musical sounds? Musically, how much are the notes in succeeding octaves really alike? If they are *really* alike, shouldn't they be interchangeable?

This has been settled with a simple demonstration (Deutsch, 1972). A very well known melody ("Yankee Doodle") was chosen in which successive notes have the same length. This melody was played with notes of the correct pitch

---

[2]This effect has since been shown to result from pitch class or spectral proximity between temporally adjacent tones. When tone pairs composed of such octave-related partials are presented, such that the tones within a pair are diametrically opposed along the pitch class circle (C–F#, D–G#, and so on) so that the principle of proximity cannot be invoked, an orderly relationship appears between the perceived height of a tone and its region along the pitch class circle: Tones lying in one region are heard as higher and those lying in the opposite region are heard as lower (Deutsch, Kuyper, & Fisher, 1987). Interestingly, the form of relationship between pitch class and perceived height here varies substantially across listeners.

class, but the octaves in which the notes lay were chosen randomly over a three-octave range. Only very, very few listeners succeed in identifying the melody under these conditions.[3]

What, then, of octave equivalence? There is clearly "something in" this concept, but the above experiment shows that Cs, Ds, and Es in different octaves just aren't necessarily interchangeable. Indeed, accuracy of melodic contour may be more important than accuracy of pitch class in evoking a known melody.

Streaming

It is remarkable how a skilled player can bring out the separate parts of Bach's works for the solo violin. Experiments concerning and demonstrations of streaming, so well discussed in Bregman's (1990) book can illustrate this only in part. But, demonstrations of streaming are simple and striking.

The simplest is the alternate, periodic playing of notes of a lower and higher pitch. When the sequence of notes is slow we hear the notes as one stream, jumping up and down in pitch. At a high enough rate we hear two streams, repeated notes of higher pitch and repeated notes of lower pitch. We lose any clear sense of the time relation of the notes in the two streams.

The phenomenon of streaming is important in getting some sense of the organization we impose on what we hear, or how we envision sounds. Proximity in pitch will link sensations together when they are close enough in time—perhaps, close enough to indicate a common source. Difference in pitch tends to differentiate sensations as to the envisioned source.

Demonstrations of streaming can be made in which the upper and lower voices do not repeat in pitch, but constitute simple melodic patterns without large jumps in pitch. These, too, are fascinating and enlightening.

It is a long way from simple streaming experiments to the skilled player creating an image of two or more sound sources in playing a Bach composition for the solo violin. But, the simplicity and inevitability of demonstrations of streaming are impressive.

The Deutsch Octave and Scale Illusions

In listening attentively we commonly listen to a sound of interest in one ear or from one direction and ignore or suppress sounds in the other ear or from another direction. This human ability is as well known as the phrase "whisper in your ear."

It would and does seem remarkable that for ingenious musical sound patterns this commonplace ability can be overridden at a high level, and the sense of

---

[3]We may note that if listeners are given clues which enable them to hypothesise the correct melody, identification becomes much easier: Listeners are able to achieve such identification by matching each incoming note to their auditory image of the untransformed version, and so confirm that each note is indeed of the correct pitch class.

sound source rearranged so as to give a sense of a "musically simpler" presentation to the two ears.

Deutsch (1974) has shown that such high-level rearrangement of sense or image of source is possible by devising binaural presentations of successive notes of different pitches which demonstrate the listener's creation of a simple sound image from a "complicated" sequence of stimuli.

In the *octave illusion,* tones are presented simultaneously to the two ears by means of headphones. The stimuli to the right and left ears and what is heard by the right and left ears are:

Stimulus to right ear	G5	G4	G5	G4	G5	G4	G5
Stimulus to left ear	G4	G5	G4	G5	G4	G5	G4
Heard by right ear	G5		G5		G5		G5
Heard by left ear		G4		G4		G4	

Somehow, one of the notes is assigned to the right ear and the other to the left ear. In this case, G5 in the right ear predominates over G4 in the left ear, but G4 in the right ear is heard in the left ear while simultaneously G5 in the left ear is not heard. The ear to which the higher note is assigned differs somewhat among individuals. For right-handed subjects the note of higher pitch is usually assigned to the right ear.

In the *scale illusion* (Deutsch, 1975b) the pitches of the notes played to the right and left ear jump up and down a great deal, but the listener produces the image of two sources, in each of which the pitch changes from note to note by no more than one step.

Stimulus to right ear	C'	D	A	F	F	A	D	C'
Stimulus to left ear	C	B	E	G	G	E	B	C
Heard by right ear	C'	B	A	G	G	A	B	C'
Heard by left ear	C	D	E	F	F	E	D	C

In this case, regardless of which ear individual notes go to, notes which form a descending and ascending scale are assigned to one ear, and notes which form an ascending and descending scale are assigned to the other ear. Again, for most right-handed subjects the higher notes are heard as in the right ear, and the lower notes as in the left ear—the reverse is true for some subjects.

These illusions show that a listener may derive a plausible musical organization or image of sound sources that seems quite at variance with the stimuli presented to the two ears.

CONCLUDING REMARKS

We have noted the unhappy climate of auditory imagery and music. Until recently, at least, psychoacousticians and cognitive psychologists have not held musicians, their art, and their technology in the esteem in which they were held through the 17th century. Even in the best of days, many ideas concerning music perception and musical imagery have been doctrinaire with little relevant foundation. Alas, musicians of the serial and post serial period appear to have put arbitrary ideas about music and perception ahead of actual musical experience. This has been bad for psychophysics and psychology, and perhaps also for music.

Happily, a new generation of musicians, skilled in the digital production and analysis of sound, have made great advances in the evocation of musical images of sound source, location, and motion. This has led to real advances in our understanding of music perception. Many or most of these advances have been motivated by a search for musically useful sounds, sound relations, sound sequences, soundscapes, if you will, rather than from an interest in psychoacoustic phenomena as such. However, compelling demonstrations have shown the scope and reality of such advances.

There is every reason to believe that new musical technology will be used to produce new and compelling effects and insights. We hope that compelling demonstrations and illustrations may be as fruitful in the psychophysics and psychology of musical sound as illustrations have long been in the field of visual perception.

REFERENCES

Aristoxenus. (1974). *The harmonics of Aristoxenus* (H. S. Macran, Ed. and Trans.). New York: Verlag.

Bekesy, G. von. (1980). *Experiments in hearing.* New York: Robert E. Krieger Publishing Company. (Original work published in 1960)

Bregman, A. S. (1990). *Auditory scene analysis.* Cambridge, MA: MIT Press.

Broadbent, D. E. (1958). *Perception and communication.* New York: Pergamon.

Chowning, J. M. (1977). The simulation of moving sound sources. *Computer Music Journal, 1,* 48–52. (Reprinted from *Journal of the Audio Engineering Society,* 1971, *19,* 2–6.

Chowning, J. M. (1977). The synthesis of complex audio spectra by means of frequency modulation. *Computer Music Journal, 1,* 46–54. (Reprinted from *Journal of the Audio Engineering Society,* 1973, *21,* 526–534.

Chowning, J. M. (1980). Computer synthesis of the singing voice. In J. Sundberg (Ed.), *Sound generation in winds, strings, and computers* (pp. 4–13). Stockholm: Royal Swedish Academy of Music.

Chowning, J. M. (1989). Frequency modulation synthesis of the singing voice. In M. V. Mathews & J. R. Pierce (Eds.), *Current directions in computer music* (pp. 57–63). Cambridge, MA: MIT Press.

Cohen, H. F. (1984). *Quantifying music.* Dordrecht: Reidel.

Cooper, F. S., Delattre, P. C., Liberman, A. M., Borst, J. M., & Gerstman, L. J. (1952). Some experiments on the perception of synthetic speech sounds. *Journal of the Acoustical Society of America, 24,* 597–606.

Deutsch, D. (1972). Octave generalization and tune recognition. *Perception and Psychophysics, 11,* 411–412.

Deutsch, D. (1974). An auditory illusion. *Nature, 1251,* 307–309.

Deutsch, D. (1975a). Auditory memory. *Canadian Journal of Psychology, 29,* 87–105.

Deutsch, D. (1975b). Two-channel listening to musical scales. *Journal of the Acoustical Society of America, 57,* 1156–1160.

Deutsch, D. (Ed.). (1982). *The psychology of music.* New York: Academic Press.

Deutsch, D., Kuyper, W. L., & Fisher, Y. (1987). The tritone paradox: Its presence and form of distribution in a general population. *Music Perception, 5,* 79–92.

Dorian, F. (1947). *The musical workshop.* London: Secker & Warburg.

Edelman, G. J., Gall, E. W., & Cowan, W. M. (Eds.). (1988). *Auditory function: Neurobiological bases of hearing.* New York: Wiley.

Fletcher, H. (1924). The physical criterion for determining the pitch of a tone. *Physical Review, 23,* 427–437.

Helmholtz, H. von. (1954). *On the sensations of tone.* (A. J. Ellis, Trans.). New York: Dover. (Original work published in 1885)

Houtsma, A. J. M., Rossing, T. D., & Wagenaars, W. M. (1987). *Auditory demonstrations* [Compact Disc, Philips 1126-061].

Knudsen, E. I. (1988). Experience shapes sound localization and auditory unit properties in the barn owl. In G. M. Edelman, W. E. Gall, & W. M. Cowan (Eds.), *Auditory Function* (pp. 721–745). New York: Wiley.

Konishi, M., Takahashi, T. T., Sullivan, W. E., Wagner, & Carr, C. (1988). Neurophysiological and anatomical substrates of sound localization in the owl. In G. M. Edelman, W. E. Gall, & W. M. Cowan (Eds.), *Auditory function* (pp. 721–745). New York: Wiley.

Licklider, J. C. R. (1951). A duplex theory of pitch perception. *Experientia, 7,* 128–133.

Mach, E. (1943). On symmetry. In *Popular Scientific Lectures.* T. J. McCormack (Trans.). La Salle: The Open Court Publishing Company. (Originally published in 1898)

Mathews, M. V. (1969). *The technology of computer music.* Cambridge, MA: MIT Press.

Mathews, M. V., Pierce, J. R., Reeves, A., & Roberts, L. (1988). Theoretical and experimental explorations of the Bohlen-Pierce scale. *Journal of the Acoustical Society of America, 84,* 1214–1222.

Miller, L., & Cohen, A. (1987). *Music in the Royal Society of London; 1660–1806.* Detroit: Detroit studies in music bibliography, No. 56.

Moog, R. A. (1977). Amplifier with multiplier. U. W. Patent 4, 117,413, filed June 21, 1977.

Neisser, U. (1967). *Cognitive psychology.* New York: Appleton-Century-Crofts.

Pierce, J. R. (1990). Rate, place, and pitch with tonebursts. *Music Perception, 7,* 205–212.

Plomp, R. (1966). *Experiments in Tone Perception.* Eindhoven, The Netherlands: Institute for Perception.

Pollack, I. (1972). Memory for auditory waveform. *Journal of the Acoustical Society of America, 51,* 1209–1215.

Risset, J.-C., & Wessel, D. L. (1982). Exploration of timbre by analysis and synthesis. In D. Deutsch (Ed.), *The psychology of music.* New York: Academic Press.

Rhode, W. S. (1970). *Measurement of the amplitude and phase of vibration of the basilar membrane using the Moessbauer Effect.* Unpublished dissertation. University of Wisconsin, Madison.

Rhode, W. S. (1971). Observations of the vibration of the basilar membrane in the squirrel monkey using the Moessbauer technique. *Journal of the Acoustical Society of America, 49,* 1218–1231.

Rodet, X., Potard, Y., & Barriere, J.-B. (1984). The CHANT project: From the synthesis of the singing voice to synthesis in general. *Computer Music Journal, 8,* 15–31.

Rossing, T. D. (1990). *The Science of Sound,* 2nd ed. New York: Addison Wesley.

Schoenberg, A. (1975). Composition with twelve tones (1). in *Style and Idea: Selected writings of Arnold Schoenberg* (pp. 214–244). (Edited by L. Stein, with translations by L. Black.) New York: St. Martin's Press.

Schreiner, C. E., & Langer, G. (1988). Coding of temporal patterns in the central auditory nervous

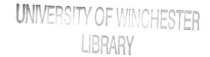

system. In G. M. Edelman, W. E. Gall, & W. M. Cowan (Eds.), *Auditory function*. New York: Wiley.

Shepard, R. N. (1964). Circularity in judgments of relative pitch. *Journal of the Acoustical Society of America, 36,* 2345–2353.

Sundberg, J. (1987). *The science of the singing voice*. DeKalb: Northern Illinois University Press.

Terhardt, E. (1974). Pitch, consonance, and harmony. *Journal of the Acoustical Society of America, 55,* 1061–1069.

Treisman, M., & Rostron, A. B. (1972). Brief auditory storage: a modification of Sperling's paradigm applied to audition. *Acta Psychologica, 36,* 161–170.

Author Index

A

Adams, J., 157, 175
Adams, K. L., 54, 69
Alba, J. W., 224, 232
Alberoni, M., 183, 196
Alegria, J., 79, 85, 92
Algom, D., 210, 232
Alpert, M., 155, 157, 158, 159, 172, 176
Anderson, J. R., 47, 63, 69, 158, 176, 201, 232
Anderson, R. A., 131, 147
Anderson, R. E., 130, 147
Annett, J., 131, 147
Arieti, S., 152, 153, 154, 172
Arixotoxenus, 239, 258
Armstrong, M. S., 155, 173
Atkinson, R. C., 121, 147, 183, 194
Attneave, F., 50, 69

B

Baddeley, A. D., 76, 78, 79, 90, 91, 96, 104, 105, 106, 107, 111, 112, 113, 115, 117, 118, 119, 121, 125, 127, 134, 137, 138, 141, 142, 147, 149, 168, 170, 172, 173, 177, 180, 181, 182, 183, 184, 185, 186, 187, 188, 189, 190, 192, 193, 194, 195, 196, 197
Baillarger, J., 158, 167, 173

Baird, J. C., 45, 70, 221, 233
Ball, T. M., 4, 7, 27, 215, 234
Bargh, J. A., 143, 147
Barriere, J.-B., 252, 259
Bartlett, J. C., 3, 26, 188, 195
Basili, A. G., 77, 91, 107, 118
Baxter, D. A., 45, 71, 99, 119, 131, 149, 161, 176
Bazhin, E. F., 160, 173
Bechtel, W., 208, 232
Beethoven, L., von, 237
Bekesy, G. von, 249, 258
Bellugi, U., 74, 76, 90, 92
Bentall, R. P., 155, 173
Berndt, R. S., 77, 91, 107, 118
Bernstein, L., 203, 232
Bertelson, P., 79, 92
Besner, D., 96, 112, 114, 115, 116, 118, 186, 190, 195
Bharucha, J. J., 205, 206, 212, 228, 231, 232
Bick, P. A., 105, 118, 164, 167, 173
Birley, J. L. T., 169, 173
Bishop, D. V. M., 80, 90, 91, 115, 118, 125, 134, 147, 183, 195
Bisiacchi, P. S., 87, 91
Bjork, R. A., 46, 54, 70
Bleuler, E., 170, 173
Block, N., 200, 207, 208, 232
Blum, M., 155, 174
Bolton, T. L., 14, 26
Borst, J. M., 253, 258

261

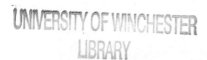